AI and Digital Innovation in Healthcare Reform:

From Policy to Practice

Kakhaber Djakeli
https://orcid.org/0000-0001-7505-5653
University of Georgia, Georgia

IGI Global
Scientific Publishing
Publishing Tomorrow's Research Today

Vice President of Editorial Melissa Wagner
Director of Acquisitions Mikaela Felty
Director of Book Development Jocelynn Hessler
Production Manager Mike Brehm
Cover Design Jose Rosado

Published in the United States of America by
IGI Global Scientific Publishing
701 East Chocolate Avenue
Hershey, PA, 17033, USA
Tel: 717-533-8845 | Fax: 717-533-7115
Website: https://www.igi-global.com E-mail: cust@igi-global.com

Library of Congress Cataloging-in-Publication Data

LCCN: (CIP Data Pending)
ISBN13: 9798260009390
Isbn13Softcover: 9798260009406
EISBN13: 9798260009413
British Cataloguing in Publication Data
A Cataloguing in Publication record for this book is available from the British Library.

Table of Contents

Detailed Table of Contents

opportunities and risks of digital mental health expansion. The chapter demonstrates how compassionate, inclusive, and accountable digital reforms can translate mental health policy into effective instruments for equity, social justice, and sustainable health system transformation.

This chapter examines the effectiveness of a culturally adapted life skills training (LST) program among marginalized Paniya tribal adolescent girls in Wayanad, Kerala. A six-month single-group pre-test–post-test intervention with 34 participants aged 11–15 years focused on key psychosocial skills, including self-awareness, communication, emotional management, decision-making, problem-solving, and interpersonal relationships. Results showed statistically significant improvements across all domains ($p \leq 0.05$), indicating enhanced psychosocial functioning. Interpreted through developmental and empowerment perspectives, the findings suggest that LST can strengthen resilience and competence, while also emphasizing the need for policy integration to address persistent structural barriers.

This chapter explores eating disorders among students in Moroccan higher education as a growing public health concern linked to healthcare reform, digital transformation, and leadership in health policy. Based on a cross-sectional study at the Higher Institute of Nursing and Health Techniques (ISPITS) of Kenitra, a synthetic Eating Disorder Risk Score (EDRS) was validated, revealing social pressure and body dissatisfaction as key predictors, with academic stress as a mediating factor. The chapter discusses the economic burden of untreated disorders—productivity loss, absenteeism, and academic dropout—and highlights the need for preventive, cost-effective strategies. It advocates for integrating mental health and nutrition into national health reform through innovative "phygital" approaches that combine digital awareness, institutional counseling, and social marketing. Finally, it underscores the importance of academic leadership in advancing inclusive, evidence-based, and sustainable student health reform in the digital age.

National health system reform is paramount to the creation of fairer and more efficient systems that meet contemporary clinical needs and advance population health in the long term. From a maternal health perspective, gestational diabetes mellitus (GDM) pinpoints the necessity of national health reform. The global prevalence of GDM has significantly risen because of maternal age, overweight, lifestyle, and genetics. GDM management was uncoordinated with variable diagnosis pathways, a lack of knowledge about GDM among women and providers, and limited follow-up post-delivery. National healthcare reform on GDM is moving away from a decreased focus on pregnancy complications to a life-course prevention strategy for chronic disease prevention by changing maternal health at the public health level. When GDM care is reformulated through an integrated phygital national framework, there will be significant improvements to maternal and child health which will also further support the national goal of reducing the intergenerational burden of non-communicable diseases.

The health care business is undergoing a high rate and unprecedented change due to the combination of new technologies and the changing societal needs. AI, telemedicine, Internet of Medical Things (IoMT), robotics, and data-driven diagnostics are all transforming the healthcare delivery, monitoring, and administration modalities. These changes in technology have become necessities in addressing increasing needs triggered by aging of the population, increase in chronic diseases, and increase in healthcare spending. However, the challenges remain, such as the lack of workforce, the unequal access to the high-quality care in both the urban and rural areas, and the complexity of the functioning of the modern healthcare structures. Considering that millions of healthcare staff spread across the globe, and the scope of service demands is rapidly expanding, there is an urgency with regard to technology-powered solutions

its performance is thoroughly examined using common metrics such as precision, recall, precision, and F1-score.

Asthma is a long-time respiratory disease that impacts millions of people across the globe with serious health threats and economic costs. Timely diagnosis and anticipation of asthma may be an important part of the plan to enhance patient outcomes, treatment plans and hospitalization. This paper discusses how machine learning algorithms can be used to predict asthma using patient data including demographic factors, lifestyle patterns, environmental issues, and clinical characteristics. Several classification models such as Decision Trees, Random Forests, Support Vector Machines and Gradient Boosting are executed and evaluated to establish the most useful method. The experimental findings indicate that prediction model based on machine learning can be highly accurate and reliable, which can serve as an important decision-support system of medical workers. The results outline the possibilities of machine learning in improving the assessment of asthma risks

Emergency department (ED) visits have been steadily increasing in recent years, making accurate prediction crucial for improving operational efficiency, quality of care, and patient outcomes. This study investigates the prediction of ED admissions using six machine learning models: Linear Regression, Fully Connected Deep Neural Network, Support Vector Regression, Extreme Learning Machine, Random Forest, and Regression Tree. Initially, base models were trained with predefined hyperparameters and evaluated using Mean Absolute Error (MAE). To enhance performance, SHAP (SHapley Additive exPlanations) and LIME (Local Interpretable Model-agnostic Explanations) were applied for model interpretation and data visualization. Insights from these methods guided model retraining, resulting in significant improvements: Linear Regression (42.73%), Neural Network (17.32%), Extreme Learning Machine (21.53%), Random Forest (32.78%), and Regression Tree (29.33%). This approach not only reduced prediction errors but also improved model interpretability, ensuring more reliable ED admission forecasts.

Preface

Healthcare systems across the globe are undergoing a profound transformation driven by rapid advancements in digital technologies and the growing integration of artificial intelligence (AI). What was once a predominantly reactive, resource-constrained sector is now evolving into a data-driven, predictive, and patient-centered ecosystem. This shift is not merely technological, it represents a fundamental re-thinking of how healthcare is delivered, governed, and experienced.

AI and Digital Innovation in Healthcare Reform: From Policy to Practice brings together interdisciplinary perspectives that examine how emerging technologies are reshaping healthcare reform agendas worldwide. From policy frameworks and ethical considerations to applied machine learning models and community-based interventions, this volume captures the breadth and complexity of contemporary healthcare transformation.

The contributions in this book highlight both the promise and the challenges of integrating AI and digital innovations into healthcare systems. While these technologies offer unprecedented opportunities to improve diagnosis, optimize resources, and enhance accessibility, they also raise critical concerns around equity, bias, governance, and implementation barriers. Importantly, the chapters emphasize that technology alone cannot solve systemic healthcare issues; rather, meaningful reform requires aligning innovation with inclusive policies, ethical safeguards, and socio-cultural realities.

This volume is structured to bridge the gap between theory and practice. It provides readers with a comprehensive understanding of how digital tools can be translated into actionable healthcare reforms that are equitable, sustainable, and evidence-based. The book will be valuable to researchers, policymakers, healthcare professionals, and technologists seeking to navigate the evolving intersection of AI and healthcare systems.

CHAPTER OVERVIEW

Chapter 1: Transforming Healthcare Reform with Artificial Intelligence – Past Insights and Future Opportunities

This opening chapter establishes the foundation for the volume by tracing the evolution of healthcare reform and the emergence of AI as a transformative force. It explores how AI enables data-driven decision-making, risk prediction, and resource optimization while also addressing regulatory frameworks, policy implications, and implementation challenges. The chapter sets the stage for understanding AI as both an enabler and a disruptor in healthcare systems.

Chapter 2: Digital Pathways to Inclusive Health Reform

Focusing on mental health inequities among informal workers, this chapter presents a "phygital" model that integrates digital and physical care systems. It emphasizes inclusivity, ethical governance, and sustainability, demonstrating how digital tools can address systemic disparities while translating policy into meaningful, equitable outcomes.

Chapter 3: Life Skills Training and Adolescent Health

This chapter highlights the importance of psychosocial interventions in healthcare reform through a case study of marginalized adolescents. It demonstrates how life skills training can improve resilience and well-being, while underscoring the need for policy integration to address structural barriers in vulnerable populations.

Chapter 4: Eating Disorders in Higher Education

Addressing a growing public health concern, this chapter examines the psychosocial and digital influences contributing to eating disorders among university students. It advocates for preventive, cost-effective strategies and emphasizes leadership's role in integrating mental health into broader healthcare reform initiatives.

Chapter 5: National Phygital Model for GDM Care

This chapter explores gestational diabetes mellitus (GDM) as a critical entry point for healthcare reform. It proposes a national "phygital" framework that integrates traditional care with digital technologies to improve maternal and child health outcomes and support long-term chronic disease prevention.

Chapter 6: New Technologies and Enduring Challenges in the Healthcare Market

Providing a systems-level perspective, this chapter examines the impact of emerging technologies such as AI, telemedicine, and IoMT on healthcare delivery. It also addresses persistent challenges, including workforce shortages, inequities in access, and the complexity of modern healthcare systems.

Chapter 7: Policy for Regulating AI in Medicine

This chapter focuses on the governance of AI in healthcare, emphasizing the need for ethical, balanced, and responsible implementation. It highlights the importance of regulatory frameworks that ensure AI supports, rather than replaces, human expertise while promoting sustainable development.

Chapter 8: Algorithmic Neutrality in Healthcare AI

Challenging the assumption that AI is inherently objective, this chapter critically examines bias and inequality in algorithmic systems. It advocates for participatory design, transparency, and accountability to ensure that AI contributes to health equity rather than reinforcing disparities.

Chapter 9: Streaming Motherhood

Through a digital ethnographic lens, this chapter explores how social media platforms serve as informal support systems for postpartum mothers. It highlights the intersection of culture, language, and digital communities in shaping maternal mental health experiences.

Chapter 10: Predicting Breast Cancer Cell Dynamics Using Bi-LSTM

This chapter presents an advanced AI modeling approach to understanding cancer cell behavior. By applying bidirectional LSTM techniques, it demonstrates how predictive analytics can enhance biomedical research and improve clinical insights into disease progression.

Chapter 11: Predictive Modeling of Asthma Risk

Focusing on chronic disease management, this chapter evaluates various machine learning algorithms for predicting asthma risk. It highlights the potential of predictive models to support clinical decision-making and improve patient outcomes.

Chapter 12: Explainable AI for Emergency Department Admissions

The final chapter addresses the critical need for transparency in AI systems. By integrating explainable AI techniques such as SHAP and LIME, it demonstrates how predictive models can become more interpretable, reliable, and actionable in real-world healthcare settings.

Together, these chapters provide a comprehensive exploration of how AI and digital innovation are reshaping healthcare reform, from conceptual foundations and ethical considerations to practical applications and future directions.

Chapter 1
Transforming Healthcare Reform With Artificial Intelligence:
Past Insights and Future Opportunities

V. Sangeetha
http://orcid.org/0000-0001-9325-7590
Ramaiah Institute of Technology, India

A. Mamatha
http://orcid.org/0000-0001-8110-5602
Ramaiah Institute of Technology, India

Kavya Natikar
http://orcid.org/0009-0000-3792-7908
Ramaiah Institute of Technology, India

ABSTRACT

With the rising wave of digital health technologies, a new dimension of global health reform agendas has evolved, where Artificial Intelligence(AI) is being branded as a revolutionary tool capable of overcoming long-existed deficiencies. AI technologies is promising in discovering hidden health patterns, health risk prediction, resource optimization, and prioritizing health reform initiatives based on empirical evidence. In this chapter, the first section discuss about the background why reform is required in healthcare, and also highlights the need for AI in healthcare and the need for AI driven transformation. The chapter throws light on the historical evolution of healthcare reform. The various applications to reform health care are discussed

DOI: 10.4018/979-8-2600-0939-0.ch001

in detail. The impact of AI on healthcare policy, regulatory framework on AI integration is described in detail. In the end, the chapter throws insights on challenges and barriers to AI driven Healthcare. The future of health will hold a new hope in using AI technologies in preparing a new wave of evidence-based individualized.

INTRODUCTION

The health care systems around the world are facing tremendous evolution with respect to changing demographics, a rise of diseases, high expenditure, and raised standards of accessibility and quality. Typical policies for health care reform have traditionally focused on service delivery improvement, approaches for financing, and policy restructuring. However, these approaches alone have not been able to address global contemporary healthcare issues such as workforce shortages, fragmented care, inequity of access, and inefficiency in both clinical and administrative processes. On that note, AI has grown to become a transformative driver that can revolutionize healthcare reform by enabling intelligent automation, predictive analytics, and data-driven decision-making.

The chapter mainly focuses on the paradigm shift represented by AI systems and discusses the emergence of healthcare reform, and also examines the technological history in relation to the paradigm shift. In this chapter, AI technology is seen as the catalyst for patient-centered, equitable, and sustainable healthcare systems by learning lessons from the past technology failures in healthcare reform.

Background of Healthcare Reform

Healthcare reform represents deliberate efforts of organizations and governments in increasing availability, effectiveness, affordability, and quality of healthcare services (Razavi et al., 2025). Social, economic, and political drivers like population growth, the increase in aged populations, outbreaks of infectious diseases, and concerns about financial sustainability have traditionally been seen in the drive for health reform.

Preventive care remained less prominent in early models of healthcare systems, which remained more hospital-based and physician-led. For making improved health outcomes a reality, public health programs, insurance-based financing systems, and health regulations made their entry. Upgrading primary health care, equity, and eventually universal coverage remained the goal of prominent global efforts led by organizations such as the World Health Organization. Yet, many healthcare systems face challenges related to concerns like:

- Prevalence of chronic diseases

- Disparities in the Accessibility of Healthcare
- Rural Community vs. Urban Community

In view of the above systemic limitations, the requirement for innovative transformation mechanisms that transcend traditional options is highlighted.

Rise of Artificial Intelligence in Healthcare

Due to the developments in computing power, the ability to analyze big data, and machine learning tools available to the medical community, the interest in the application of AI in the medical industry began to gain momentum (Dangi et al., 2025). Applications of AI that were restricted to research labs soon made their entry into practical medical settings.

Natural Language Processing, Computer Vision, Deep Learning, Machine Learning, and many fields in Artificial Intelligence technologies are now been integrated in healthcare service delivery processes such as:

- Diagnosis of medical images using AI assistance
- Using Predictive analytics to anticipate the outbreak of diseases
- Intelligent EHR Systems
- Intelligent Electronic Health Record
- Personal Care & Pharmaceuticals

Adoption of AI has gained speed due to the large amount of health data provided by the use of wearables, genomics, EHRs, and medical imaging. People have become more informed about the enabling role of AI in the transformation of the health care system rather than the enabling role of the technology itself.

Need for AI-Driven Transformation

Where digitization made data more accessible, the digital systems per se did not correct the fundamentals amiss with healthcare (Faiyazuddin et al., 2025). The problems persisted-manual data interpretation, too many clinicians in the chain, and too much time before a decision is taken. AI-driven transformation addresses these gaps by facilitating automation, prediction, and real-time intelligence.

The main factors for AI-powered change in the medical care industry are:

- Efficiency: Automating administrative processes and resource allocation
- Quality of Care: Enhancing Diagnostic Accuracy and Clinical Decision Support

- Equity: Improving health care access for underserved communities with telemedicine and artificial intelligence triage tools
- Sustainability: Cost savings due to Predictive and Preventive Care

AI enables healthcare reform to shift from reacting to changes in the system to proactive redesign, making healthcare systems more resilient.

Early Healthcare Policies and Delivery Models

Early systems of the delivery of health care were almost completely dependent on charity support or private financing without much governmental intervention(El-Jerjawi et al., 2024). This later changed as the governmental system took up the responsibility for health care through sanitation campaigns, inoculation campaigns, and the maintenance of levels in hospitals. The adoption of social health insurance schemes in Europe and the later adaptation of public health care systems is an important turning point in the delivery of health care in an organized manner after World War II, which brought about:

- Accessibility to universal healthcare
- Availability of universal healthcare
- Government financing and oversight

However, many of these models tended to support treatment rather than prevention and thus were more expensive and incapable of using resources effectively.

Technological Interventions Before AI

Prior to the advent of AI, there had been healthcare reforms in the form of technological initiatives aimed at improving the efficiency and quality of healthcare. These included:

- Electronic Health Records (EHRs)
- Hospital Information Systems-HIS
- Telehealth platforms
- Healthcare imaging technologies

Although these step-by-step developments were helpful in improving the area of documentation and communication, these were essentially passive stores of data. A lot of human data interpretation had to be done, causing mental fatigue and lack of usage of existing data. Lack of interoperability, therefore, restricted their reformist potency.

Such pre-AI technologies formed the backbone of digital medicine but were not intelligent, flexible, or innovative enough to bring about a paradigm shift.

Takeaways from Previous International Healthcare Reform

AI-driven reforms can learn a lot from global health reform projects(Salehi F, 2024). Experiences with strengthening primary care, implementing value-based care systems, and expanding national health insurance have demonstrated that policy change is insufficient without technology assistance.

Key lessons include:

- Making decisions based on data is essential to long-lasting transformation.
- Technology must align with standards, policy goals, and clinical procedures.
- Equity and inclusivity should be the cornerstones of reform growth.
- Flexibility and ongoing evaluation are also crucial.

APPLICATIONS RESHAPING HEALTHCARE REFORM

Around the globe, systems of healthcare have changed significantly, medical costs are increasing, novel illnesses are developing, and patients need better care. Healthcare is being forced to operate by such factors. AI is a major factor in this upheaval, helping to improve health related situations in terms of preventing illness, treatment, and decision-making. AI systems use information from data to help create healthcare plans that work ahead of time(Sutton et al., 2020). These new ways of dealing things are more productive and get things right more often. Take a look at Figure 1 to get a feel for the different AI applications that are driving healthcare reform across a range of areas - prevention, diagnosis, public health, operations, personalised medicine & remote care. In this section a closer look at some of the AI applications that are having a real impact in some key areas are discussed.

Figure 1. Overview of major Artificial Intelligence applications reshaping healthcare reform

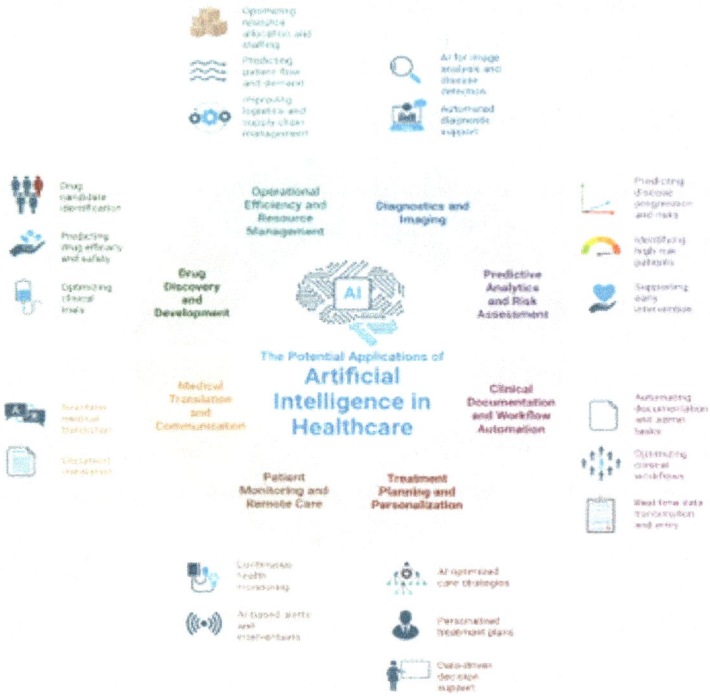

AI in Preventive and Predictive Healthcare

Artificial intelligence(AI) driven preventive & predictive healthcare is all about spotting potential health problems long before they turn into full-blown illnesses. By digging through electronic health records, data from wearable gadgets & people's daily habits, AI systems can zero in on early warning signs of chronic conditions that are still in their infancy. AI models then crunch the numbers to figure out the likelihood of disease occurring, how fast it might progress & what kind of complications could arise - all of which makes for a perfect opportunity for early intervention(Herrera-Poyatos A, 2025). This approach is basically a winner when it comes to stopping unnecessary hospital trips & making a bigger positive impact on community health. Figure 2 gives you a rundown of some of the wearable health gadgets that get used in AI-driven preventive & predictive healthcare - that includes smartwatches, smart rings, sensor stickers, and on-going health tracking devices that keep gathering vital stats.

Figure 2. Examples of wearable health devices used in AI-driven preventive and predictive healthcare

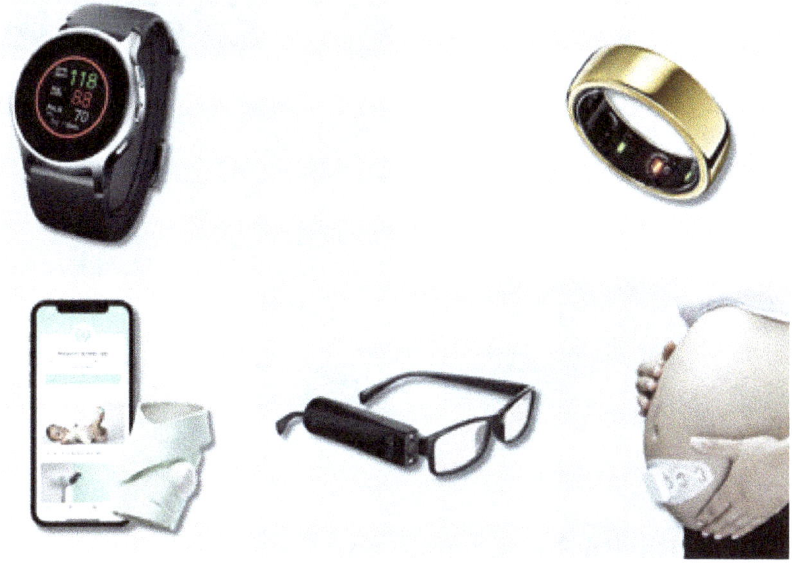

AI-Powered Diagnostics and Clinical Decision Support

AI diagnostic systems help doctors, nurses and other healthcare professionals make sense of complicated medical images, lab results and patient data with a lot more accuracy. They help doctors spot conditions like cancer, infections and organ problems right from the start. These systems also help with clinical decision making by providing doctors with solid evidence based treatment plans and alerts if there's a potential for a bad drug reaction(Gagnon et al., 2024). By using AI they can make sure diagnoses are consistent and help doctors make informed decisions about care. Figure 3 shows a sample workflow of an AI-based clinical decision support system for generating treatment recommendations.

Figure 3. Workflow for a clinical decision support system using AI to recommend treatments.

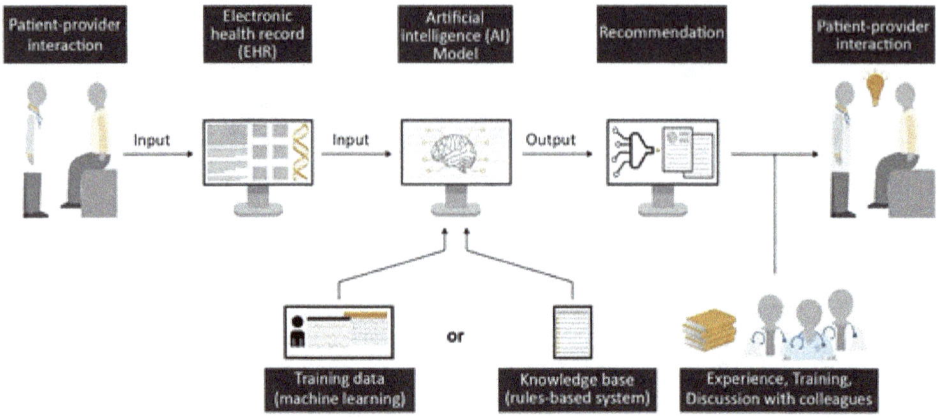

AI in Public Health Surveillance and Epidemiology

By merging different types of data from hospitals, labs, the environment, and population movements, a powerful AI system can help with public health monitoring. They are able to watch developments in health patterns over time and identify the initial stages of new outbreaks owing to this real-time data. Thanks to artificial intelligence models in disease prediction research, they can even forecast the chances that a disease will become widespread and the potential effectiveness of specific public health interventions. This helps them to prepare and allows the concerned authority to plan for everyone's health safety during the crisis in the community. Figure 4 illustrates how all of the information is used to support public health choices by identifying the source of illness outbreaks and determining the best course of action.

Figure 4. AI-powered healthcare monitoring system.

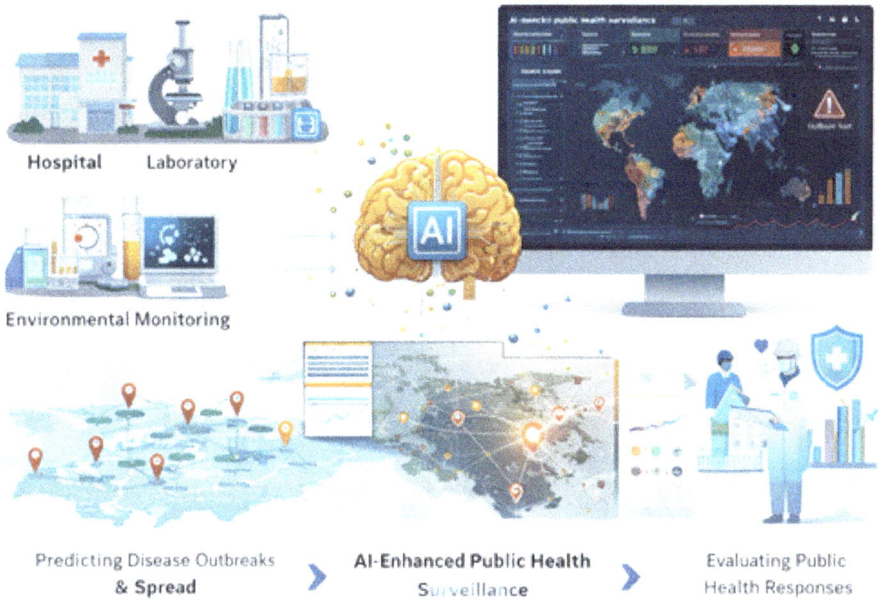

AI-Enabled Operational Efficiency (Triage, Scheduling, Hospital Management)

Artificial intelligence is advantageous for healthcare organizations because it eliminates the hurdles in both administrative and medical operations also promotes overall productivity. AI-powered triage systems are excellent at classifying patients based on the urgency of their care, taking into account all of the important symptoms, vital signs, and medical histories(Li et al., 2025) This prevents the emergency department from being overcrowded. Additionally, scheduling algorithms play a significant role in ensuring that patients see the appropriate physician at the appropriate time, sending the appropriate staff to the appropriate location, and optimizing operating room time. Hospital administrators also profit greatly from all of this since predictive analytics gives them a heads-up on potential developments. This allows them to anticipate patient admissions, bed occupancy, and needed resources in order to provide healthcare to those in need as rapidly as achievable. Figure 5 makes it fairly evident how the AI-based patient triage process determines which patients require the highest degree of care and where they should be assigned.

Figure 5. Artificial intelligence-powered patient triage system for prioritized care and gauging risk.

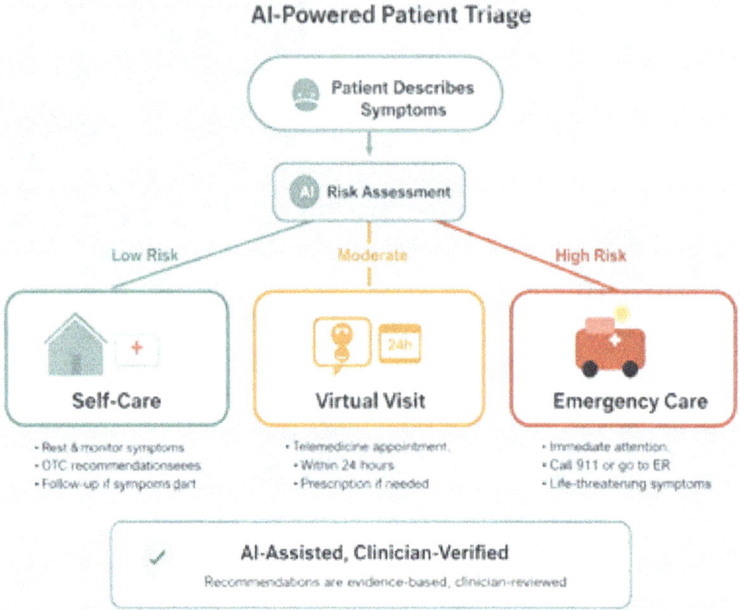

AI in Personalized and Precision Medicine

Personalized and precision medicine focuses therapies based on each patient's specific traits rather than following one-size-fits-all therapeutic recommendations. AI plays a significant role in this. It looks into elements like your lifestyle, medical history, genes, and past response to therapy. With all that information, physicians can actually forecast the patient's response to specific treatments. This implies that they are able to decide on the safest and most efficient choices, rather than just those that work for the majority of people. AI additionally speeds up the search for many different diagnostics and supports the creation of personalized drugs. When applying this approach, patients have more favorable results and fewer negative consequences. AI's role in precision medicine is depicted in Figure 6, which highlights from genetic evaluation and personalized treatment plans to grouping patients and monitoring their progress.

Figure 6. Artificial Intelligence's contribution to personalized medicine

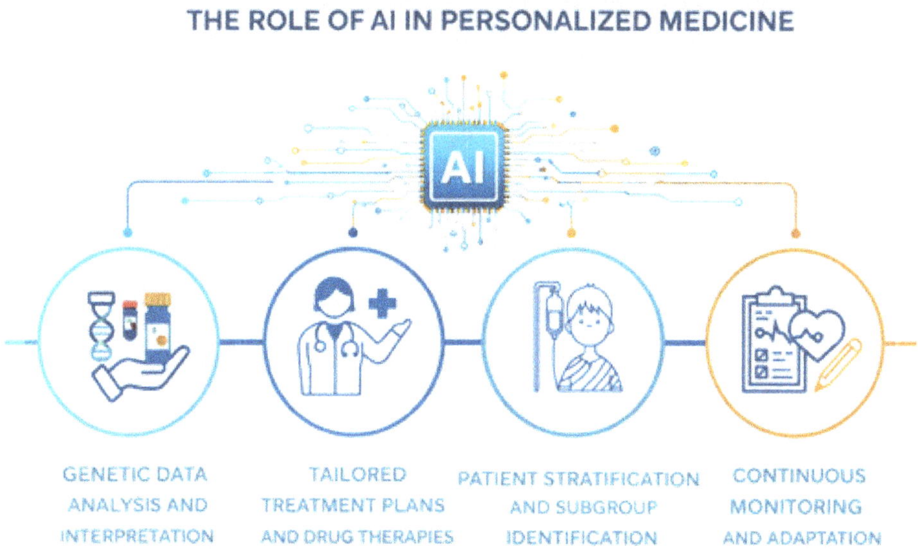

AI for Remote Care: Telemedicine, Virtual Assistants, and Home Monitoring

AI is not only transforming healthcare, but also making it much more convenient and individualized. Thanks to modern technology that maintains operating even when a patient is far away from hospital zone, patients can readily get medical treatment and support at home. AI-powered telemedicine facilities allow people to completely avoid waiting rooms. From the comfort of the patient seat, patients can deal with examinations and have their symptoms evaluated, or consult a physician.. Additionally, seeking doctor's advice is not the only option. Virtual health assistants can converse or chat with patients, providing them advice, encouraging them to take their medications, or guiding them in managing chronic conditions. Smart devices and wearables monitor things like blood pressure and heart rate, providing real-time updates so medical professionals can act quickly if something is wrong. Combine all of the information together to create a system that assists patients who live far from clinics, keeps people more involved in their own health care, and makes life easier for elderly people or anyone suffering with chronic issues. Figure 7 portrays a futuristic robot supporting an elderly person at household work.

Figure 7. A futuristic robot assisting an elderly person.

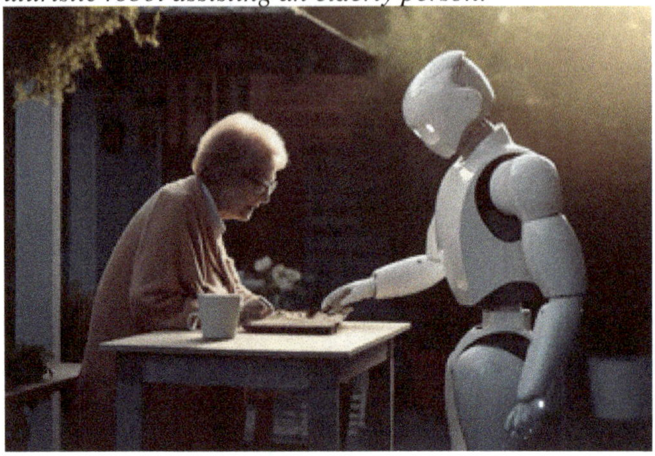

Impact of AI on Healthcare Policy and Governance

The swift advancement of artificial intelligence (AI) is transforming healthcare policies and governance. It entails preparation and enables data-driven decision-making (Blanco et al., 2025). AI provides helpful tools for wise policy making as healthcare systems grapple with problems like expanding health needs, limited resources, and escalating costs. AI is essential for maximizing resource usage and guaranteeing moral and legal adherence. This section examines how AI can affect international policy integration, cost reduction, regulatory supervision, and analytics in healthcare policy.

AI-Driven Policy Analytics and Decision Modeling

Healthcare professionals can make better decisions by utilizing information and artificial intelligence. Instead of concentrating only on the past events, they may swiftly analyze a vast amount of data. Artificial intelligence tracks expenses, keeps track of illnesses, computes the frequency of healthcare service usage, and carries out population health research. This enables policymakers to learn about the problems they were previously unaware of and identify the places where regulations are not being applied. Certain tools can show what can happen in the future if legislators decide to change healthcare spending, decide who is eligible for insurance, or choose which disease prevention initiatives.. By utilizing these instruments and considering all the data, artificial intelligence is capable of aiding healthcare policymakers in their decision making process. This capability to foresee consequences is a strong support for evidence- based policymaking, which leads to better policy effectiveness and transparency in healthcare governance.

AI for Cost Reduction and Resource Allocation

Governments and healthcare organizations are increasingly concerned about the rising healthcare expenses, especially in systems with inadequate funding and workforce capacity. Data-driven analytical tools are being utilized more frequently to assist supply chain operations, personnel planning, bed occupancy, and patient flow management in response to growing demand and the limited infrastructure. Inefficiencies including unnecessary diagnoses, extended hospital stays, avoidable readmissions, fraud, and medical errors can all be found with the aid of these instruments. When combined with the value-based healthcare models, analytics-driven approaches allow more efficient consumption of resources while preserving acceptable standards of service quality and accessibility. The main data-driven methods for reducing healthcare costs are shown in Figure 8. These actions include streamlining processes, boosting employee productivity, reducing readmissions, spotting fraud, improving the manufacturing process, and getting rid of medical errors.

Figure 8. Key data analytics driven strategies for reducing healthcare costs.

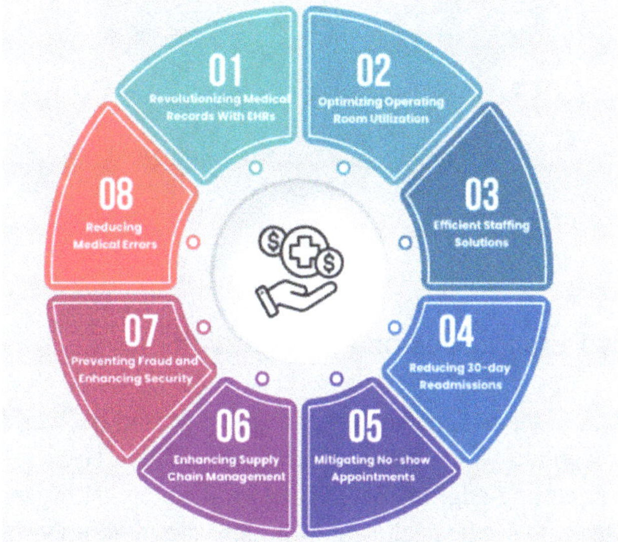
01
Revolutionizing Medical Records With EHRs
02
Optimizing Operating Room Utilization
03
Efficient Staffing Solutions
04
Reducing 30-day Readmissions
05
Mitigating No-show Appointments
06
Enhancing Supply Chain Management
07
Preventing Fraud and Enhancing Security
08
Reducing Medical Errors

Regulatory Frameworks, Data Governance, and Ethical Standards

For the application of AI in healthcare systems in order to guarantee moral and secure procedures, certain laws and regulatory frameworks are to be framed and maintained. Data security, privacy, sharing, and permissions must all be governed by the data governance policies. This preserves patient rights and encourages innovation. Ethical standards tackle bias in algorithms, transparency, accountability, and the explainability of AI systems. Regulatory agencies must approve and evaluate AI technologies for health care. They ensure that these solutions uphold moral and legal obligations and promote public trust. Figure 9 depicts the AI governance architecture, which integrates accountability, transparency, and justice.

Figure 9. AI governance framework

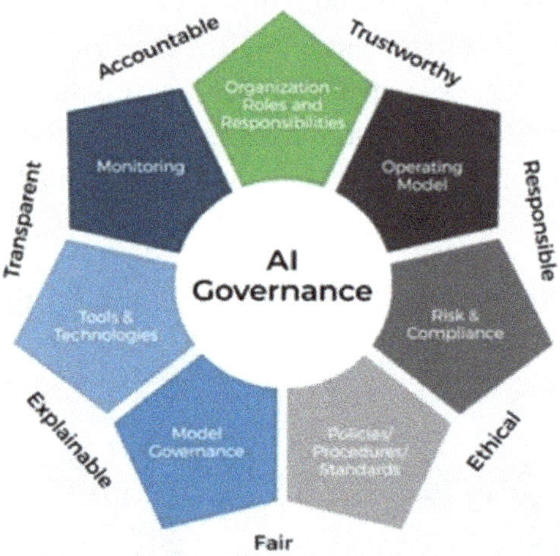

Global Policy Perspectives on AI Integration

AI integration in the healthcare systems differs around the world due to differences in funds, regulatory maturity, and technical facilities. High-income countries usually focus on cutting-edge AI healthcare applications. However, scalable and affordable wellness to public health care solutions are more important in low- and moderate-income countries. Through the exchange of moral principles, suggestions for policies, and capability-building applications the international organizations foster collaboration. Global policy perspectives highlight the requirement for the uniform standards with broad policies to guarantee fair access to the healthcare advantages made possible by AI across the globe.

CHALLENGES AND BARRIERS TO AI-DRIVEN HEALTHCARE REFORM

Addressing difficulties related to healthcare data is necessary for improving the efficiency and quality of healthcare services. As we investigate the complexities of storing healthcare data, a number of critical issues become apparent. Another key issue in AI development is AI bias, which is linked with unequal representation and access to opportunities. When AI models are trained on large data sets, they may inherit biases found in previous medical data, resulting in discrepancies in treatment recommendations or diagnosis accuracy. AI must eventually become the benchmark for safe, inclusive, and responsible conduct.

Technical Challenges (Bias, Explainability, Data Quality)

- Data Security and Privacy: Data, which frequently includes sensitive personal information, serves as the foundation for AI in healthcare. Strong encryption techniques, secure data-sharing processes, and compliance with legislation such as the GDPR in the EU and the HIPAA (Health Insurance Portability and Accountability Act) in the United States are all required to safeguard the privacy and security of this data (Bertl et al., 2023).
- Bias and Ethical Concerns: AI systems are only as unbiased as their training data. If the training data is uneven, the AI may draw biased conclusions, perhaps leading to unequal treatment outcomes for particular demographic groups. Addressing these preconceptions and ensuring that ethical considerations are built into AI systems is a difficult task.
- Interoperability: Healthcare data is challenging to collect and evaluate because it is fragmented across many systems and formats. Software engineers must address the interoperability barrier in order to enable smooth data transmission and semantic integration, as well as ensure that AI systems can use a range of data sources for full analysis. The fact that data is regularly processed but the representation format remains consistent adds another layer of complexity. Thus, semantics serves as a refinement of the concept of type, as shown in semantic data types. This must also fall within the scope of AI tools.
- Regulatory Compliance: Navigating the medical industry's regulatory environment can be difficult. AI-based healthcare systems must comply with numerous rules governing medical equipment and patient data. A detailed understanding of both the technological and regulatory realms is required to ensure that these systems are efficient and legally compliant.
- Trust and Adoption: In order to use AI-based technology, patients and healthcare personnel must first establish trust. This includes demonstrating the ef-

ficacy, safety, and dependability of AI therapies. To develop technologies that complement rather than replace human judgment in clinical operations, software engineers must work closely with healthcare experts.

Table 1. Challenges and Solutions in AI Healthcare Implementation

Challenge	Description	Proposed Solutions
Data Privacy and Security	Concerns over patient data confidentiality and unauthorized access	Implement secure AI systems, using encryption and decentralized data management systems like blockchain
Algorithmic Bias	AI models may inherit biases from historical data, leading to inequitable outcomes	Develop bias-mitigation techniques and ensure AI systems are trained on diverse, representative data
Integration with Legacy Systems	Difficulty integrating AI technologies with existing healthcare infrastructure	Adopt open standards and modular AI systems that are inoperable with legacy healthcare systems.
Lack of Explainability	AI's "black box" nature creates challenges in understanding decision-making processes	Develop Explainable AI (XAI) models that provide clear rationale for AI-generated decisions in clinical contexts.

As a result represented in Table 1, incorporating AI into healthcare systems presents a great opportunity to improve healthcare delivery, make tailored medicine a reality, and improve access to care. However, the trip is laden with difficulties, ranging from data privacy and bias to regulatory impediments and the requirement for interoperability.

Ethical, Legal, and Privacy Concerns

There are still numerous unanswered problems regarding algorithmic bias, data privacy, and accountability. Healthcare executives encounter uncertainty since the legal framework governing AI and healthcare is constantly evolving, albeit US standards such as HIPAA provide a basis (Hassan et al., 2024). AI adoption in the healthcare industry frequently lacks clear lines of accountability, especially in critical cases involving life-or-death decisions. Who is in charge of AI findings is frequently unknown. Medical errors, wrong diagnoses, and difficulty in regulating ethical AI in critical health decisions may emerge from a failure to give responsibility in AI applications.

Organizational and Workforce Readiness Barriers

Clinical interviews revealed significant concerns regarding the state of their institutions' IT infrastructure and digital preparedness. Many people believe that the slowness and age of their current IT systems is a key impediment to digital transformation and the adoption of AI-driven solutions. They also stressed the importance of having a sufficient number of computers and competent maintenance services to ensure the security and continuity of the digital system. Radiologists in the Netherlands raised similar concerns, claiming that the present healthcare infrastructure is insufficient to adopt and grow AI technologies. These findings were backed by a number of studies, which identified a lack of AI-compatible gear and software, outdated IT infrastructure, and limited computing resources as major hurdles to AI adoption in healthcare. The successful implementation and long-term viability of AI technologies in healthcare are significantly reliant on organizational and financial support, in addition to technological infrastructure. One of the main issues highlighted by healthcare practitioners is that the deployment of AI and other digital technology is typically done from the top down, with little input from frontline staff. Clinicians reported unhappiness with not being included in the decision-making processes for AI implementation, resulting in resistance and disengagement.

Socioeconomic and Equity Implications

Artificial intelligence (AI) assists healthcare providers in improving patient outcomes and resource efficiency by analyzing massive amounts of medical data and facilitating informed decision-making. AI has the potential to totally alter healthcare by enabling more precise diagnosis, personalized treatment regimens, and efficient resource utilization. However, when building, deploying, and using AI, it is critical to establish fair expectations and consider ethical problems such as duty, justice, and transparency.

EMERGING AI TRENDS DRIVING FUTURE OPPORTUNITIES

Generative AI in Healthcare

In the healthcare industry, generative artificial intelligence (Gen AI) has the ability to revolutionize patient care, tailor treatment options, conduct medical research, and teach healthcare staff (Vallée, 2023). This research has examined a number of clinical and non-clinical uses of Zen AI. Customized treatment plans, synthetic data generation, medical image analysis, nurse workflow management, risk prediction, pandemic preparedness and population health management are all supported by General AI in clinical settings. General AI has the potential to reduce physicians' stress by automating administrative duties such as medical recording, freeing up more time for direct patient care.

In addition, by automating specific tasks in the operating room and providing real-time feedback, General AI can improve surgical outcomes. The production of synthetic data improves research capacity and prediction accuracy by opening up new avenues for disease model training and simulation. General AI improves medical education, public relations, revenue cycle management, health care marketing, and other non-clinical applications. Because of its ability to constantly learn and adapt, it can support long-term gains in clinical and operational efficiency, leading in more proactive, accurate, and predictable healthcare delivery.

Federated Learning and Privacy-Preserving AI

Federated learning allows several businesses to collaborate to train AI models while protecting the privacy and security of sensitive data across all platforms as shown in Figure 10. Instead of aggregating all data in one place, only model updates are shared, ensuring privacy while generating powerful AI. This solution addresses one of the most pressing issues in modern AI development: acquiring various forms of real-world data while maintaining anonymity. Smartphone users, for example, can help developers improve keyboard predictions without disclosing their private messages, and hospitals can work together to produce better diagnostic tools without disclosing patient information. Federated learning represents a dramatic shift in our view of data ownership and artificial intelligence development.

Figure 10. Federated Learning and Privacy-preserving AI

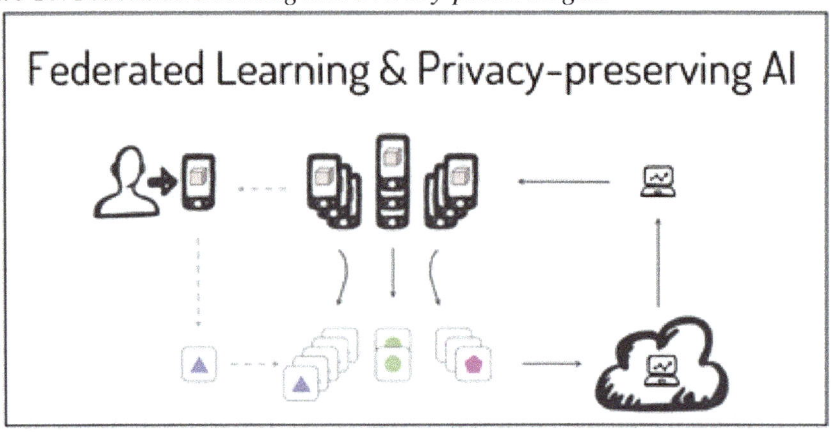

The increasing amount of personal data being collected and used by AI systems necessitates privacy-preserving AI. AI that respects privacy ensures that people have control over their data and can trust that it will be handled responsibly. Federated learning significantly improves privacy by storing raw data on users' devices. Only model updates are transferred over networks, not private data to central servers. This design protects personal data from exposure while it is being sent or stored. Studies show that model tweaks can still leak information. Attackers could utilize inference attacks to extract private information from these updates. Recent research suggests that sophisticated attackers may be able to identify specific users or reconstitute training samples.

Digital Twins of Patients, Hospitals, and Communities

Digital twin technology is transforming health-care systems by harnessing real-time data integration and virtual simulation, allowing for predictive analytics and aiding training and simulation. Digital twins can collect and analyze enormous volumes of patient data from many sources to deliver individualized therapy suggestions based on patient traits, medical history, and real-time physiological data. Digital twins can improve clinical operations by analyzing workflow and resource allocation, leading in more efficient processes and improved patient care. Digital twin technology has the potential to dramatically improve patient outcomes, increase patient safety, and promote healthcare innovation. Digital twin technologies have the ability to significantly improve clinical operations in health care systems. Digital twins assist health care providers in examining and optimizing workflows, allocating resources, and increasing operational efficiency by constructing virtual duplicates of physical systems and combining real-time data.

The utilization of digital twins can offer healthcare staff a platform for ongoing professional growth. Digital twins give healthcare personnel access to case studies, simulation scenarios, and virtual training modules, allowing them to learn new ways, keep up with the latest breakthroughs, and acquire specialized abilities. Because of this self-paced learning and continual training, health care personnel are better prepared to offer high-quality care, which promotes lifelong learning.

AI-Blockchain Integration for Trust and Security

As artificial intelligence (AI) spreads across industries, businesses struggle to trust its outputs, while regulators demand more openness and auditability from algorithms. Chief information officers (CIOs) are under unprecedented pressure to implement AI governance policies in order to maintain their businesses and jobs, particularly given the rapid adoption of generative AI (GAI) in organizations (Kumar et al., 2025). Regardless of existing institutions, CIOs will need to update internal policies to keep up with the rapid pace of innovation. Although many organizations have begun to implement governance initiatives, not all components are in place. Others have not yet prioritized AI governance and risk management, but this is not due to a lack of interest; rather, they are unsure where to begin.

Blockchain and AI offer enormous potential for protecting sensitive data, particularly in industries such as healthcare and finance. There are already various cutting-edge techniques for managing sensitive medical data that utilize blockchain and artificial intelligence. For example, Medical Chain, a UK-based health technology business, leverages blockchain technology to deliver a transparent, secure medical records system that protects both patients' and doctors' privacy.

Edge AI and 6G-Enabled Smart Healthcare Ecosystems

The combination of AI and upcoming 6G wireless connectivity promises to transform healthcare delivery by providing ultra-fast, dependable, and intelligent medical services. The convergence of cutting-edge breakthroughs in edge computing, 6G communication networks, and artificial intelligence is expected to usher in a technological revolution in the healthcare industry . These advancements are transforming the delivery, analysis, and optimization of healthcare services, enabling faster, more accurate, and tailored care. The healthcare industry is fast changing due to rising prices and a growing shortage of competent staff. Innovative approaches, such as the use of cutting-edge 6G technology and AI-driven algorithms, are critical for tackling these difficulties. These technologies are revolutionizing health care by improving overall therapy, automating alarms, and offering improved patient monitoring.

Figure 11. Flowchart of 6G integration with smart healthcare

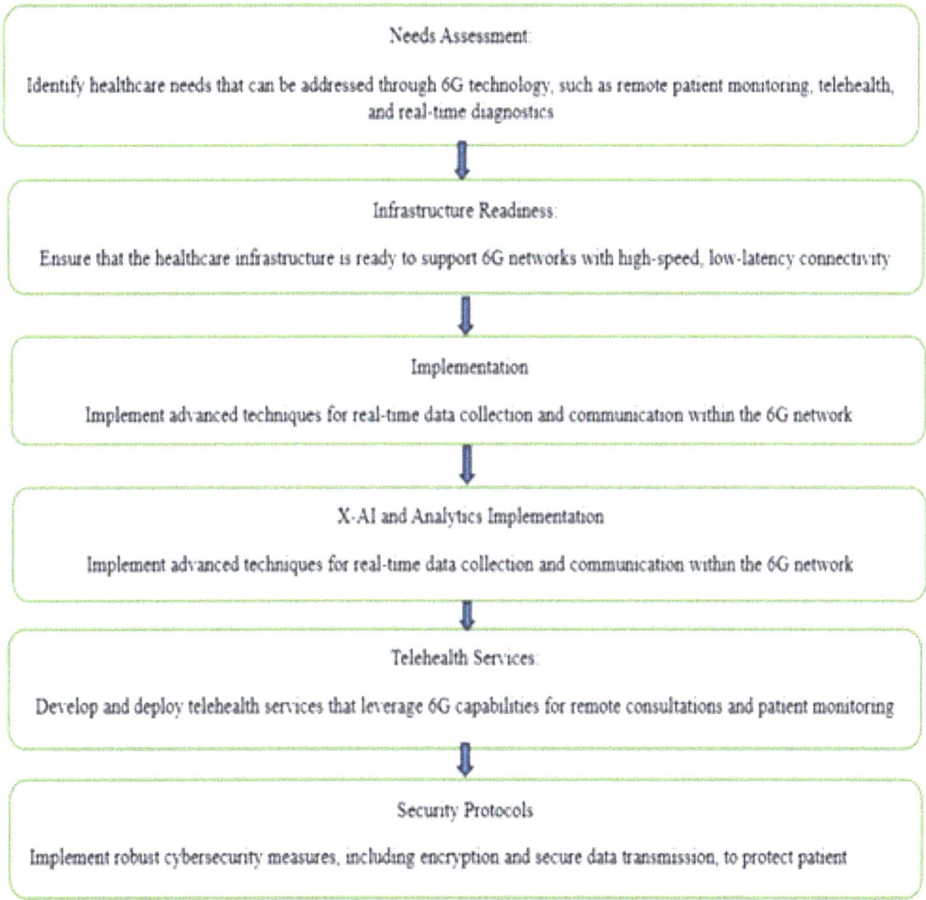

6G networks' rapid speeds and low latency lay the groundwork for instantaneous communications, allowing the integration of a variety of healthcare sensors and equipment as shown in Figure 11. Healthcare professionals can make data-driven choices faster because to 6G's rapid connectivity, which allows for real-time data sharing. Furthermore, 6G's capacity to provide high-quality, low-latency video communications enables telemedicine applications. Telehealth services, like as remote patient monitoring and virtual consultations, are becoming more effective and accessible, particularly in remote or low-income communities. In brief, 6G and smart healthcare collaborate to create a dynamic ecosystem that offers dependable, fast connectivity and cutting-edge medical solutions. By boosting efficiency, accessibility, and healthcare capabilities, our alliance ushers in a new era of patient-centered care.

CASE STUDIES AND GLOBAL BEST PRACTICES

AI-Enabled Health Systems (US, EU, India, Singapore, UK)

Artificial intelligence (AI) has drastically changed access, efficiency, and health care systems all around the world. AI-managed health systems emerge as a game-changing option for addressing these complex difficulties as healthcare systems around the world struggle with aging populations, workforce shortages, growing costs, and the persisting problem of health inequities. This in-depth analysis investigates the state of AI application in global health systems by assessing successful case studies, calculating performance measurements, and providing a strategic roadmap for future development. Real-world applications, such as Singapore's nationally implemented diabetic retinopathy screening system and the UK's AI-enhanced ambulance triage guidelines, show how AI may increase healthcare access for underprivileged populations, lower costs, and improve diagnostic accuracy.

One of the most advanced uses of AI in healthcare is diagnostic imaging. Currently, the most popular use of AI is the automated classification of medical images. More than half (58%) of the AI/ML-based medical devices certified in the USA and Europe between 2015 and 2020 were CE designated or approved for radiological use, according to a recent assessment.

AI systems rely on Electronic Health Records (EHRs) as their data source, yet regional differences in EHR quality and standardization are substantial. Medical Imaging analysis, Remote Monitoring & Wearables, Predictive analytics, Virtual Health Assistants and Chatbots, AI-driven robots help a lot for analysis of patient data. CNNs have proven to be quite good at diagnosing diabetic retinopathy from fundus photos, pneumonia from chest X-rays, and different types of cancer from medical imaging as shown in Figure 12. These systems process images much more quickly while frequently achieving diagnosis accuracy on par with or higher than that of human experts.

Pandemic-Driven AI Innovation Lessons (e.g., COVID-19)

Figure 12. Application of AI to tackle COVID-19

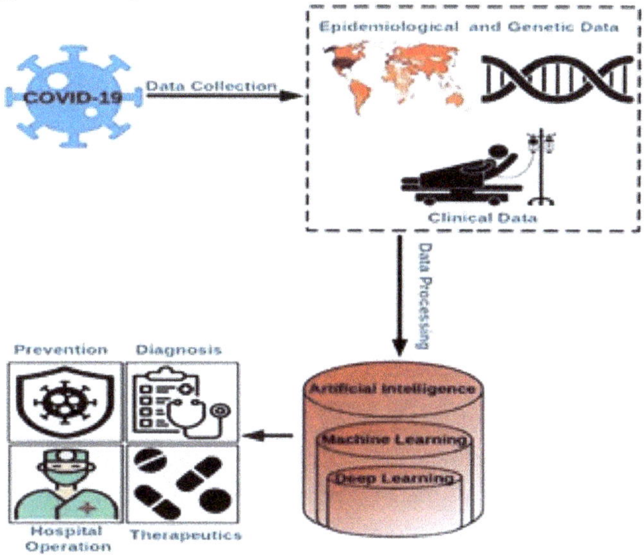

In considering the health sector's history, it has been noted that artificial intelligence is essential in combating the viruses that were common at the time. This observation inspired developers to develop AI applications that minimize human intervention in healthcare during the pandemic. As of right now, it has been discovered that artificial intelligence plays a major role in vaccine research, tracking, monitoring, and projections.

The COVID-19 pandemic has pushed the application of artificial intelligence (AI) in a variety of sectors, including public sentiment analysis, healthcare, and pandemic management. AI systems processed massive quantities of data to track and anticipate transmission pathways, resulting in a considerable decline in local transmission rates within the first month. To successfully identify sick individuals and implement quarantine measures, major cities deployed AI-based thermal imaging and facial recognition in transit centers. This helped to stop the spread in densely populated areas. AI was utilized to monitor and predict COVID-19 infection through dashboards and data visualization methods. They provided a comprehensive picture of patients from all around the world who were at risk. The two main types of data visualization systems are local and global dashboards. The datasets fall into a number of general categories, including text, social media, biomedical, speech, and case studies.

Successful AI-Policy Integration Models

The organization's present situation, its current capabilities, and level of readiness must all be carefully taken into account for AI implementation in healthcare to be successful. Before incorporating AI technology into their operations, healthcare organizations must thoroughly evaluate their internal workflows, data management procedures, and technical infrastructures. Some of these supply-and-demand issues may be resolved by the use of technology and artificial intelligence (AI) in the healthcare industry. A moment of convergence between healthcare and technology to fundamentally transform models of healthcare delivery through AI-augmented healthcare systems is heralded by the growing availability of multi-modal data (genomics, economic, demographic, clinical, and phenotypic) combined with technological advancements in mobile, internet of things (IoT), computing power, and data security.

A thorough evaluation of the existing technical infrastructure is a critical step in incorporating AI into healthcare. Healthcare businesses must determine whether their present IT systems can support advanced AI applications, including network capacity, picture storage, laboratory information systems, and electronic health records (EHRs). Processing capacity, the availability of graphic processing units (GPUs) for real-time data analysis and model training, computing capabilities (cloud-based or on-premises), and adequate data storage should all be taken into account during these evaluations.

CONCLUSION

Healthcare Challenges in Developing Countries: A lack of healthcare services is a major issue in many developing countries. This includes a scarcity of critical medical supplies, inadequate healthcare facilities, and a paucity of medical professionals. Many developing countries struggle with the availability of hospitals, clinics, and medical equipment. Educating people about illness prevention, diet, and hygiene can be quite helpful. Collaborations between the public and private sectors can help close gaps in healthcare infrastructure and service delivery. Engaging the private sector can help achieve public health objectives by contributing resources and encouraging innovation. Telemedicine and mobile health applications can improve healthcare access, particularly in rural regions, by allowing patients to consult with healthcare professionals remotely, hence increasing ease and accessibility.

- *Equitable Access to Healthcare:* One key concern is the difference in health-care access between socioeconomic categories and between urban and rural communities.
- *Affordable Healthcare Delivery:* Many patients struggle to receive high-quality care due to high treatment expenses, pricey drugs, and restricted insurance coverage.
- *Lack of Skilled Healthcare Workforce:* A dearth of trained doctors, nurses, and other healthcare professionals, particularly in remote areas, makes it difficult to provide timely and high-quality care.
- *Technology Integration in Healthcare:* The adoption of technologies such as telemedicine and artificial intelligence is limited due to high costs, insufficient infrastructure, and a lack of digital literacy.

Opportunities for Future Research

It is widely acknowledged that shifting demographics and an increased emphasis on community-based care will place unprecedented strains on health-care systems. Although the combination of scientific and technical achievements with new and emerging care pathways has the potential to significantly improve clinical results, the risk of rising health inequities must also be considered. Although interdisciplinary approaches may be better suited to dealing with some of the more difficult ethical dilemmas that arise, the advancements made by interdisciplinary research will surely present challenges.

REFERENCES

Bertl, M., Lamo, Y., Leucker, M., Margaria, T., Mohammadi, E., Mukhiya, S. K., & Rabbi, F. (2023). Challenges for ai in healthcare systems. In International Conference on Bridging the Gap between AI and Reality (pp. 165-186). Cham: Springer Nature Switzerland.

Blanco, J., Ferreras, M., & Cosido, O. (2025). Predictive modeling of hospital emergency department demand using artificial intelligence: A systematic review. *International Journal of Medical Informatics*, •••, 106215. PMID: 41401760

Dangi, R. R., Sharma, A., & Vageriya, V. (2025). Transforming healthcare in low-resource settings with artificial intelligence: Recent developments and outcomes. *Public Health Nursing (Boston, Mass.)*, *42*(2), 1017–1030. DOI: 10.1111/phn.13500 PMID: 39629887

El-Jerjawi, N. S., Murad, W. F., Harazin, D., Qaoud, A. N., Jamala, M. N., Abunasser, B. S., & Abu-Naser, S. S. (2024). The role of artificial intelligence in revolutionizing health: Challenges, applications, and future prospects.

Faiyazuddin, M., Rahman, S. J. Q., Anand, G., Siddiqui, R. K., Mehta, R., Khatib, M. N., & Sah, R. (2025). The impact of artificial intelligence on healthcare: A comprehensive review of advancements in diagnostics, treatment, and operational efficiency. *Health Science Reports*, *8*(1), e70312. DOI: 10.1002/hsr2.70312 PMID: 39763580

Gagnon, M. P., Ouellet, S., Attisso, E., Supper, W., Amil, S., Rhéaume, C., & Sasseville, M. (2024). Wearable devices for supporting chronic disease self-management: Scoping review. *Interactive Journal of Medical Research*, *13*(1), e55925. DOI: 10.2196/55925 PMID: 39652850

Hassan, M., Kushniruk, A., & Borycki, E. (2024). Barriers to and facilitators of artificial intelligence adoption in health care: Scoping review. *JMIR Human Factors*, *11*, e48633. DOI: 10.2196/48633 PMID: 39207831

Herrera-Poyatos, A., Del Ser, J., López de Prado, M., Wang, F.-Y., Herrera-Viedma, E., & de Prado, M. (2025). Responsible artificial intelligence systems: A roadmap to society's trust through trustworthy AI, auditability, accountability, and governance. *arXiv*.

Kumar, A., Masud, M., Alsharif, M. H., Gaur, N., & Nanthaamornphong, A. (2025). Integrating 6G technology in smart hospitals: Challenges and opportunities for enhanced healthcare services. *Frontiers in Medicine*, *12*, 1534551. DOI: 10.3389/fmed.2025.1534551 PMID: 40255587

Li, J. H., Tseng, Y. J., Chen, S. H., & Chen, K. F. (2025). Artificial Intelligence in Infection Surveillance: Data Integration, Applications and Future Directions. *Biomedical Journal*, •••, 100929. DOI: 10.1016/j.bj.2025.100929 PMID: 41205676

Razavi, J., Dhafar, H. O., & BaHammam, A. S. (2025). Transforming health care with artificial intelligence: Regulations, challenges, and future directions. *Saudi Journal for Health Sciences*, *14*(1), 11–22. DOI: 10.4103/sjhs.sjhs_26_25

Salehi, F. (2024). The transformative role of artificial intelligence in the healthcare industry: A comprehensive analysis. *Asian Journal of Research in Medicine and Medical Science*, *6*(1), 62–70.

Sutton, R. T., Pincock, D., Baumgart, D. C., Sadowski, D. C., Fedorak, R. N., & Kroeker, K. I. (2020). An overview of clinical decision support systems: Benefits, risks, and strategies for success. *NPJ Digital Medicine*, *3*(1), 17. DOI: 10.1038/s41746-020-0221-y PMID: 32047862

Vallée, A. (2023). Digital twin for healthcare systems. *Frontiers in Digital Health*, *5*, 1253050. DOI: 10.3389/fdgth.2023.1253050 PMID: 37744683

Chapter 2

Digital Pathways to Inclusive Health Reform:

Addressing Mental Health Inequities Among Informal Workers in India

Jince George
http://orcid.org/0000-0003-3371-7334
Christ University, India

Sheeja B. Karalam
Christ University, India

ABSTRACT

This chapter examines how digital transformation can address mental health inequities among informal workers in India, focusing on discrimination, labor precarity, and unequal access to care. Using empirical insights from Kerala within broader national and global contexts, it analyzes how psychological distress among native and migrant workers emerges from intersecting socioeconomic, institutional, and digital factors. Drawing on psychology, public health, economics, and digital governance, the chapter proposes a phygital mental health framework integrating physical services with digitally enabled care pathways. Emphasis is placed on ethical leadership, data governance, and economic sustainability, highlighting both opportunities and risks of digital mental health expansion. The chapter demonstrates how compassionate, inclusive, and accountable digital reforms can translate mental health policy into effective instruments for equity, social justice, and sustainable health system transformation.

DOI: 10.4018/979-8-2600-0939-0.ch002

INTRODUCTION

India's transition toward a digitally integrated healthcare ecosystem presents a critical opportunity to address long-standing inequities in access, quality, and continuity of care. National initiatives such as the Ayushman Bharat Digital Mission (ABDM) and the National Mental Health Programme (NMHP) reflect a strong policy commitment to digital modernization. Yet, despite this momentum, a substantial proportion of India's informal workforce—nearly 93% of total employment—remains structurally excluded from formal healthcare systems. Daily-wage laborers, agricultural workers, street vendors, and migrant construction workers continue to face intersecting challenges of economic precarity, social marginalization, and unmet mental health needs.

Mental health inequities within the informal sector are not merely clinical concerns but are produced through layered structural conditions, including discrimination, insecure employment, migration-related stress, and weak institutional protection. Empirical research from Kerala provides important insight into these dynamics. Findings from the study by Fr. Jince George and Dr. Sheeja Karalam indicate that perceived discrimination is a major contributor to psychological distress among informal workers, with particularly adverse effects observed among migrant populations. These findings align with broader psychological and public health literature that identifies discrimination as a chronic psychosocial stressor capable of undermining self-esteem, coping capacity, and overall well-being.

Kerala represents a revealing yet paradoxical context for examining these issues. Despite its comparatively strong welfare orientation, high literacy rates, and advanced healthcare infrastructure, significant gaps persist in migrant inclusion, linguistic accessibility, and mental health outreach. This paradox underscores a key limitation of welfare- and technology-led development: institutional capacity and digital expansion alone do not guarantee equitable outcomes. Without explicit attention to ethics, governance, and participation, digital health reforms risk reinforcing existing social hierarchies rather than dismantling them.

Within this landscape, digital health technologies—particularly when implemented through a *phygital approach* that integrates physical service delivery with digital platforms—offer promising pathways to inclusion. Telepsychiatry, mobile counseling, AI-assisted screening, and community-based digital interventions have the potential to extend mental health services to underserved populations, reduce opportunity costs, and improve continuity of care. However, their effectiveness depends not only on technological availability but also on digital literacy, trust, ethical data governance, workforce readiness, and accountable leadership.

Building on these concerns, this chapter develops a policy-oriented framework for inclusive mental health reform grounded in interdisciplinary perspectives from psychology, public health, economics, and digital governance. While Kerala serves as an empirical anchor, the analysis is situated within broader national and global debates on digital public goods, ethical innovation, and health equity. The chapter advances a *phygital mental health model* that foregrounds ethical leadership, participatory governance, and economic sustainability as prerequisites for meaningful digital transformation.

Accordingly, the chapter asks: *How can India's digital health transformation be leveraged to create inclusive, ethical, and sustainable mental health systems for informal workers?* By integrating empirical evidence, theoretical insights, and policy analysis, it offers a roadmap for phygital health reform that reframes mental health equity not only as a human rights imperative but also as a foundational requirement for inclusive development and resilient health governance.

BACKGROUND

The informal sector constitutes the backbone of India's labour economy, employing nearly 93% of the workforce and contributing substantially to national productivity (Government of India, 2020). Despite this central economic role, informal workers—including daily-wage labourers, construction workers, domestic helpers, agricultural workers, street vendors, and migrant labourers—remain largely excluded from formal healthcare systems. The absence of social security, health insurance, and institutional protection exposes this population to chronic insecurity and heightened psychological vulnerability. Informality is therefore not merely an employment category but a structural condition shaped by low wages, job precarity, legal invisibility, and limited access to welfare mechanisms (Srivastava, 2011).

Globally, more than two billion people are engaged in informal work, with South Asia accounting for a disproportionately high share (ILO, 2018). Across low- and middle-income countries, precarious employment conditions—characterized by unsafe workplaces, unstable incomes, long working hours, and social marginalization—have been consistently linked to elevated risks of anxiety, depression, and psychosomatic distress (Li et al., 2020). Mental health inequities thus emerge as one of the most pervasive yet under-addressed consequences of informality, reinforced by stigma, policy neglect, and fragmented service delivery. In India, these vulnerabilities are further intensified by intersecting axes of caste, gender, migration status, and linguistic identity, which shape access to psychosocial support and healthcare engagement.

Empirical evidence from Kerala offers critical insight into these dynamics. The study by Fr. Jince George and Dr. Sheeja Karalam demonstrates that perceived discrimination functions as a chronic psychosocial stressor among informal workers, accounting for a substantial proportion of psychological distress. Migrant workers reported significantly higher levels of anxiety, depression, and stress than native workers, underscoring how institutional exclusion and social marginalization undermine self-esteem, belonging, and perceived control—key dimensions of psychological well-being (Ryff & Keyes, 1995; Williams & Mohammed, 2009). Importantly, the study also highlights a dual burden within informal labour markets: while migrants face exclusion, exploitation, and cultural alienation, native workers often experience economic displacement and identity insecurity. This coexistence of privilege and vulnerability reflects the layered nature of informality rather than a simple migrant–native dichotomy.

Kerala represents a revealing paradox within India's development trajectory. Despite strong literacy rates, welfare-oriented governance, and relatively advanced healthcare infrastructure, the state continues to struggle with migrant inclusion, linguistic barriers, and uneven access to mental health services (Rajan & Zachariah, 2019). This paradox illustrates a broader limitation of welfare-led development models: institutional capacity and technological advancement do not automatically ensure equitable outcomes. Similar patterns have been documented across other regions in India and in LMICs globally, where informal workers experience distress linked to discrimination, income insecurity, and lack of institutional recognition (Aguilar-Gaxiola et al., 2011).

Migration further compounds mental health vulnerability by producing what Bhugra (2004) describes as "triple exclusion"—disconnection from the place of origin, marginalization within host communities, and limited access to formal support systems. The COVID-19 pandemic starkly exposed these structural weaknesses, as millions of migrant workers in India faced abrupt job loss, displacement, and psychological trauma amid restricted access to care (Thomas et al., 2020). While digital innovations such as telemedicine and AI-enabled triage expanded healthcare reach during this period, they also revealed a growing "phygital divide" rooted in unequal digital access, literacy gaps, language barriers, and trust deficits (NITI Aayog, 2021).

These developments highlight a critical policy blind spot. Although untreated mental health conditions impose an estimated global economic cost of nearly US$1 trillion annually (WHO, 2022), mental health among informal workers remains weakly integrated into national health and labour policies. Bridging this gap requires reframing mental health distress and discrimination as systemic governance challenges rather than individual pathologies. Kerala's relatively strong infrastructure and participatory governance structures make it a valuable laboratory for examining how inclusive, phygital mental health systems might be designed—provided that ethical leadership, data governance, and community engagement are embedded into digital reform.

This background establishes the necessity of an equity-oriented digital health approach that addresses not only service delivery gaps but also the structural, ethical, and intersectional determinants of mental health. It provides the contextual foundation for the theoretical, economic, and policy frameworks developed in subsequent sections, situating India's digital health transformation within a broader agenda of inclusive governance and sustainable health system reform.

THEORETICAL FRAMEWORK

Understanding mental health inequities among informal workers in India requires a theoretically integrated approach that connects psychological processes, structural discrimination, and digital governance. Mental health outcomes among native and migrant informal workers are not shaped by individual factors alone but emerge from the interaction of social hierarchies, labor precarity, institutional exclusion, and unequal access to digital resources. To capture this complexity, the chapter synthesizes four complementary theoretical perspectives: the Stress–Appraisal–Coping Model (Lazarus & Folkman, 1984), the Discrimination and Mental Health Framework (Williams & Mohammed, 2009), the Psychological Well-being Model (Ryff & Keyes, 1995), and Digital Inclusion and Equity Models (WHO, 2022; NITI Aayog, 2021).

The Discrimination and Mental Health Framework conceptualizes discrimination as a chronic psychosocial stressor that affects cognitive, emotional, and physiological functioning over time. Rather than isolated incidents, discriminatory experiences accumulate, undermining self-esteem, perceived control, and social belonging—key determinants of mental health. Empirical evidence from informal labor contexts, including Kerala, supports this framework by demonstrating strong associations between perceived discrimination and elevated levels of anxiety, depression, and stress, particularly among migrant workers. This perspective situates mental distress within structural and institutional conditions rather than individual pathology.

The Stress–Appraisal–Coping Model further explains how individuals interpret and respond to such stressors. According to Lazarus and Folkman (1984), psychological outcomes depend on primary appraisal (perceived threat), secondary appraisal (available coping resources), and coping strategies. In informal work settings, limited social protection, economic insecurity, linguistic barriers, and low institutional trust often constrain adaptive coping responses, increasing vulnerability to sustained distress. This model highlights how unequal access to resources transforms discrimination from a stressor into a persistent mental health risk.

Ryff and Keyes' Psychological Well-being Model expands the analysis beyond distress to positive mental health by emphasizing six dimensions of well-being: self-acceptance, autonomy, environmental mastery, purpose in life, positive relations, and personal growth. Discrimination and precarity systematically erode these domains, while protective factors such as self-esteem, social recognition, and supportive environments can buffer adverse effects. From a policy perspective, this framework underscores that mental health reform must focus not only on symptom reduction but also on restoring dignity, agency, and psychosocial resilience.

In the digital era, these psychosocial processes are increasingly mediated by access to technology, introducing digital inclusion as a critical determinant of mental health equity. Digital Inclusion and Equity Models emphasize three interdependent pillars: access, literacy, and trust. Access reduces spatial and financial barriers to care; digital literacy enhances self-efficacy and help-seeking capacity; and trust—shaped by ethical data governance, privacy protections, and cultural sensitivity—determines sustained engagement. Without these conditions, digital health interventions risk reproducing exclusion rather than alleviating it.

Integrating these perspectives produces a multi-level theoretical model of inclusive mental health reform. At the micro level, individual appraisal, coping, and well-being processes shape psychological outcomes. At the meso level, discrimination and institutional practices influence community-level access and social support. At the macro level, digital governance, policy design, and ethical leadership define the structural conditions for equity. The interaction of these levels supports a *phygital approach*, in which physical and digital systems are jointly deployed to address both psychological distress and structural exclusion.

This integrated framework clarifies that digitalization without social inclusion lacks ethical depth, while social reform without digital integration lacks scalability. By aligning psychological theory, structural analysis, and digital governance, the framework provides a coherent foundation for designing inclusive, ethical, and sustainable mental health systems for informal workers. It also establishes the conceptual basis for the chapter's subsequent economic, policy, and leadership analyses, positioning mental health equity as a systemic governance challenge rather than an individual deficit.

CONCEPTUAL FRAMEWORK

The conceptual framework for *Digital Pathways to Inclusive Health Reform* integrates psychosocial theory, digital inclusion principles, and governance perspectives to explain how mental health inequities among informal workers are produced and how they can be addressed through inclusive digital transformation. Rather than treating mental distress as an individual deficit, the framework conceptualizes it as an outcome of structural discrimination, labor precarity, and uneven access to institutional and digital resources. Digital inclusion and ethical leadership are positioned as enabling forces that can interrupt these pathways and support equitable reform.

At its core, the framework advances a *phygital mental health model*, which integrates physical health services with digitally enabled pathways to care. This hybrid approach is designed to enhance accessibility, continuity, and dignity for marginalized labor groups whose mobility, income insecurity, and social exclusion limit engagement with conventional healthcare systems. The framework operates across four interrelated domains:

1. *Psychosocial determinants*,
2. *Digital inclusion*,
3. *Economic and policy conditions*, and
4. *Leadership and governance*.

Within the psychosocial domain, discrimination is conceptualized as a multidimensional structural stressor encompassing institutional, interpersonal, and internalized forms of exclusion. These experiences undermine self-esteem, social belonging, and perceived control, thereby increasing vulnerability to psychological distress. Coping capacity and psychological well-being function as mediating mechanisms in this relationship. Drawing on stress–coping and well-being theories, the framework distinguishes between adaptive coping strategies—such as help-seeking, problem-solving, and social support—and maladaptive responses that exacerbate distress. Strengthening self-esteem, recognition, and psychosocial resources is therefore central to mitigating mental health inequities.

Digital inclusion constitutes the enabling environment through which psychosocial interventions can be scaled and sustained. Building on national and global digital health equity frameworks, the model identifies *access*, *digital literacy*, and *trust* as foundational pillars. Access reduces geographic and financial barriers to care; literacy enhances confidence, autonomy, and help-seeking behavior; and trust—shaped by ethical data governance, privacy safeguards, and cultural sensitivity—determines sustained engagement with digital mental health services. Without these conditions, digital tools risk reinforcing exclusion rather than alleviating it.

Economic and policy dimensions shape the feasibility and sustainability of reform. Mental health inclusion is framed not only as a rights-based obligation but also as an economic imperative, given the productivity losses associated with untreated psychological distress. Policies that integrate mental health into digital health missions, labor protections, and social welfare schemes create the structural conditions necessary for scalable impact. Phygital systems reduce opportunity costs for informal workers while improving efficiency and data-informed planning.

Leadership and governance operate at the macro level as catalytic forces that institutionalize equity. Drawing from transformational and servant leadership principles, the framework emphasizes ethical accountability, empathy, and participatory decision-making as prerequisites for inclusive digital health reform. Governance mechanisms—such as grievance redressal systems, cross-sector coordination, and transparent data stewardship—reinforce trust and accountability across digital ecosystems.

Structurally, the framework functions as a multi-level system: individual coping and digital literacy shape resilience at the micro level; community norms and institutional practices influence access at the meso level; and leadership, policy, and digital governance define equity at the macro level. Feedback loops link these levels, illustrating how ethical leadership strengthens digital inclusion, which in turn enhances coping, well-being, and civic trust.

In application, the framework informs initiatives under the Ayushman Bharat Digital Mission and the National Mental Health Programme by embedding psychosocial sensitivity, digital ethics, and participatory governance into program design. Overall, the conceptual model rests on five core propositions: mental health inequities are structurally produced; coping and well-being mediate distress; digital inclusion moderates access and outcomes; ethical leadership sustains reform; and phygital integration offers a scalable pathway to equity. By aligning psychological, technological, and institutional systems, the framework translates empirical insights into actionable strategies for inclusive, ethical, and resilient digital mental health governance in India.

PURPOSE AND CONTRIBUTION OF THE CHAPTER

The primary purpose of this chapter is to examine mental health inequities among informal workers in India through an integrated lens that combines psychology, public health, digital transformation, economics, and governance. While existing scholarship has extensively documented either informal labour conditions or mental health outcomes, few studies systematically connect discrimination, digital exclusion, and governance structures to mental health inequities within the informal sector. This chapter addresses that gap by positioning mental health distress among informal workers not as an individual or clinical problem, but as a structural outcome shaped by labor precarity, migration, social exclusion, and uneven access to institutional and digital resources.

Anchored in empirical evidence from Kerala and situated within broader national and global contexts, the chapter aims to reinterpret existing findings for policy and system-level reform. Rather than presenting Kerala as an exceptional case, it uses the state as an analytical anchor to illustrate how mental health inequities persist even within welfare-oriented and digitally progressive settings. This approach allows the chapter to identify transferable lessons while avoiding context-bound generalizations.

The chapter makes four key contributions. *First*, it offers a conceptual contribution by advancing a *phygital mental health framework* that integrates physical healthcare infrastructure with digitally enabled pathways to care, emphasizing that digital innovation must be ethically governed and socially embedded to achieve equity. *Second*, it contributes theoretically by synthesizing stress–coping models, discrimination frameworks, psychological well-being theory, and digital inclusion perspectives into a unified, multi-level explanatory model of mental health inequity. *Third*, it provides policy-relevant insight by reframing mental health inclusion as both a governance imperative and an economic investment, demonstrating how discrimination and untreated distress function as systemic inefficiencies within large informal economies. *Fourth*, it contributes to practice by translating interdisciplinary evidence into actionable recommendations spanning leadership, institutional design, community engagement, and digital ethics.

By foregrounding issues of intersectionality, digital governance, and implementation constraints, the chapter moves beyond technology-centric narratives of health reform. Its central argument is that inclusive mental health reform requires human-centered digital transformation—where leadership, ethics, and participation mediate the relationship between innovation and outcomes. In doing so, the chapter seeks to inform scholars, policymakers, and practitioners engaged in health equity, digital public infrastructure, and labor governance, while offering a scalable framework relevant to other low- and middle-income contexts with large informal workforces.

Overall, the chapter contributes to ongoing debates on digital health reform by demonstrating that mental health equity is not a peripheral concern but a foundational requirement for inclusive development, resilient health systems, and sustainable economic growth.

INFORMAL SECTOR MENTAL HEALTH — LESSONS FROM KERALA

Kerala occupies a distinctive position within India's development landscape. Internationally recognized for its high literacy rates, welfare orientation, and comparatively strong public health infrastructure, the state nonetheless reveals persistent mental health inequities within its informal workforce. Empirical research on informal workers in Kerala demonstrates that progressive social indicators do not automatically translate into psychosocial inclusion, particularly for migrant and precariously employed populations. This paradox makes Kerala a valuable, though not exceptional, case for examining how structural inequities persist within otherwise advanced welfare regimes.

Kerala's informal economy relies heavily on migrant labour from states such as Bihar, Odisha, Assam, and West Bengal, resulting in a stratified workforce shaped by nativity, language, and class (Rajan & Zachariah, 2019). Migrant workers frequently remain outside formal policy frameworks, with limited access to health insurance, welfare databases, and institutional grievance mechanisms. Studies consistently document overcrowded living conditions, social isolation, and cultural alienation among migrants—conditions that heighten psychological vulnerability (Thomas et al., 2020; Devassy & George, 2021). At the same time, native informal workers experience a different but related form of distress linked to economic displacement, wage competition, and identity insecurity. This dual burden underscores that mental health inequities within informality are systemic rather than confined to a single demographic group.

Empirical evidence from Kerala illustrates how discrimination operates as a key structural determinant of mental health. Research by George and Karalam demonstrates strong associations between perceived discrimination and psychological distress among informal workers, with migrant workers exhibiting disproportionately higher levels of anxiety, depression, and stress. These findings align with broader evidence that discrimination undermines self-esteem, social belonging, and perceived control, thereby intensifying mental health risks. Importantly, coping mechanisms mediate these outcomes: adaptive strategies such as social support and community engagement reduce distress, while maladaptive responses amplify vulnerability. This pattern reinforces theoretical models that situate mental health outcomes within broader social and institutional contexts rather than individual pathology.

Despite Kerala's welfare architecture, significant institutional gaps remain. Mental health services are unevenly distributed, with counseling and psychiatric support rarely reaching informal labour clusters or migrant settlements. Policy initiatives such as migrant insurance schemes have had limited impact due to low awareness, administrative complexity, and linguistic barriers. The absence of systematic mental health surveillance among informal workers further perpetuates what has been described as institutional invisibility—where universal welfare frameworks mask the exclusion of marginalized populations. Language barriers and cultural stigma compound these challenges, often discouraging help-seeking and undermining effective communication between workers and healthcare providers.

At the same time, Kerala offers important lessons in resilience and participatory governance. Decentralized institutions such as panchayats, women's collectives, and civil society organizations have demonstrated their capacity to mobilize community-based responses during public health crises, including the Nipah outbreak and the COVID-19 pandemic. These grassroots networks highlight the potential of locally embedded, culturally adaptive interventions for mental health outreach. Integrating such community capacity with digital tools—through multilingual telepsychiatry, mobile counseling platforms, and digitally supported community hubs—illustrates the promise of a *phygital approach* that combines technological reach with human mediation.

The Kerala experience yields several transferable insights for national health reform. First, empirical evidence on discrimination and distress must inform policy design rather than remain confined to academic discourse. Second, digital expansion must be accompanied by investments in literacy, trust, and ethical data governance to avoid reinforcing exclusion. Third, physical and digital infrastructures must be integrated to ensure continuity of care for mobile and informal populations. Finally, inclusive leadership and sustained community partnerships are essential for translating digital innovation into equitable outcomes.

Viewed in this light, Kerala functions less as an exception and more as a diagnostic case for India's broader health reform agenda. It demonstrates that even welfare-oriented systems can reproduce mental health inequities if structural discrimination, institutional gaps, and digital divides remain unaddressed. Incorporating Kerala's lessons into national initiatives such as the Ayushman Bharat Digital Mission and the National Mental Health Programme can support the development of a scalable, inclusive model of mental health governance—one that places dignity, participation, and ethical digital transformation at its core.

EMPIRICAL EVIDENCE SNAPSHOT ACROSS CONTEXTS

Empirical research across India and other low- and middle-income countries (LMICs) consistently demonstrates that mental health inequities among informal workers are widespread, structurally produced, and closely linked to discrimination, labor precarity, and limited access to care. While Kerala provides a robust empirical anchor for this chapter, evidence from other regions confirms that the patterns observed are neither unique nor exceptional, but reflective of broader national and global trends.

Across Indian states, studies on construction workers, domestic workers, agricultural laborers, street vendors, and platform-based gig workers reveal elevated levels of anxiety, depression, substance use, and psychosomatic distress. Research from urban centers such as Delhi, Mumbai, Bengaluru, and Hyderabad highlights how informal workers experience chronic stress arising from income insecurity, unsafe working conditions, long hours, and weak social protection. Migrant workers, in particular, report higher psychological distress due to linguistic barriers, social isolation, discrimination, and limited access to public services. Gendered patterns further intensify vulnerability, with women informal workers facing compounded stress linked to unpaid care work, workplace harassment, and restricted mobility.

Comparative evidence from other LMICs reinforces these findings. Studies from South and Southeast Asia—including Sri Lanka, Bangladesh, Vietnam, and Indonesia—show that informal employment is strongly associated with poor mental health outcomes, especially among migrants and urban poor populations. In Latin America and Sub-Saharan Africa, informal workers similarly report high levels of distress linked to economic volatility, lack of institutional recognition, and exposure to discrimination. Across these contexts, discrimination—whether based on migration status, ethnicity, caste, or gender—emerges as a recurring determinant of psychological distress, mediating the relationship between precarious employment and mental health outcomes.

Digital mental health initiatives across LMICs provide mixed but instructive evidence. Telepsychiatry programs in India, Brazil, and South Africa have demonstrated improved access and reduced treatment gaps, particularly in underserved areas. Mobile health (mHealth) interventions offering psychoeducation, stress management, and counseling support have shown positive short-term outcomes in reducing symptoms of anxiety and depression. However, these benefits are unevenly distributed. Studies consistently report barriers related to digital literacy, language accessibility, trust in digital platforms, and concerns about data privacy—especially among informal and migrant workers. These findings underscore that digital tools alone do not guarantee inclusion; governance, ethics, and contextual adaptation are decisive factors.

Evidence from public health and labor economics further illustrates the systemic implications of untreated mental health conditions. Across countries, poor mental health among informal workers is associated with reduced productivity, increased absenteeism, higher injury rates, and lower labor retention. Economic analyses from the World Bank and the World Health Organization indicate that investments in mental health yield substantial returns through improved workforce participation and reduced healthcare costs, reinforcing the argument that mental health inequity constitutes both a social injustice and an economic inefficiency.

Taken together, empirical evidence across contexts converges on three key insights. First, mental health inequities among informal workers are structurally embedded and closely tied to discrimination, migration, and institutional exclusion. Second, digital mental health interventions can expand access, but only when embedded within inclusive governance frameworks that address literacy, trust, and ethics. Third, the consequences of neglecting informal workers' mental health extend beyond individual suffering to broader economic and social costs.

This cross-contextual snapshot situates the Kerala findings within a wider empirical landscape, strengthening the chapter's generalizability and policy relevance.

It demonstrates that the challenges and opportunities identified are shared across regions, making the proposed phygital and governance-oriented reforms applicable not only within India, but across diverse settings characterized by large informal economies and growing digital health infrastructures.

ECONOMIC AND POLICY DIMENSIONS OF HEALTH REFORM

Inclusive digital health reform in India is not only a moral or social imperative but also an economic necessity. The mental health of informal workers—who constitute the majority of the national labour force—directly affects productivity, labour efficiency, and long-term economic resilience. Systemic neglect of mental health within this population generates hidden economic costs through reduced work performance, absenteeism, and increased healthcare expenditure. Viewed through a policy–economic lens, discrimination and psychosocial distress among informal workers represent both a human rights concern and a source of macroeconomic inefficiency.

The informal sector contributes close to half of India's gross domestic product while employing approximately 93% of its workforce (Government of India, 2020). Yet it remains largely disconnected from formal healthcare and insurance systems, resulting in significant productivity losses. Globally, depression and anxiety account for an estimated economic cost of nearly US$1 trillion annually (WHO, 2022), and similar burdens can be inferred for India's informal economy. Evidence from Kerala illustrates how discrimination and untreated psychological distress translate into reduced labour participation, occupational fatigue, and diminished well-being. These patterns align with labour economics research showing that exclusion and insecurity constrain innovation and labour efficiency, whereas inclusion yields measurable economic returns (Banerjee & Duflo, 2007).

From a public health economics perspective, investment in mental health produces high social and economic returns. The World Bank estimates that every dollar invested in mental health generates approximately four dollars in improved productivity and reduced healthcare costs. Digital mental health interventions—such as telecounselling, mobile screening, and community-based digital support—offer cost-effective mechanisms to extend care to informal workers while reducing opportunity costs associated with travel and lost wages. However, economic efficiency alone does not ensure equitable outcomes; digital interventions must be embedded within supportive policy and governance structures.

India's health policy landscape has evolved from predominantly welfare-oriented approaches toward data-driven digital reform, particularly through initiatives such as the Ayushman Bharat Digital Mission. Despite this shift, mental health remains peripheral within broader digital health planning, even though legal frameworks such as the National Mental Health Policy (2014) and the Mental Healthcare Act (2017) establish the right to care. Bridging this gap requires aligning three interdependent principles: *equity in access, efficiency through digital systems*, and *empathy in implementation*. Together, these principles underpin *phygital governance*, a hybrid model that integrates physical and digital service delivery to reduce transaction costs, overcome geographic barriers, and improve continuity of care.

Experiences from Kerala illustrate the potential of phygital approaches, where mobile-based mental health services are linked to local health infrastructure and community institutions. While these experiences are context-specific, they highlight transferable policy insights: digital health systems can improve access and affordability when combined with local mediation, multilingual outreach, and trust-building mechanisms. Without investments in digital literacy, cultural contextualization, and ethical data governance, however, technological efficiency risks excluding those it is intended to serve.

Achieving sustainable reform requires coordinated governance and cross-sector collaboration. Public–private–community partnerships can integrate government agencies, technology providers, civil society organizations, and labour groups to design worker-centered digital mental health solutions. Such partnerships enable innovation while maintaining accountability and social legitimacy. Framed within the shared value perspective, mental health inclusion strengthens both economic performance and social well-being, reinforcing the interdependence of equity and growth.

Ultimately, equitable health reform demands a balance between economic rationality and social justice. Discrimination and psychological distress are not only ethical failures but structural inefficiencies that weaken economic resilience. As India advances toward a digital-first healthcare paradigm, mental health inclusion must be recognized as a core indicator of national progress. A resilient health economy treats mental well-being as productive capital, leverages digital systems to expand equity, and grounds reform in ethical leadership and participatory governance. Through phygital integration—where technology complements rather than replaces human care—India can build a mental health system that is both economically sustainable and socially inclusive.

DIGITAL INNOVATION AND PHYGITAL MENTAL HEALTH DELIVERY

The rapid digitalization of healthcare in India presents both a significant opportunity and a critical governance challenge: how to deploy technology not merely for efficiency, but for equity and inclusion. For informal workers—who are often excluded from institutional healthcare systems—digital innovation offers one of the few scalable pathways to expand access to mental health services. However, digital expansion alone is insufficient. Effective reform requires a *phygital approach* that integrates digital tools with physical health infrastructure, community mediation, and ethical oversight.

The phygital paradigm, articulated in national digital health frameworks, combines online platforms with offline service delivery to preserve trust, relational care, and continuity. Unlike purely virtual models, phygital systems recognize that mental health care depends on human connection, cultural sensitivity, and contextual support. For informal workers, this means ensuring that digital technologies strengthen community-based care rather than displacing it. Telepsychiatry, mobile counseling platforms, and AI-assisted screening tools can be embedded within primary health centres, community hubs, NGOs, and labour collectives to create integrated care pathways that are both technologically enabled and socially grounded.

Telepsychiatry has emerged as a particularly promising intervention, offering reduced travel costs, greater confidentiality, and improved access to qualified professionals. When integrated into existing public health infrastructure—such as Health and Wellness Centres or mobile clinics—it can mitigate geographic and time constraints that often prevent informal workers from seeking care. Evidence from multiple low-resource contexts suggests that such hybrid delivery models are most effective when supported by local facilitators, multilingual interfaces, and clear referral mechanisms.

Alongside telepsychiatry, AI-driven and mobile health (mHealth) technologies represent an expanding frontier in mental health delivery. Digital tools capable of detecting early signs of distress through behavioural or interactional data offer opportunities for preventive care and early intervention. National initiatives in digital mental health training and telemedicine demonstrate the feasibility of embedding such tools within public systems. However, the deployment of AI in mental health raises critical ethical concerns related to algorithmic bias, informed consent, data privacy, and surveillance—risks that are particularly acute for informal workers with limited legal and digital protection.

Digital literacy and trust therefore emerge as decisive enabling conditions. Many informal workers face barriers related to language, education, and confidence in navigating digital platforms. Without targeted capacity-building, digital mental health tools risk reinforcing exclusion. Community-based digital literacy initiatives, supported by local institutions and civil society organizations, are essential to ensure meaningful participation. Equally important is ethical data governance. Transparent consent mechanisms, culturally sensitive design, and clear accountability structures are necessary to foster trust and psychological safety, transforming digital systems from sources of apprehension into instruments of empowerment.

From an economic perspective, phygital mental health delivery offers efficiency gains through reduced service costs, optimized clinician workloads, and lower opportunity costs for workers. Teleconsultations minimize income loss associated with travel and waiting times, while digital triage tools enable more targeted allocation of scarce mental health resources. Yet economic efficiency must be balanced with institutional integration. Digital innovations should complement, not replace, existing healthcare systems. Embedding digital mental health services within primary care, local governance structures, and welfare mechanisms ensures continuity and avoids fragmentation.

Experiences from states such as Kerala illustrate both the promise and limits of phygital innovation. Strong public health infrastructure, community networks, and crisis governance capacity provide favourable conditions for experimentation, but these experiences are not universally replicable without adaptation. The broader lesson lies not in replication, but in transferability: scalable phygital models must be flexible, multilingual, ethically governed, and locally anchored.

In practice, a phygital mental health system may enable a migrant worker in a remote worksite to access counseling through a mobile interface in their native language, supported by a trained community mediator and linked to a nearby health facility. Such models demonstrate how technology, when embedded within ethical governance and community participation, can reduce invisibility and restore dignity. Ultimately, digital innovation guided by compassion and accountability can transform mental health delivery for informal workers—ensuring that technology functions as a bridge to care rather than a barrier to inclusion.

LEADERSHIP FOR INCLUSIVE HEALTHCARE TRANSFORMATION

Digital health reform in India ultimately depends not on technological sophistication alone, but on the quality of leadership that shapes its vision, ethics, and execution. Technology can expand reach and efficiency, but without inclusive and accountable leadership it cannot correct entrenched inequities. In the context of informal workers—where discrimination, invisibility, and mental health vulnerabilities persist—leadership functions as the critical mechanism through which policy intent is translated into lived inclusion.

Global health governance frameworks emphasize that digital health leadership must be grounded in trust, transparency, and accountability (WHO, 2022). For India, this requires leadership that is sensitive to social hierarchies, cultural diversity, and the structural marginalization of informal and migrant workers. Evidence from Kerala illustrates both the potential and the limitations of existing leadership models. While decentralized governance and community participation have enabled effective public health responses, migrant and informal labourers continue to remain underrepresented in decision-making and service design, revealing gaps between institutional capacity and inclusive outcomes.

Transformational leadership provides an important foundation for addressing these gaps by articulating a shared vision, mobilizing commitment, and integrating mental health equity into digital health agendas (Burns, 1978; Bass, 1985). Such leadership is essential for aligning digital innovation with public values and for motivating healthcare workers to engage marginalized populations. Complementing this, servant leadership emphasizes empathy, ethical responsibility, and empowerment, repositioning leadership as service rather than authority (Greenleaf, 1977). In healthcare systems, servant leadership supports trust-building, cultural sensitivity, and patient-centered care—qualities that are particularly relevant for informal workers who often experience institutional neglect.

Adaptive leadership further strengthens reform by enabling leaders to navigate uncertainty, resistance, and multi-sector complexity (Heifetz, 1994). Digital mental health reform presents both technical challenges—such as data integration and platform interoperability—and adaptive challenges, including stigma, low digital literacy, and fear of surveillance. Leaders must therefore balance technological problem-solving with social learning and dialogue. Distributed leadership complements this approach by diffusing responsibility across governance levels and stakeholder groups (Bolden, 2011). In digital health ecosystems, this includes collaboration among policymakers, health professionals, community organizations, and local digital facilitators who mediate access and build trust at the grassroots level.

Across these leadership models, certain competencies emerge as indispensable for inclusive digital health transformation. These include equity orientation, ethical data literacy, cultural intelligence, collaborative problem-solving, and emotional awareness (Boyatzis & McKee, 2005). Such competencies counteract the structural discrimination and institutional invisibility identified in studies of informal workers, fostering psychological safety and institutional trust. Importantly, leadership must also be embedded within governance structures through clear accountability mechanisms, grievance redressal systems, and transparent data stewardship.

Lessons from Kerala's public health experience point toward transferable principles rather than direct replication. Decentralized authority, community partnerships, and data-informed decision-making can support inclusive outcomes when aligned with ethical leadership. Translating these principles into digital mental health reform requires institutional mechanisms such as district-level coordination units, participatory planning forums, and leadership training focused on digital ethics and inclusion. Academic and training institutions can play a critical role by integrating digital governance, mental health ethics, and reflective leadership practices into professional curricula.

Ultimately, leadership for inclusive healthcare transformation must humanize digital innovation. Rather than treating technology as an end in itself, leaders must act as ethical stewards who ensure that digital systems serve dignity, participation, and care. This shift—from bureaucratic control to compassionate governance—marks a fundamental reorientation of health reform. When leadership at all levels embraces inclusion as a strategic and moral imperative, digital health reform can move beyond efficiency to become genuinely humane. In this sense, leadership is the moral and operational fulcrum of phygital health transformation, ensuring that technological progress heals systems as well as the people they are designed to serve.

DIGITAL ETHICS AND DATA GOVERNANCE IN MENTAL HEALTH

As digital technologies increasingly shape mental health service delivery, ethical considerations and data governance emerge as foundational determinants of trust, inclusion, and effectiveness—particularly for informal and migrant workers who occupy structurally vulnerable positions within health and labour systems. Digital mental health interventions generate, process, and store highly sensitive personal data, including psychological states, behavioural patterns, and socio-demographic information. Without robust ethical safeguards, such systems risk reproducing discrimination, deepening exclusion, and exposing marginalized populations to surveillance, misuse, or harm.

A central ethical concern relates to *privacy and informed consent*. Informal workers often possess limited digital literacy and constrained bargaining power, raising questions about the voluntariness and comprehension of consent within digital platforms. Consent mechanisms must therefore move beyond formalistic "click-through" agreements toward context-sensitive, multilingual, and comprehensible processes that clearly explain data use, storage, and sharing. Ethical governance requires that consent be ongoing, revocable, and proportionate to the sensitivity of mental health data.

Algorithmic bias and fairness constitute a second critical challenge. AI-driven mental health tools—such as risk screening, symptom detection, or triage systems—are trained on datasets that may underrepresent informal workers, migrants, women, or caste-marginalized groups. This can result in misclassification, exclusion from services, or stigmatizing risk profiles. Ethical digital mental health governance must therefore mandate bias auditing, transparency in model design, and regular evaluation of algorithmic outcomes across demographic groups. Human oversight and explainability are essential to ensure that automated systems support, rather than replace, professional judgment.

Data sovereignty and ownership are particularly salient for mobile and migrant populations. Informal workers frequently move across districts and states, complicating questions of who controls their health data and how continuity of care is maintained without exposing individuals to surveillance or discrimination. Ethical data governance frameworks must ensure that individuals retain meaningful control over their mental health records, with clear limits on secondary data use by employers, insurers, or other third parties. Interoperability under national digital health systems must be balanced with strict purpose limitation and access controls.

Trust is the ethical currency of digital mental health systems. For populations historically excluded from institutional care, mistrust of data collection can deter help-seeking and undermine program effectiveness. Ethical governance therefore requires *transparency, accountability, and grievance redressal mechanisms*. Independent oversight bodies, clear accountability structures, and accessible complaint processes can help build confidence in digital platforms. Ethical stewardship also entails culturally sensitive design, including language accessibility and respect for local norms surrounding mental illness and disclosure.

Importantly, digital ethics in mental health cannot be treated as an abstract regulatory concern; it must be embedded in everyday practice and leadership. Training programs for health administrators, technologists, and frontline workers should include ethical data literacy, human rights perspectives, and participatory design principles. Ethical leadership plays a decisive role in aligning innovation with values, ensuring that efficiency gains do not come at the expense of dignity or justice.

In the Indian context, ethical digital mental health governance must align with emerging data protection legislation and labour protections while addressing the specific vulnerabilities of informal workers. This includes explicit safeguards against discrimination based on mental health data, protections against coercive data sharing, and mechanisms to ensure that digital inclusion does not become a precondition for accessing care. Ethical governance should thus be understood as an enabling condition for inclusion rather than a constraint on innovation.

In sum, ethical and data governance frameworks are not peripheral to digital mental health reform; they are central to its legitimacy and sustainability. By foregrounding privacy, fairness, consent, transparency, and accountability, digital mental health systems can function as instruments of empowerment rather than exclusion. For informal workers, ethical digital governance represents the difference between technology as a tool of surveillance and technology as a pathway to care, dignity, and psychological well-being.

POLICY FRAMEWORK FOR MENTAL HEALTH REFORM IN INDIA

India's health policy landscape is undergoing a structural transition—from centralized, hospital-centric care toward digitally enabled, community-oriented systems that increasingly recognize mental health as a core component of universal healthcare. Despite this shift, informal workers—who constitute the economic backbone of the country—remain at the margins of mental health reform. Existing legal and policy instruments, including the National Mental Health Policy (2014) and the Mental Healthcare Act (2017), establish the right to care, yet their implementation has been uneven, particularly within informal labour clusters. This gap underscores the need for a policy framework that moves beyond welfare provision to address mental health as a governance priority and an economic necessity.

The proposed framework conceptualizes mental health inequities not as isolated clinical outcomes but as indicators of systemic inefficiency arising from discrimination, institutional fragmentation, and unequal access to digital resources. Drawing on empirical insights from informal labour contexts, the framework integrates digital innovation, economic rationality, and participatory leadership to support inclusive reform. It is guided by five core principles: *equity and justice*, *phygital integration*, *ethical leadership and accountability*, *community participation*, and *data ethics*. Together, these principles translate into four operational pillars that structure policy action.

The first pillar, *institutional integration*, emphasizes embedding mental health across all levels of the healthcare system. This includes integrating digital counseling and referral mechanisms within Health and Wellness Centres, establishing district-level telepsychiatry networks, and mandating mental health literacy and anti-discrimination training for frontline health workers. Such integration ensures that mental health services are not siloed but coordinated with primary care, labour welfare, and social protection systems.

The second pillar, *digital infrastructure*, focuses on building inclusive and interoperable systems under initiatives such as the Ayushman Bharat Digital Mission. Key measures include multilingual mobile health applications for informal and migrant workers, AI-assisted screening tools embedded within public telemedicine platforms, and interoperable data standards that enable continuity of care while safeguarding privacy. Importantly, digital expansion must be accompanied by ethical data governance to prevent exclusion, surveillance, or misuse of sensitive mental health information.

The third pillar, *economic incentives and sustainability*, recognizes mental health inclusion as a high-return investment rather than a welfare cost. Policy instruments such as targeted public financing under the National Health Mission, tax incentives and CSR-linked grants for digital mental health initiatives, and outcome-based funding mechanisms can encourage both public and private participation. By reducing absenteeism, improving productivity, and lowering long-term healthcare costs, inclusive mental health reform contributes directly to economic resilience.

The fourth pillar, *leadership and governance*, institutionalizes accountability and participation. This includes the creation of national and state-level coordination mechanisms for digital mental health, independent oversight bodies to address ethical concerns, and grievance redressal systems accessible to informal workers. Participatory governance is essential for sustainability: local governments, civil society organizations, labour unions, and women's collectives should be actively involved in outreach, awareness, and service design to ensure cultural relevance and trust.

Community engagement remains a cross-cutting requirement across all pillars. Locally embedded interventions—such as community mental health committees, mobile counseling units, and regionally tailored awareness programs—enhance legitimacy and uptake. These approaches reflect global evidence that culturally grounded, community-defined solutions are more effective in addressing mental health disparities among marginalized populations.

Legally, the framework must align with emerging data protection and labour regulations by embedding privacy, consent, and non-discrimination into digital health governance. Monitoring and accountability mechanisms—including equity audits, digital mental health dashboards, and the inclusion of psychosocial well-being indicators in health performance metrics—enable real-time evaluation and adaptive policymaking. Alignment with global frameworks such as the WHO Comprehensive Mental Health Action Plan (2021–2030) and the Sustainable Development Goals further situates India's reform agenda within international best practices.

Experiences from states such as Kerala illustrate the feasibility of piloting integrated digital mental health initiatives within decentralized governance structures. However, the policy value of such cases lies in transferability rather than replication. Scalable reform requires flexible models that can be adapted to diverse regional, linguistic, and institutional contexts across India.

The overarching goal of this policy framework is to create a *phygital mental health ecosystem* in which digital technologies function as connectors, policies act as equalizers, and leadership serves as an ethical anchor. By integrating economic logic, digital innovation, and human-centered governance, India can advance a model of mental health reform that is inclusive, sustainable, and just—positioning mental well-being not merely as a health outcome, but as a foundation for equitable development and national resilience.

DISCUSSION

The findings discussed in this chapter confirm that mental health inequities among India's informal workers are not isolated psychological conditions but systemic outcomes of discrimination, institutional neglect, and fragmented governance. Rather than individual vulnerability alone, psychological distress emerges from structurally embedded disadvantages associated with labor precarity, migration, social exclusion, and uneven access to care. Empirical evidence from Kerala illustrates how discrimination functions as a chronic stressor shaping mental health outcomes among both migrant and native informal workers, reinforcing the argument that inequity operates across multiple social layers rather than within a single group.

The Kerala-based findings demonstrate that perceived discrimination is strongly associated with anxiety, depression, and stress, with distinct but interconnected mechanisms affecting different worker groups. Migrant workers experience exclusion through linguistic, cultural, and institutional barriers, while native workers often confront economic insecurity and perceived displacement within informal labor markets. This dual burden underscores that mental health inequity is systemic in nature, requiring policy responses that address structural drivers rather than relying solely on clinical or individual-level interventions. In this sense, discrimination functions as a structural determinant of health, comparable to poverty, housing insecurity, or unemployment, and must be treated as a central concern of public policy and governance.

Psychological resources such as self-esteem, coping capacity, and overall well-being play an important mediating role in this relationship. Consistent with stress–appraisal–coping and psychological well-being frameworks, individuals with stronger coping mechanisms and social support experience lower levels of distress even under adverse conditions. However, access to such resources is unevenly distributed. Migrant and informal workers often lack stable social networks, institutional recognition, and culturally appropriate mental health services, which amplifies vulnerability. These patterns highlight the need for interventions that strengthen resilience while simultaneously addressing the structural conditions that constrain coping capacity.

Digital inclusion emerges in the discussion as a key transformative pathway, but one that is contingent on governance, ethics, and trust. Telepsychiatry, mobile counseling platforms, and AI-assisted screening tools have the potential to expand access and continuity of care for informal workers, particularly when geographic mobility and opportunity costs limit engagement with traditional services. However, the effectiveness of these tools depends on digital literacy, cultural adaptation, language accessibility, and ethical data governance. Without these safeguards, digital expansion risks reproducing existing inequalities or creating new forms of exclusion.

Leadership plays a critical mediating role in translating digital potential into inclusive outcomes. Transformational, servant, adaptive, and distributed leadership models collectively highlight the importance of vision, empathy, flexibility, and shared responsibility in reform processes. Decentralized governance structures, community participation, and cross-sector coordination enable context-sensitive responses that align technology with lived realities. Leadership is therefore not an auxiliary factor but a central mechanism through which ethical digital health reform is operationalized.

From an economic perspective, the discussion reinforces that mental health inclusion is both a moral and fiscal imperative. Untreated depression and anxiety generate substantial productivity losses, and these costs are magnified in economies where informal labor predominates. Integrating mental health into digital health policy yields returns in the form of improved productivity, reduced absenteeism, and enhanced workforce stability. The phygital model—integrating digital platforms within physical and community-based infrastructures—offers a pragmatic approach by connecting micro-level psychological processes with meso-level community engagement and macro-level policy governance.

At the same time, the discussion acknowledges persistent implementation challenges. Digital divides, language barriers, workforce shortages, privacy concerns, and stigma continue to constrain equitable reform. These challenges underscore the need for incremental, participatory, and evidence-driven policy design, supported by iterative evaluation rather than one-time technological deployment. Pilot initiatives must therefore be scaled cautiously, with continuous feedback from informal worker communities.

While Kerala provides a useful empirical anchor, the broader relevance of these findings extends beyond a single state. Many low- and middle-income countries face similar challenges arising from large informal labor markets, migration, and uneven digital capacity. The Kerala experience illustrates how equity and innovation can coexist under certain conditions, offering transferable lessons rather than a universal template. These insights contribute to emerging South–South dialogues on inclusive digital health governance.

Three overarching insights emerge from this discussion. First, mental health inequity among informal workers is fundamentally a governance challenge rather than an individual pathology. Second, digital innovation becomes socially meaningful only when guided by inclusion, ethics, and participation. Third, leadership serves as the connective force aligning empathy with efficiency across policy, technology, and practice. Together, these insights suggest that India's health reform agenda must move beyond a narrow focus on technological modernization toward a human-centered, ethically governed digital transformation.

In conclusion, the discussion highlights that discrimination, when addressed through inclusive governance and ethical leadership, can become a catalyst for systemic reform rather than a persistent source of harm. Phygital innovation—rooted in compassion, accountability, and community engagement—offers a pathway toward a more equitable mental health system. Such a transformation reframes digital health not merely as a technical upgrade, but as a collective commitment to dignity, justice, and sustainable social well-being.

IMPLEMENTATION CHALLENGES AND SYSTEMIC CONSTRAINTS

While digital and phygital mental health reforms offer significant promise for addressing inequities among informal workers, their implementation is constrained by a range of systemic, institutional, and socio-cultural challenges. Recognizing these constraints is essential to avoid technology-driven optimism and to design reforms that are realistic, equitable, and sustainable. The barriers outlined below highlight why mental health reform must be incremental, participatory, and context-sensitive rather than uniform or purely technocratic.

A primary constraint lies in *digital access and infrastructure variability*. Although national digital health initiatives have expanded connectivity, significant disparities persist between urban and rural regions, across states, and within informal labour clusters. Many informal workers lack consistent access to smartphones, stable internet connectivity, or private spaces to engage in tele-mental health services. For migrant workers residing in temporary or overcrowded housing, digital access is often shared, insecure, or intermittent, limiting confidentiality and continuity of care.

Closely related is the challenge of *digital literacy and usability*. A substantial proportion of informal workers possess limited experience with digital platforms, low functional literacy, or unfamiliarity with health-related applications. Complex interfaces, English-dominated platforms, and procedural requirements such as multi-step authentication can deter engagement. Without targeted digital literacy initiatives and simplified, multilingual design, digital mental health services risk reinforcing exclusion rather than expanding access.

Workforce capacity and readiness represent another significant constraint. India faces a chronic shortage of mental health professionals, particularly in public and rural settings. Expecting digital platforms to compensate for workforce gaps without parallel investments in training, supervision, and task-sharing is unrealistic. Frontline health workers often lack training in mental health, digital tools, or culturally responsive care, while community volunteers may face burnout or role ambiguity without adequate institutional support.

Language and cultural barriers further complicate implementation. India's linguistic diversity means that standardized digital platforms often fail to accommodate regional languages and culturally specific expressions of distress. Migrant workers may be unable to communicate symptoms effectively to providers who do not share their language or cultural context, leading to misdiagnosis or disengagement. Cultural stigma surrounding mental illness also suppresses help-seeking behavior, particularly among men and marginalized communities.

Governance and coordination challenges constitute a major systemic constraint. Responsibilities for mental health, labour welfare, digital health, and migration are distributed across multiple ministries and administrative levels, often operating in silos. This fragmentation results in overlapping mandates, unclear accountability, and inconsistent implementation across states. Without integrated governance mechanisms, digital mental health initiatives risk duplication, inefficiency, or policy drift.

Ethical and legal uncertainties also impede implementation. While data protection frameworks are evolving, ambiguity remains regarding data ownership, consent, secondary data use, and cross-platform interoperability. Informal workers may fear that disclosure of mental health information could affect employment, mobility, or access to welfare benefits. Without explicit safeguards and grievance redressal mechanisms, such fears undermine trust and participation.

Economic constraints cannot be overlooked. Although digital mental health is often framed as cost-effective, initial investments in infrastructure, training, localization, and governance are substantial. States with limited fiscal capacity may struggle to sustain digital platforms beyond pilot phases, particularly if funding is project-based rather than institutionalized. Informal workers themselves face opportunity costs, such as time away from work, that can deter participation even when services are nominally free.

Finally, *monitoring and evaluation limitations* constrain learning and scale-up. Many digital mental health initiatives lack robust outcome measurement, equity indicators, or feedback loops from users. Without systematic evaluation, it is difficult to identify what works, for whom, and under what conditions. This limits adaptive learning and risks scaling ineffective or inequitable models.

Together, these challenges underscore that digital and phygital mental health reform is as much an institutional and social transformation as a technological one. Addressing systemic constraints requires coordinated governance, sustained investment, ethical leadership, and continuous community engagement. By acknowledging and actively managing these barriers, policymakers can move beyond pilot-driven reform toward scalable, inclusive, and resilient mental health systems for informal workers.

RECOMMENDATION AND SOLUTIONS

Effective mental health reform for India's informal workforce requires a shift from fragmented, clinic-centered responses toward a coordinated, system-level transformation grounded in inclusion, ethical digital integration, and accountable leadership. Persistent inequities arising from discrimination, digital exclusion, and governance gaps cannot be resolved through isolated interventions; instead, they demand multi-level strategies spanning policy design, institutional capacity, economic incentives, community engagement, and continuous research and evaluation.

Policy and Governance Interventions

At the national level, mental health should be embedded as a core objective within the National Health Mission and the Ayushman Bharat Digital Mission through a *National Phygital Mental Health Plan*. This plan should formally integrate telepsychiatry, hybrid counseling models, and digital screening into public health delivery for informal and migrant workers. A dedicated regulatory body for digital mental health governance is recommended to coordinate cross-sector implementation, enforce data protection and privacy standards, and oversee ethical compliance across platforms. Legal reform should include the introduction of a *digital equity provision* within existing mental health legislation to ensure that informal and migrant workers receive equitable access to multilingual, accessible digital services.

Leadership reform is central to effective implementation. Mandatory training in inclusive leadership, ethical data governance, and participatory decision-making should be institutionalized for health administrators and digital health managers, supported by collaboration with academic and professional training institutions. These measures would help translate policy commitments into ethical and context-sensitive practice.

Institutional and System-Level Solutions

At the state and district levels, *Phygital Health Hubs* should be established as integrated service points combining physical care spaces with telepsychiatry kiosks, digital screening tools, and structured digital literacy programs. These hubs should be linked with Primary Health Centres and local governance institutions to ensure continuity of care and community trust. National telemedicine platforms should incorporate AI-assisted triage for early identification of stress and discrimination-related risks, while interoperable registries can support continuity of care without compromising privacy.

Regional telepsychiatry clusters with multilingual helplines and trained community facilitators can further enhance access, particularly for mobile and migrant populations. Importantly, institutional design must prioritize language accessibility, cultural adaptation, and clear referral pathways to avoid technological exclusion.

Economic and Workforce Measures

Mental health inclusion should be incentivized through targeted public financing, tax benefits, and outcome-based grants for organizations delivering digital mental health services to informal workers. Allocating a defined proportion of public health expenditure toward mental health infrastructure, training, and digital tools would signal policy commitment and sustainability. A new cadre of *Digital Mental Health Facilitators* can be trained to act as intermediaries between communities and digital systems, supporting navigation, trust-building, and follow-up care.

Community-Based and Cultural Interventions

Community engagement is essential for legitimacy and uptake. Civil society organizations, women's collectives, and labour groups should be formally integrated into outreach, peer-support initiatives, and mental health literacy campaigns. Culturally grounded interventions—such as peer counseling, stress management workshops, and locally meaningful resilience practices—can strengthen coping capacity and reduce stigma when combined with professional support. Ensuring access to multilingual helplines and low-bandwidth communication options is critical for reaching the most marginalized workers.

Research, Monitoring, and Accountability

Sustainable reform must be anchored in robust research and evaluation. Longitudinal and implementation-focused studies should assess the impact of discrimination, digital inclusion, and phygital interventions on mental health outcomes and productivity. A *Digital Mental Health Index* measuring access, affordability, trust, and equity can serve as a benchmarking tool across regions. Independent equity audits and anonymous user feedback mechanisms should be institutionalized to identify disparities and inform adaptive policy refinement.

Phased and Collaborative Implementation

To ensure feasibility and accountability, digital mental health reform should follow a phased approach. Initial stages should prioritize capacity building and ethical system design through multidisciplinary task forces that integrate mental health expertise, digital technology, social science, and economics. Subsequent stages should emphasize community co-creation, involving worker representatives and local organizations in service design and evaluation. Strategic public–private partnerships can support scalable infrastructure, while academic institutions validate effectiveness through pilot studies.

International collaboration can further strengthen reform by facilitating knowledge exchange, funding, and benchmarking with global best practices. However, global engagement should complement—not substitute—locally grounded solutions tailored to India's diverse informal workforce.

Integrative Vision

Collectively, these recommendations emphasize a phygital approach that combines digital reach with human mediation, ethical governance, and community participation. Mental health reform must be designed inclusively, governed transparently, measured ethically, and sustained collaboratively. When implemented holistically, these strategies can transform India's fragmented mental health landscape into a resilient ecosystem that advances equity, dignity, and social justice.

Ultimately, redefining mental health as both a technological and moral frontier enables India to move beyond symbolic reform toward meaningful inclusion. By aligning digital innovation with compassionate leadership and participatory governance, India can pioneer a model of mental health reform that is scalable, ethical, and human-centered—ensuring that no informal worker remains invisible, unheard, or untreated.

LIMITATIONS OF THE STUDY

While this chapter offers a comprehensive and interdisciplinary analysis of mental health inequities among informal workers in India, several limitations must be acknowledged to contextualize its findings and interpretations.

First, the chapter relies primarily on *empirical evidence from Kerala* as its central analytical anchor. Although Kerala provides a valuable case due to its relatively advanced welfare systems and digital readiness, the findings may not fully capture the diversity of institutional capacity, cultural contexts, and digital infrastructure present across other Indian states. As such, the transferability of insights requires cautious interpretation and contextual adaptation rather than direct replication.

Second, much of the analysis is based on *secondary empirical data and synthesis of existing studies*, rather than original primary data collection on digital mental health interventions. While this approach enables broad theoretical and policy integration, it limits the ability to draw causal inferences about the effectiveness of specific phygital or AI-driven mental health solutions in real-world informal work settings.

Third, the chapter emphasizes *structural and governance determinants* of mental health inequity, which may underrepresent individual-level variability such as personal resilience, informal support networks, and coping styles that differ across communities and cultural groups. Although these factors are discussed conceptually, they are not empirically disaggregated in detail.

Fourth, the discussion of *digital innovation and AI-enabled mental health tools* is necessarily prospective in parts. Many proposed digital interventions are at early stages of deployment or remain unevenly implemented across regions. As a result, the analysis may overestimate scalability or readiness in contexts where digital literacy, workforce capacity, or infrastructure are limited.

Fifth, *intersectional dimensions* such as gender, caste, disability, and tribal identity are addressed analytically but not empirically examined in depth due to data constraints in existing studies. More granular empirical work is required to understand how these intersecting identities shape mental health outcomes and access to digital care.

Finally, the chapter does not include a *formal cost–benefit or experimental evaluation* of proposed policy and governance models. Economic arguments are drawn from global evidence and secondary sources rather than context-specific trials within India's informal sector.

Acknowledging these limitations does not diminish the chapter's contributions; rather, it clarifies the scope of interpretation and highlights areas where future empirical, experimental, and longitudinal research is needed. These limitations reinforce the importance of cautious generalization, phased implementation, and evidence-driven scaling of digital mental health reforms.

FUTURE RESEARCH DIRECTIONS

As India progresses toward a digitally enabled healthcare ecosystem, future research must play a central role in ensuring that mental health reform for informal workers is evidence-based, equitable, and ethically governed. The complex interplay of discrimination, psychological distress, labor precarity, and digital exclusion demands a multidisciplinary research agenda that integrates psychology, public health, economics, digital governance, and cultural studies.

Building on empirical insights from Kerala, future studies should expand beyond single-state analyses to include *multi-state and sectoral comparisons* across construction, agriculture, domestic work, and urban informal services. Mixed-methods designs that combine psychometric measurement with qualitative and ethnographic approaches can deepen understanding of how discrimination, migration, and institutional invisibility shape mental health outcomes across diverse contexts. Longitudinal research is particularly necessary to examine how digital inclusion, leadership practices, and community participation influence psychological well-being over time and across life stages.

As digital and AI-enabled mental health interventions become more widespread, rigorous evaluation of their *effectiveness, accessibility, and ethical implications* is essential. Future research should assess algorithmic bias, cultural appropriateness, explainability, and user trust in AI-assisted screening and telepsychiatry platforms, especially among populations with limited digital literacy. Collaborative research involving behavioral scientists, technologists, and ethicists can support the development of transparent, human-centered digital mental health systems that do not reproduce structural inequities.

Leadership and governance constitute another critical research frontier. Empirical studies should examine how different leadership models—transformational, servant, adaptive, and distributed—shape inclusion, trust, and implementation outcomes within decentralized health systems. Research at the level of local governance, NGOs, community health workers, and digital intermediaries can illuminate how collaborative leadership practices enable or constrain reform. Gender-sensitive leadership research may further reveal how women-led initiatives contribute to empathetic and community-centered mental health delivery.

Economic research is also required to quantify the costs of discrimination and untreated psychological distress among informal workers, as well as the returns on investment from phygital mental health models. Behavioral economics approaches can examine help-seeking behavior, stigma reduction, and incentives for digital engagement. Developing measurable indicators—such as productivity gains, household income stability, and labor retention—can strengthen the economic case for inclusive mental health reform.

Culturally grounded research remains essential in India's pluralistic context. Future studies should develop and validate *multilingual digital tools and psychometric instruments* to assess stress, resilience, and discrimination among migrant, tribal, and marginalized workers. Investigating indigenous and faith-based coping practices—including meditation, yoga, prayer, and collective mindfulness—can inform culturally responsive intervention design without compromising scientific rigor. Comparative research on stigma, spirituality, and mental health literacy across regions can further refine outreach strategies.

Interdisciplinary collaboration will be crucial to sustain innovation. Universities, policy institutes, and public health agencies can establish *Digital Mental Health Research and Innovation Hubs* that integrate psychology, AI, anthropology, and governance studies. Such platforms can support participatory research models that involve informal workers as stakeholders rather than passive subjects, enhancing relevance and ethical validity.

Finally, future research should prioritize *implementation science and sustainability*, examining how digital mental health systems perform during crises such as pandemics, economic shocks, or migration surges. Long-term evaluations—including intergenerational impacts on education, aspiration, and resilience—can reveal the broader social dividends of inclusive reform. Comparative Global South research collaborations can further situate India's experience within shared developmental challenges, contributing to global knowledge on equitable digital mental health governance.

In summary, future research must move beyond siloed inquiry to adopt a systems-oriented, human-centered approach that integrates empirical rigor with ethical reflection and cultural sensitivity. While Kerala provides an important empirical reference point, the next phase of scholarship must broaden its scope to ensure generalizability, policy relevance, and global contribution. Such an agenda will support the evolution of digital mental health reform not only as a technical innovation, but as a sustained commitment to inclusion, dignity, and social justice.

CONCLUSION

India's pursuit of inclusive health reform unfolds at the intersection of digital innovation, governance, and social equity. Evidence drawn from informal labour contexts illustrates that mental health inequities are not isolated clinical conditions but outcomes of structural discrimination, labour precarity, migration-related stress, and institutional invisibility. These forces undermine psychological well-being and economic participation, indicating that mental health inequity must be addressed as a systemic governance challenge rather than an individual deficit.

This chapter has argued that a *phygital approach*—integrating physical health infrastructure with digitally enabled mental health services—offers a pragmatic and scalable pathway to reform. By combining telepsychiatry, mobile counseling, AI-assisted screening, and community-based mediation, phygital systems can extend access across geographic, linguistic, and social boundaries. However, the analysis also underscores that digital expansion alone is insufficient. Without ethical leadership, participatory governance, and attention to digital literacy, trust, and data protection, technological solutions risk reinforcing existing exclusions.

Leadership emerges as a central mediating force in translating digital potential into inclusive outcomes. Compassionate, adaptive, and accountable leadership models are essential for aligning policy design, technological innovation, and lived realities. When leadership embeds empathy, transparency, and participation into digital health governance, reform moves beyond efficiency toward equity. The economic dimension further reinforces this argument: investments in mental health inclusion yield measurable returns in productivity, workforce stability, and long-term resilience, positioning mental well-being as both a social and economic priority.

Kerala's experience provides a valuable empirical anchor, illustrating both the possibilities and limitations of welfare-oriented and digitally ready systems. While decentralized governance and community engagement enable innovation, persistent inequities reveal that progress must be deliberately inclusive to be meaningful. The policy relevance of Kerala's case lies not in replication but in its transferable lessons for designing context-sensitive, ethically governed digital health systems across diverse regions.

In conclusion, India's digital health transformation must prioritize the human dimensions of reform. Humanizing the digital—by embedding equity, ethical governance, and participatory leadership into technological systems—offers a pathway toward sustainable mental health inclusion for informal workers. Such an approach reframes digital health not merely as a technical advancement, but as a collective commitment to dignity, justice, and national well-being. By aligning technology with compassion and governance with accountability, India can advance a model of health reform that is both inclusive and resilient, ensuring that no segment of the workforce remains unseen or underserved.

REFERENCES

Aayog, N. I. T. I. (2021). *National digital health blueprint.* Government of India. https://www.nhp.gov.in/NDHM/Documents/National_Digital_Health_BluePrint.pdf

Aguilar-Gaxiola, S., Loera, G., Méndez, L., Sala, M., & Kopelowicz, A. (2011). *Community-defined solutions for Latino mental health care disparities: Workgroup report.* University of California. https://health.ucdavis.edu/media-resources/crhd/documents/pdfs/community-defined-solutions-latino-mental-health-care-disparities-exec-summary.pdf

Banerjee, A. V., & Duflo, E. (2007). The economic lives of the poor. *The Journal of Economic Perspectives, 21*(1), 141–167. https://www.aeaweb.org/articles?id=10.1257/jep.21.1.141. DOI: 10.1257/jep.21.1.141 PMID: 19212450

Bass, B. M. (1985). *Leadership and performance beyond expectations.* Free Press. https://books.google.com/books/about/Leadership_and_Performance_Beyond_Expect.html?id=NCd-QgAACAAJ

Bhugra, D. (2004). Migration and mental health. *Acta Psychiatrica Scandinavica, 109*(4), 243–258. DOI: 10.1046/j.0001-690X.2003.00246.x PMID: 15008797

Bolden, R. (2011). Distributed leadership in organizations: A review of theory and research. *International Journal of Management Reviews, 13*(3), 251–269. DOI: 10.1111/j.1468-2370.2011.00306.x

Boyatzis, R., & McKee, A. (2005). *Resonant leadership: Renewing yourself and connecting with others through mindfulness, hope, and compassion.* Harvard Business School Press. https://books.google.com/books/about/Resonant_Leadership.html?id=ViVX3O9YP6oC

Burns, J. M. (1978). *Leadership.* Harper & Row.

Devassy, R., & George, A. (2021). Interstate migration and health disparities in Kerala: A sociological overview. *Economic and Political Weekly*, *56*(45), 41–49. DOI: 10.4103/ijmr.IJMR_2217_20

George, J., & Karalam, S. B. R. (in progress). Research work related to migrant workers in Kerala [Unpublished working thesis]. Department of social work, Christ University, Bengaluru.

Greenleaf, R. K. (1977). *Servant leadership: A journey into the nature of legitimate power and greatness.* Paulist Press. https://books.google.com/books/about/Servant_Leadership.html?id=AfjUgMJlDK4C&utm_source=chatgpt.com

Heifetz, R. A. (1994). *Leadership without easy answers*. Harvard University Press. DOI: 10.4159/9780674038479

International Labour Organization. (2018). *Women and men in the informal economy: A statistical picture* (3rd ed.). International Labour Office. https://www.ilo.org/global/publications/books/WCMS_626831/lang--en/index.htm

International Labour Organization. (2018). *Women and men in the informal economy: A statistical picture* (3rd ed.). International Labour Office. https://www.ilo.org/global/publications/books/WCMS_626831/lang--en/index.htm

Lazarus, R. S., & Folkman, S. (1984). *Stress, appraisal, and coping*. Springer. https://link.springer.com/book/10.1007/978-1-4419-1006-9

Li, J., Theng, Y. L., & Foo, S. (2020). Game-based digital interventions for depression therapy: A systematic review and meta-analysis. *Cyberpsychology, Behavior, and Social Networking*, *23*(8), 543–552. DOI: 10.1089/cyber.2019.0700 PMID: 24810933

Rajan, S. I., & Zachariah, K. C. (2019). *Emigration and remittances: New evidences from the Kerala migration survey 2018*. Centre for Development Studies. https://cds.edu/wp-content/uploads/2019/03/KMSReport2018.pdf

Ryff, C. D., & Keyes, C. L. M. (1995). The structure of psychological well-being revisited. *Journal of Personality and Social Psychology*, *69*(4), 719–727. DOI: 10.1037/0022-3514.69.4.719 PMID: 7473027

Srivastava, R. (2011). Labour migration in India: Recent trends, patterns and policy issues. *The Indian Journal of Labour Economics : the Quarterly Journal of the Indian Society of Labour Economics*, *54*(3), 411–440. https://www.researchgate.net/publication/319253996_Labour_migration_in_India_Recent_trends_patterns_and_policy_issues

Thomas, L., Rajeev, P. V., & Philip, S. (2020). Health crises and migrant vulnerabilities in Kerala: Lessons from COVID-19. *The Indian Journal of Social Work*, *81*(4), 523–540. DOI: 10.1177/0020872820951150

Williams, D. R., & Mohammed, S. A. (2009). Discrimination and racial disparities in health: Evidence and needed research. *Journal of Behavioral Medicine*, *32*(1), 20–47. DOI: 10.1007/s10865-008-9185-0 PMID: 19030981

World Bank. (2016). *Making mental health a global development priority*. World Bank. https://documents1.worldbank.org/curated/en/270131468187759113/pdf/105052-WP-PUBLIC-wb-background-paper.pdf

World Health Organization. (2021). *Comprehensive mental health action plan 2013–2030*. WHO. https://www.who.int/publications/i/item/9789240031029

World Health Organization. (2022). *Global report on effective access to assistive technology*. WHO. https://www.who.int/publications/i/item/9789240049451

KEY TERMS AND DEFINITIONS

Compassionate Leadership: Compassionate leadership refers to a leadership approach that combines empathy, ethical awareness, and action-oriented concern for others' well-being. It involves understanding the challenges faced by individuals or communities, responding with sensitivity, and taking decisions that prioritize human dignity alongside institutional performance. In the context of digital health reform, compassionate leadership ensures that technological innovation is guided by empathy, inclusion, and fairness, making systems more humane and equitable.

Digital Health: Digital health encompasses the use of information and communication technologies (ICTs)—such as mobile health (mHealth) applications, telemedicine, artificial intelligence (AI), and electronic health records (EHRs)—to enhance healthcare delivery, monitoring, and accessibility. It represents a shift toward data-driven, patient-centered care. Within this chapter's framework, digital health serves as a transformative tool to expand mental health access among informal workers, enabling efficiency, transparency, and scalability in service provision.

Discrimination: Discrimination is the unjust or prejudicial treatment of individuals based on attributes such as caste, gender, ethnicity, migration status, or occupation. In mental health contexts, discrimination acts as a *structural determinant of psychological distress*, limiting access to care and fostering chronic stress, anxiety, and reduced self-esteem. For informal workers in India, discrimination manifests both socially and institutionally—reinforcing marginalization and perpetuating mental health inequities.

Economic Inclusion: Economic inclusion refers to the process of ensuring equitable access to economic opportunities, resources, and social protection for all individuals, especially marginalized populations. It seeks to reduce income inequality and promote participation in the formal economy. In healthcare, economic inclusion implies that financial and employment structures support mental well-being by integrating mental health benefits, digital access, and workplace wellness programs into labor policy frameworks.

Informal Workers: Informal workers are individuals engaged in economic activities that are not regulated by formal labor laws or protected by social security systems. This includes daily wage earners, domestic workers, street vendors, and migrant laborers. Lacking stable employment, healthcare coverage, or legal safeguards, they are often excluded from institutional support systems. The mental health of informal workers is affected by precarious work conditions, discrimination, and limited access to healthcare, making them a critical focus group for inclusive policy reform.

Mental Health: Mental health is a state of emotional, psychological, and social well-being in which individuals can cope with stress, work productively, and contribute to their communities. It is not merely the absence of mental illness but the presence of resilience, self-esteem, and meaningful engagement. Within the reform framework, mental health is treated as a *fundamental human right* and a public health priority, integral to economic productivity and social justice.

Phygital Governance: Phygital governance is a hybrid model that integrates *physical (offline)* service delivery with *digital (online)* systems to enhance accessibility, efficiency, and inclusivity in public administration. In healthcare, it involves combining digital platforms such as telemedicine and AI screening with physical touchpoints like local health centers and community workers. This "technology-with-human-touch" model ensures that digital health systems remain empathetic, participatory, and context-sensitive.

Policy Reform: Policy reform refers to the systematic redesign of governmental or institutional policies to improve equity, efficiency, and accountability. In the context of this chapter, policy reform entails integrating mental health into national missions (e.g., NHM, ABDM), establishing ethical digital governance structures, and promoting leadership accountability. Effective reform transforms mental health care from a fragmented service into an inclusive, sustainable ecosystem guided by compassion, data ethics, and participatory governance.

Chapter 3
Life Skills Training and Adolescent Health:
Evidence From the Paniya Community Study and Its Implications for Healthcare Reform

Jishamol Thomas
http://orcid.org/0000-0002-2912-9188
Christ College of Science and Management, India

ABSTRACT

This chapter examines the effectiveness of a culturally adapted life skills training (LST) program among marginalized Paniya tribal adolescent girls in Wayanad, Kerala. A six-month single-group pre-test–post-test intervention with 34 participants aged 11–15 years focused on key psychosocial skills, including self-awareness, communication, emotional management, decision-making, problem-solving, and interpersonal relationships. Results showed statistically significant improvements across all domains ($p \leq 0.05$), indicating enhanced psychosocial functioning. Interpreted through developmental and empowerment perspectives, the findings suggest that LST can strengthen resilience and competence, while also emphasizing the need for policy integration to address persistent structural barriers.

INTRODUCTION

Adolescence represents a critical stage in the human life course, marked by rapid and interconnected changes across physical, cognitive, emotional, and social

DOI: 10.4018/979-8-2600-0939-0.ch003

domains. Beyond biological maturation, this developmental period involves profound psychosocial transitions that shape identity formation, emotional regulation, decision-making capacity, and social competence (Shearer et al., 2021; Graber & Petersen, 2017). As adolescents negotiate autonomy and develop enduring behavioral patterns, their trajectories are deeply influenced by family contexts, peer networks, educational institutions, and broader socio-economic and political structures (Fearon et al., 2014; Tavares et al., 2020). Supportive environments can promote resilience and well-being, whereas adverse conditions may intensify vulnerability and long-term disadvantage.

For adolescents living in contexts of social marginalization, developmental challenges are significantly compounded. Structural inequalities including poverty, social exclusion, limited educational access, and discriminatory institutional practices disrupt normative developmental processes and heighten psychosocial risk. Emotional dysregulation, low self-esteem, school disengagement, and restricted aspirations often emerge not as individual deficits, but as consequences of constrained opportunity structures. Understanding adolescent health in marginalized settings therefore requires integrating developmental analysis with attention to socio-structural determinants.

India's Scheduled Tribe population, comprising over 104 million individuals (Census, 2011), reflects immense cultural diversity alongside enduring structural disadvantage. Despite constitutional protections and targeted welfare policies, many tribal communities continue to experience inequities in education, health access, employment, and political representation. These disparities are rooted not in cultural inadequacy but in historical processes of land dispossession, social exclusion, and uneven integration into mainstream development frameworks. Limited educational quality, language barriers, under-resourced healthcare infrastructure, and culturally insensitive service delivery models continue to shape intergenerational disadvantage.

Kerala presents a notable paradox. Although widely recognized for strong social development indicators, significant disparities persist among tribal populations, particularly in Wayanad district. Tribal households in this region experience chronic poverty, precarious livelihoods, and educational marginalization. Among these communities, the Paniya tribe represents one of the most historically disadvantaged groups, having endured bonded labor, land alienation, and systemic denial of autonomy under feudal and colonial systems (Mohindra et al., 2010; Shijina, 2020). These structural legacies continue to shape adolescent experiences through intergenerational poverty, limited educational capital, and persistent social stigma.

Gender intensifies these vulnerabilities. Evidence indicates pronounced disparities in literacy, school retention, and decision-making autonomy among Paniya girls (Asha, 2020; SCERT Kerala, 2020). Early marriage, school dropout, and constrained agency reflect the intersection of tribal marginalization and gendered norms. Importantly, these outcomes cannot be reduced to cultural practices alone; research documents experiences of discrimination and exclusion within educational systems that further erode confidence, emotional regulation, and motivation (Joy & Sreehari, 2014). While welfare initiatives provide material support, psychosocial dimensions of adolescent development often remain insufficiently addressed.

Within this context, life skills training (LST) has emerged as a preventive and promotive psychosocial strategy. The World Health Organization defines life skills as cognitive, social, and emotional competencies that enable individuals to manage everyday challenges effectively (WHO, 1994; 2003). Skills such as self-awareness, communication, decision-making, problem-solving, and emotional regulation are particularly salient for adolescents navigating structural constraints. UNICEF further conceptualizes life skills education as a holistic process that integrates knowledge, attitudes, and competencies to strengthen resilience and social participation (UNICEF, 2005).

Although empirical evidence supports the effectiveness of life skills interventions in mainstream populations, research among highly marginalized tribal communities remains limited. Few studies have systematically evaluated culturally adapted psychosocial interventions for indigenous adolescents, particularly girls. Moreover, existing research often fails to situate intervention outcomes within broader sociopolitical realities, limiting policy relevance.

Responding to these gaps, the present study develops and evaluates a culturally adapted life skills training program for Paniya tribal adolescent girls in Wayanad, Kerala. Focusing on six core competencies self-awareness, communication, decision-making, problem-solving, interpersonal relationships, and emotional management the intervention employs a structured, participatory design and assesses outcomes across pre-intervention, post-intervention, and follow-up time points.

Importantly, the study does not position life skills training as a substitute for structural reform. Rather, it conceptualizes LST as a supportive and enabling intervention that strengthens internal capacities within environments marked by persistent inequality. By integrating empirical evaluation with structural analysis, this chapter contributes to equity-oriented adolescent health scholarship and highlights the relevance of culturally responsive psychosocial interventions within broader community-based health reform frameworks.

BACKGROUND

Adolescence is widely recognized as a pivotal developmental stage during which individuals acquire cognitive, emotional, and social capacities that shape long-term health, well-being, and life trajectories. This period involves rapid neurobiological development alongside heightened sensitivity to environmental influences, making adolescents particularly responsive to both protective and risk factors. Life skills acquired during adolescence influence not only psychological adjustment but also sexual and reproductive health, educational engagement, social participation, and future socio-economic outcomes (Mahanta et al., 2021). Consequently, adolescence represents a critical window for preventive and promotive interventions aimed at strengthening psychosocial competence and resilience.

A substantial body of developmental and mental health research indicates that adolescents' transitions are often accompanied by increased vulnerability to anxiety, emotional dysregulation, identity confusion, and behavioral difficulties. These vulnerabilities are especially pronounced in contexts marked by poverty, social exclusion, and limited institutional support (Hankin, 2006; Rockhill et al., 2010; Pao & Bosk, 2011). In such environments, adolescents frequently encounter cumulative stressors including academic pressure, family instability, exposure to discrimination, and constrained future prospects that interfere with healthy psychosocial development. Without adequate support, these challenges can translate into school disengagement, risk behaviors, and long-term mental health concerns.

Within this context, interventions that strengthen psychosocial competencies have gained increasing prominence. Life skills training (LST) has emerged as a globally endorsed approach aimed at enhancing adolescents' capacity to cope with developmental challenges and everyday stressors. Empirical studies across educational and community settings suggest that experiential learning strategies such as role-play, group discussions, problem-based activities, and reflective exercises are particularly effective in strengthening self-awareness, emotional regulation, communication, and decision-making (Bhaskaran, 2023; Saravanakumar, 2020). These competencies are foundational for adolescents' ability to manage interpersonal relationships, navigate academic demands, and respond adaptively to adversity.

Evidence further suggests that deficits in life skills are associated with low self-esteem, poor emotional control, academic disengagement, and maladaptive coping behaviors (Seema et al., 2018; Prajapati et al., 2017). Conversely, adolescents who demonstrate stronger psychosocial skills tend to exhibit greater emotional resilience, improved peer relationships, and enhanced motivation for learning. As a result, life skills education has increasingly been positioned as both a preventive and promotive strategy within adolescent mental health and development frameworks, particularly in low-resource and marginalized settings.

International agencies have played a key role in conceptualizing and promoting life skills education. The World Health Organization defines life skills as a set of cognitive, social, and emotional abilities that enable individuals to effectively manage the demands and challenges of everyday life (World Health Organ World Health Organization, 1994; World Health Organ World Health Organization, 2003).

These skills include self-awareness, critical and creative thinking, decision-making, problem-solving, communication, interpersonal relationships, empathy, and coping with emotions and stress. UNICEF further conceptualizes life skills education as a holistic process that integrates knowledge, attitudes, and practical competencies to promote resilience, positive behavior, and social inclusion (UNICEF, 2017). Together, these frameworks emphasize that life skills education extends beyond academic achievement to foster adaptive functioning, motivation, and psychosocial well-being.

Despite the growing global emphasis on life skills education, much of the empirical literature has focused on mainstream school-based populations, often within urban or semi-urban contexts. There remains limited attention to how life skills interventions function within structurally marginalized and culturally distinct communities, particularly indigenous and tribal populations. This gap is significant, as psychosocial development among marginalized adolescents is shaped not only by individual characteristics but also by historical, socio-economic, and political conditions that constrain opportunities and shape lived experiences.

For tribal and indigenous adolescents, psychosocial development is profoundly influenced by intersecting structural determinants, including poverty, educational exclusion, discrimination, and historical marginalization. Studies from India consistently highlight that tribal adolescents especially girls experience disproportionately high rates of school dropout, early marriage, adolescent pregnancy, substance exposure, and restricted decision-making autonomy (Joy & Srihari, 2014; Ministry of Tribal Affairs, 2013; State Council of Educational Research and Training, 2016). These outcomes are not simply reflections of individual vulnerability or cultural practices but are rooted in entrenched socio-political and economic inequalities that limit access to quality education, healthcare, and psychosocial support across generations.

Importantly, these structural constraints interact with educational systems in ways that further disadvantage tribal adolescents. Language barriers, culturally incongruent curricula, discriminatory attitudes, and inadequate institutional support often undermine tribal students' engagement and sense of belonging within formal schooling environments. Research indicates that experiences of stigma and exclusion within schools can erode self-esteem, emotional regulation, and motivation, contributing to higher dropout rates and poorer psychosocial outcomes (Joy & Srihari, 2014). While welfare schemes and residential schooling initiatives aim to address access-related barriers, they often fall short in addressing the psychosocial dimensions of adolescent development.

The Paniya tribe of South India represents one of the most marginalized tribal communities, both historically and in contemporary contexts. The Paniya people have endured extreme forms of social and economic exclusion, including bonded labor, land dispossession, and systematic denial of autonomy under feudal and colonial systems (Mohindra et al., 2010). These historical injustices have produced enduring "vulnerability traps," characterized by chronic poverty, low educational attainment, and limited access to health and social services. Such structural disadvantages continue to shape the everyday realities of Paniya adolescents, influencing their educational experiences, psychosocial well-being, and future aspirations.

Empirical evidence from Kerala indicates that Paniya adolescents face multiple psychosocial challenges, including low self-esteem, poor academic performance, emotional distress, and limited life opportunities (Saranya et al., 2022; Rahna & Nithya, 2022). Gender further compounds these vulnerabilities. Adolescent girls within the Paniya community are particularly disadvantaged due to gendered norms, early life transitions, and restricted agency, which amplify their exposure to educational discontinuation, early marriage, and psychosocial stress. These patterns highlight the need for interventions that address not only material deprivation but also the internal capacities required for navigating adversity and asserting agency.

Despite growing recognition of these challenges, the literature reveals a significant gap in empirically evaluated, culturally responsive life skills interventions for Paniya tribal adolescents. Existing studies tend to document vulnerability, deprivation, and risk behaviors without systematically examining whether psychosocial skill-building interventions can enhance resilience, agency, and well-being within this population. Moreover, few intervention studies engage critically with the cultural and structural contexts that shape both the need for and the outcomes of life skills training. This lack of contextualized intervention research limits the development of evidence-based programs tailored to the realities of highly marginalized tribal communities.

In addition, many life skills interventions reported in the literature adopt short-term or generalized approaches that may not adequately account for the lived experiences of indigenous adolescents. Without cultural adaptation, participatory engagement, and sensitivity to structural constraints, such interventions risk limited relevance and sustainability. Scholars increasingly argue that psychosocial interventions in marginalized contexts must be grounded in local realities, incorporate community knowledge systems, and acknowledge the broader socio-political forces shaping adolescent lives.

Responding to these gaps, the present study develops and evaluates a culturally adapted life skills training program for Paniya tribal adolescent girls in Wayanad, Kerala. Drawing on the World Health Organization's life skills framework, the intervention focuses on six core competencies self-awareness, communication, decision-making, problem-solving, interpersonal relationships, and emotional regulation identified through a population-specific needs assessment. These domains were selected to align with the psychosocial challenges most salient to the participants' lived experiences.

By employing a structured, participatory intervention design and quantitatively assessing changes across pre-intervention, post-intervention, and follow-up assessments, the study seeks to examine the potential of life skills training as a psychosocial intervention that strengthens resilience and well-being among a highly marginalized adolescent population. At the same time, the study adopts a critical perspective that situates intervention outcomes within broader structural constraints, recognizing that psychosocial skill development operates alongside, rather than in place of, systemic reform.

Through this approach, the study contributes to a more nuanced understanding of adolescent health promotion in marginalized tribal contexts. It extends the literature by providing empirical evidence on culturally responsive life skills training among Paniya tribal adolescent girls and informs equity-oriented strategies for community-based healthcare reform. By integrating psychosocial capacity-building with structural awareness, the chapter offers insights relevant to researchers, practitioners, and policymakers seeking to support holistic adolescent development within indigenous and marginalized communities.

THEORETICAL FRAMEWORK

This study is guided by an integrative theoretical framework that brings together Social Learning Theory (Bandura), Psychosocial Development Theory (Erikson), Empowerment Theory (Zimmerman), Bronfenbrenner's Ecological Systems Theory, and contemporary resilience scholarship. Together, these perspectives help explain how life skills training (LST) may influence psychosocial development among marginalized Paniya tribal adolescent girls while remaining embedded within structural realities.

Bandura's Social Learning Theory explains how life skills are acquired through observation, modeling, feedback, and reinforcement. The intervention relied heavily on role-plays, peer interaction, and guided reflection. These activities created opportunities for participants to observe adaptive behaviors and practice them in a supportive setting. For adolescents who may have limited exposure to positive role models, such structured rehearsal is important. Improvements in communication and emotional regulation can therefore be understood as products of socially mediated learning and increasing self-efficacy.

Erikson's theory provides a developmental lens. Adolescence is marked by the tension between identity and role confusion. For tribal girls facing stigma, poverty, and school discontinuity, identity formation is often complicated by restricted agency. Skills such as self-awareness and decision-making support reflection on personal strengths and aspirations. From this perspective, gains observed in the study are not only behavioral improvements but signs of emerging identity consolidation and emotional maturity.

Empowerment Theory extends the analysis beyond individual development. Empowerment involves increased participation, critical awareness, and perceived control over one's circumstances. Within the intervention, dialogue-based activities encouraged girls to express opinions, reflect collectively, and explore solutions to everyday challenges. These processes foster psychological empowerment greater confidence and voice even though broader structural constraints remain.

To situate these changes within wider systems, the study also draws on Bronfenbrenner's Ecological Systems Theory. At the microsystem level, the hostel and peer group served as the immediate environment where skill-building occurred. The mesosystem connections between school and family may be strengthened as girls gain confidence in communication. The exosystem includes tribal welfare institutions and educational governance structures that shape opportunities indirectly. At the macrosystem level, caste hierarchies, gender norms, and histories of land dispossession frame adolescent development. The chronosystem reminds us that present challenges are rooted in intergenerational poverty and bonded labor histories. LST operates within these layered systems; it does not remove structural inequality but may enhance adolescents' capacity to respond to it.

Resilience theory further clarifies this process. Masten describes resilience as "ordinary magic," emerging from adaptive systems such as self-regulation and supportive relationships. Ungar emphasizes that resilience is ecological and culturally embedded. In this study, life skills training strengthened both internal capacities (emotional regulation, problem-solving) and relational resources (peer support). For Paniya girls, resilience may mean sustaining school participation, managing stigma, or negotiating family responsibilities forms of adaptation shaped by context.

Finally, principles of culturally responsive pedagogy informed implementation. The curriculum was adapted through needs assessment, translated into Malayalam, and grounded in participants' lived experiences. Although not formally co-designed with community elders, sessions encouraged dialogue and local reflection. Adolescents were treated as knowledge contributors rather than passive recipients.

Taken together, this framework positions life skills training as a context-sensitive, multi-level intervention that strengthens psychosocial competence while acknowledging enduring structural inequality.

CONCEPTUAL FRAMEWORK

The conceptual framework guiding this study is anchored in the World Health Organization's Life Skills Framework (World Health Organization, 1994; World Health Organ World Health Organization, 2003) and operationalized through an input–process–output (IPO) model that is explicitly situated within the socio-structural realities of tribal marginalization. Rather than conceptualizing life skills training as an isolated or individualistic intervention, the framework positions it as a mediating psychosocial process through which adolescents develop internal capacities that enable them to respond more effectively to structurally constrained environments. This approach reflects an understanding that adolescent development particularly among marginalized tribal populations is shaped by the interaction between individual competencies and broader socio-economic, cultural, and institutional conditions.

At the input level, the framework foregrounds the characteristics and contextual realities of the study population, namely adolescent girls from the Paniya tribal community in Wayanad, Kerala, aged 11 to 15 years. These adolescents are situated within intersecting vulnerabilities, including poverty, educational exclusion, gender-based disadvantage, historical marginalization, and limited access to psychosocial support services. These vulnerabilities are not treated as background variables but as constitutive conditions that shape adolescents' developmental experiences and opportunities. The framework also incorporates the intervention curriculum as a critical input, emphasizing its culturally adapted design and alignment with the WHO life skills domains. The curriculum focuses on six core competencies self-awareness, communication, decision-making, problem-solving, interpersonal relationships, and emotional management identified through a population-specific needs assessment. This needs-based approach ensures that the selected skills correspond to the lived experiences, psychosocial challenges, and developmental gaps observed among Paniya tribal adolescent girls. Facilitation constitutes a third key input, with the intervention delivered through researcher-led sessions validated by subject experts to ensure developmental relevance, ethical sensitivity, and contextual appropriateness. Facilitation is conceptualized not merely as content delivery but as a relational and pedagogical process that shapes learning, engagement, and internalization of skills.

The process component of the framework delineates how these inputs are transformed into psychosocial outcomes through structured intervention mechanisms. Central to this process is a six-month life skills training program implemented through experiential and participatory methods, including role-plays, group discussions, games, storytelling, and guided reflection. These methods are grounded in principles of active learning and social interaction, recognizing that psychosocial skills are best acquired through practice, observation, feedback, and shared meaning-making rather than didactic instruction alone. The framework emphasizes the importance of a supportive and culturally sensitive learning environment, designed to encourage peer interaction, dialogue, and safe emotional expression. Such an environment is particularly significant for tribal adolescent girls, whose voices are often marginalized within both familial and institutional settings. The process also includes systematic assessment at three time points pre-intervention, post-intervention, and follow-up using a modified Life Skills Assessment Scale (LSAS). These assessments are not viewed solely as measurement tools but as integral components of the intervention process, enabling reflection, reinforcement, and monitoring of change over time.

At the output level, the framework conceptualizes multiple layers of outcomes emerging from participation in the life skills training process. The most immediate outputs are improvements in psychosocial competencies across the six targeted domains, including enhanced self-awareness, more effective communication, improved decision-making and problem-solving abilities, stronger interpersonal skills, and greater emotional regulation. These competencies are understood as foundational capacities that support adolescents' ability to manage daily stressors, navigate social relationships, and engage constructively with educational and community environments. Beyond these skill-specific outcomes, the framework identifies broader psychosocial outcomes, such as increased self-efficacy, confidence, and sense of belonging. These outcomes reflect changes in how adolescents perceive themselves and their capacity to act within their social worlds, signaling shifts in internalized beliefs and emotional orientation rather than merely observable behaviors.

Crucially, the framework extends beyond individual-level outcomes to conceptualize emergent empowerment as a longer-term and more complex output of the intervention. Empowerment is understood here not as an immediate or absolute state but as a gradual and relational process involving enhanced resilience, perceived agency, and the ability to make informed choices within constrained contexts. For Paniya tribal adolescent girls, empowerment may manifest in subtle but meaningful ways, such as increased willingness to express opinions, greater confidence in decision-making, improved emotional coping, and more active engagement with educational opportunities. These manifestations are shaped by both individual capacities and the availability of supportive structures, underscoring the relational nature of empowerment.

The conceptual linkage at the core of the framework explicitly positions life skills training as a mediating mechanism between structural marginalization and psychosocial empowerment outcomes. Structural marginalization encompassing poverty, educational exclusion, gendered constraints, historical dispossession, and fragmented governance is treated as a distal but pervasive influence on adolescent development. Rather than assuming that psychosocial interventions can eliminate these structural inequities, the framework acknowledges their persistence and constraining effects. Life skills training is thus conceptualized as an enabling intervention that operates within these constraints, enhancing adolescents' internal capacities to cope with adversity, engage more effectively with available opportunities, and navigate institutional systems. In this sense, the framework avoids over-claiming causal transformation at the structural level while still recognizing the meaningful role of psychosocial capacity-building.

Importantly, the framework adopts a multi-level perspective that integrates individual, relational, and structural dimensions of change. At the individual level, life skills training strengthens cognitive, emotional, and social competencies. At the relational level, it fosters improved peer interactions, communication, and emotional expression within supportive group settings. At the structural level, the framework recognizes that the effectiveness and sustainability of psychosocial gains are contingent upon alignment with broader educational, health, and welfare systems. This positioning underscores the necessity of embedding life skills interventions within multi-sectoral support frameworks, including schools, hostels, community institutions, and policy initiatives.

The framework also incorporates a temporal dimension, recognizing that psychosocial change unfolds over time and may not follow linear trajectories. By including follow-up assessment, the framework allows for examination of the short-term sustainability of intervention effects, while acknowledging that longer-term outcomes depend on continued reinforcement, supportive environments, and structural opportunities. This temporal sensitivity reflects a developmental perspective that views adolescence as a dynamic period of growth influenced by ongoing interactions between individuals and their environments.

If visually represented, the conceptual framework may be depicted as a flow model illustrating the progression from socio-structural constraints through life skills training processes to cognitive, emotional, and social skill development, culminating in psychosocial empowerment and well-being. However, the narrative articulation of the framework emphasizes that this progression is neither automatic nor deterministic. Instead, it is mediated by contextual factors, facilitation quality, cultural relevance, and institutional support.

Overall, this conceptual framework provides a coherent and context-sensitive structure for understanding how life skills training can contribute to adolescent psychosocial development within marginalized tribal settings. It aligns theoretical principles with intervention design and outcome evaluation, ensuring conceptual consistency across the study. By explicitly situating psychosocial interventions within structural realities, the framework advances a balanced and ethically grounded approach to adolescent empowerment one that recognizes both the potential and the limits of life skills training. In doing so, it contributes to broader discussions on equity-oriented adolescent health promotion, emphasizing that sustainable well-being emerges from the interaction between internal capacities and supportive social systems rather than from isolated interventions alone.

OBJECTIVES

1. To analyze the extent of life skills based on knowledge and practice among tribal adolescent girls in the Wayanad district.
2. To design and implement the life skills intervention program among the Paniya adolescent girls.
3. To assess the efficacy of the life skills intervention program among Paniya adolescent girls.

METHOD

This study adopted a *single-group pre-test–post-test experimental design* to evaluate the effectiveness of a culturally adapted life skills training intervention among Paniya tribal adolescent girls. The design did not include a control group, as the study was implemented within a constrained and vulnerable community setting where withholding intervention was not ethically or practically feasible. Accordingly, findings are interpreted as indicative of intervention-related change rather than causal attribution.

Data collection and intervention implementation were conducted across *four sequential phases*. The first phase involved a *baseline (pre-intervention) assessment* to establish participants' initial levels of life skills. The second phase focused on the *development and expert validation of the life skills training module*, informed by a population-specific needs assessment. The third phase comprised the *six-month implementation of the structured life skills intervention*, delivered using participatory and experiential methods. The final phase involved *post-intervention assessment*, conducted using the same standardized measures to evaluate changes in psychosocial competencies following program completion.

This phased approach ensured systematic implementation, alignment between assessment and intervention content, and consistency in outcome measurement.

Conducting psychosocial interventions within indigenous communities requires attention to cultural respect, informed participation, and contextual sensitivity. The intervention design emphasized participatory methods, linguistic accessibility, and community-based delivery to minimize harm and enhance relevance. Future studies should further strengthen co-design approaches with community stakeholders to ensure ethical engagement and cultural legitimacy. During facilitation, several participants initially hesitated to speak in group discussions. Over time, increased peer trust appeared to support greater participation.

Figure 1. Single Group Pre-test and Post-test Research Design

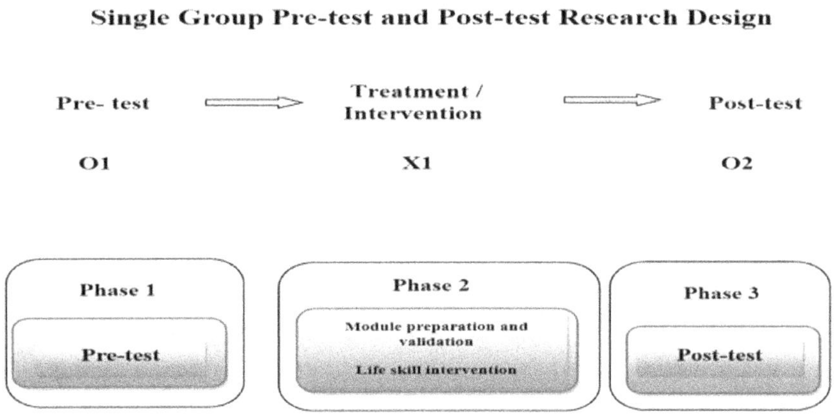

Sample

Participants were recruited from a *tribal residential hostel in Wayanad district, Kerala*, which predominantly serves students from the Paniya tribal community. The study sample comprised *34 adolescent girls aged 11–15 years*, enrolled in grades 6 to 10. *Convenience sampling* was employed due to the limited accessibility of the population and the institutional setting in which the intervention was implemented; this sampling strategy is acknowledged as a limitation with respect to generalizability.

Participant selection was guided by clearly defined *inclusion and exclusion criteria*. Adolescents were eligible to participate if they (a) belonged to the Paniya tribal community, (b) scored below the established cut-off on a ten-item life skills screening inventory administered prior to the intervention, (c) expressed willingness to participate, and (d) had not previously undergone any formal life skills training. Participants were required to have *functional proficiency in Malayalam* to ensure comprehension of the intervention content and assessment tools.

Adolescents with *known or self-reported diagnosed psychological or psychiatric conditions* were excluded to avoid confounding intervention effects and to ensure participant well-being. The intervention spanned *six months and consisted of 25 structured sessions*. Participants who were absent for more than two training sessions were excluded from the final analysis to maintain intervention fidelity and consistency of exposure.

All selected participants met the inclusion criteria and completed the intervention protocol. Demographic characteristics of the study sample are presented in *Table 2*.

Intervention

The life skills training intervention was developed through a *systematic, needs-based approach* tailored to the psychosocial context of Paniya tribal adolescent girls. During the preliminary phase, a broader screening assessment was conducted among adolescents from the Paniya community using a life skills inventory to identify domains requiring targeted intervention. Findings from this needs assessment informed the selection of six core life skills self-awareness, communication, decision-making, problem-solving, interpersonal relationships, and emotional management as priority areas for program development.

Based on these identified needs, a *structured six-month intervention module* was designed, incorporating culturally sensitive content and developmentally appropriate activities. The module was subjected to *expert validation by five subject specialists* with expertise in adolescent development, psychology, and social work to ensure content relevance, clarity, and suitability for a tribal adolescent population. Revisions were made based on expert feedback prior to implementation.

The intervention was delivered *in person by the researcher* at a tribal residential hostel in Wayanad. Training sessions were conducted *once weekly*, each lasting approximately *two hours*, resulting in a total of *25 structured sessions* over the six-month period. The sessions employed *experiential and participatory methods*, including games, role-plays, group discussions, and guided reflection, to facilitate engagement, peer learning, and skill practice within a supportive environment. This delivery approach was intended to promote active participation and reinforce skill acquisition through observation and practice.

An overview of the intervention structure and session content is presented in *Table 1*.

Life Skills Intervention Schedule

The life skills intervention was implemented over a *six-month period* and was systematically structured to address six core psychosocial competencies identified through the needs assessment. Each month focused on a specific life skill domain, allowing sufficient time for skill introduction, practice, and consolidation through experiential learning methods.

During the *first month*, the intervention focused on *self-awareness*, utilizing structured questionnaires, reflective exercises, and guided activities aimed at helping participants identify personal strengths, values, emotions, and aspirations. These activities were designed to support identity exploration and self-reflection.

The *second month* targeted *effective communication skills*, with emphasis on verbal and non-verbal expression, active listening, and assertiveness. Group activities and role-playing scenarios were employed to facilitate peer interaction and real-life communication practice.

In the *third month*, the focus shifted to *interpersonal relationship skills*, addressing cooperation, empathy, and conflict management. Interactive discussions, group games, and collaborative tasks were used to enhance social connectedness and relational competence.

The *fourth month* emphasized *decision-making skills*, incorporating storytelling, situational analysis, and group-based activities that encouraged participants to evaluate alternatives, anticipate consequences, and make informed choices relevant to everyday life.

The *fifth month* concentrated on *problem-solving skills*, employing role-plays, case scenarios, and guided group discussions to strengthen analytical thinking, adaptability, and constructive coping strategies in challenging situations.

The *final month* addressed *emotional management*, focusing on recognizing, understanding, and regulating emotions. Mindfulness-based exercises, relaxation techniques, and group reflection activities were used to promote emotional awareness and adaptive emotional responses.

This phased and skill-specific structure ensured progressive learning, reinforcement, and integration of psychosocial competencies across the intervention period, supporting sustained skill development among the participants.

Measures

Data were collected using two instruments: a *socio-demographic questionnaire* and a standardized *Life Skills Assessment Scale (LSAS).*

A researcher-developed socio-demographic questionnaire was used to obtain background information on participants, including age, grade level, family characteristics, and parental occupation. This information was used to describe the study sample and contextualize the findings.

Life skills were assessed using the *Life Skills Assessment Scale (LSAS)* developed by the Rajiv Gandhi National Institute of Youth Development (Subasree & Nair, 2014). The original LSAS consists of 100 items rated on a *5-point Likert scale* ranging from 1 (*always true*) to 5 (*never true*), with selected items reverse-scored to minimize response bias. The scale has demonstrated satisfactory psychometric properties, with a reported reliability coefficient of *0.84* and established content validity (*89%*).

For the purposes of the present study, a *reduced and domain-specific version of the LSAS* was employed, retaining only those items relevant to the six targeted life skills: self-awareness, communication, decision-making, problem-solving, interpersonal relationships, and emotional management. This adaptation was undertaken to ensure alignment between the intervention content and outcome measurement.

To enhance *cultural and linguistic appropriateness*, the selected items were translated into Malayalam by qualified language professionals and subsequently reviewed and validated by subject matter experts with experience in adolescent and tribal research. This process aimed to ensure conceptual equivalence, clarity, and suitability for the study population.

Procedure

Prior to data collection, *formal permission* was obtained from the relevant government authorities to conduct the study at a residential tribal hostel located in *Panamaram Panchayath, Wayanad district, Kerala.* Institutional consent was secured, and participants were informed about the purpose and procedures of the study in age-appropriate language before participation.

The study commenced with a *baseline screening and pre-intervention assessment*, during which participants completed the reduced version of the Life Skills Assessment Scale (LSAS) to establish initial levels of psychosocial competencies. This assessment also served to confirm eligibility based on the predefined inclusion criteria.

Following the baseline assessment, the *life skills training intervention was implemented over a six-month period*, with sessions delivered weekly by the first author using structured and participatory methods. The intervention adhered to the validated module and maintained consistency in content and delivery throughout the program duration.

To evaluate intervention outcomes, life skills were assessed at *two post-intervention time points* using the same reduced LSAS instrument. The *post-assessment* was conducted two weeks after completion of the intervention to capture immediate effects, and a *follow-up assessment* was administered three months later to examine the short-term sustainability of observed changes.

This sequential assessment design enabled systematic comparison of pre-, post-, and follow-up measures, facilitating evaluation of intervention-related changes over time.

Analyses

Data were analyzed using *IBM SPSS Statistics version 29.0*, in accordance with the study objectives. Prior to inferential analysis, the *Shapiro–Wilk test of normality* was conducted to assess the distribution of scores for each life skills domain across assessment points. Results indicated that scores for *self-awareness* ($W = .957$, $p >$

.05), *communication* ($W = .949$, $p > .05$), *decision-making* ($W = .979$, $p > .05$), and *emotional management* ($W = .967$, $p > .05$) met assumptions of normality. In contrast, *problem-solving* ($W = .932$, $p < .05$) and *interpersonal relationship skills* ($W = .895$, $p < .05$) deviated from normal distribution.

Based on these distributional characteristics, *repeated measures analysis of variance (ANOVA)* was employed to examine differences across pre-intervention, post-intervention, and follow-up assessments for variables that met normality assumptions. For variables violating normality assumptions, the *Friedman non-parametric test* was used to assess changes across the three assessment points.

This analytical strategy ensured appropriate alignment between data characteristics and statistical techniques, enabling robust evaluation of changes in life skills following the intervention. Statistical significance was evaluated at conventional alpha levels, and effect sizes were calculated where applicable to support interpretation of intervention effects.

RESULTS

The effects of the life skills training intervention were examined across **three assessment points pre-intervention, post-intervention, and follow-up **using appropriate *repeated-measures statistical analyses.* For life skills domains that met assumptions of normality, *repeated measures ANOVA* was employed, while the *Friedman non-parametric test* was used for domains that violated normality assumptions. These analyses were conducted to evaluate changes in psychosocial competencies following the intervention.

Table 2. Demographics of the study participants

Variable	Groups	Frequency (N=34)	Percent	Total percent
Age	11	6	17.6	100
	13	7	20.6	
	14	8	23.5	
	15	13	38.2	
Grade	6	6	17.6	100
	8	10	29.4	
	9	7	20.6	
	10	11	32.4	

continued on following page

Table 2. Continued

Variable	Groups	Frequency (N=34)	Percent	Total percent
Type of family	Nuclear family	25	73.5	100
	Joint-family	09	26.5	
Number of siblings	Without siblings	2	5.9	100
	One- Two	12	35.3	
	Three- four	15	44.1	
	Five & above	5	14.7	
Employment of parents	Daily wages	26	76.4	100
	Govt employee	1	2.9	
	Private employee	7	20.7	

The differences between pre-, post, and follow-up assessments on life-skills intervention

Tables 3 and 4 summarize the results of the repeated-measures analyses examining differences in the six life skills domains across *pre-intervention, post-intervention, and follow-up assessments*. Repeated measures ANOVA was used for variables that met normality assumptions, while the Friedman test was applied to variables that violated these assumptions.

The null hypothesis tested was that *no statistically significant differences* would be observed across the three assessment points for any of the life skills domains self-awareness, communication, emotional management, decision-making, problem-solving, and interpersonal relationship skills among the participating tribal adolescent girls.

Table 3. Descriptive Statistics of the Repeated Measures ANOVA test of pre-, post, and follow-up assessments

Variable	Test	Mean	*SD*	*F*	Sig.	ηp^2
Self- Awareness	Pre-test	29.88	3.4	281.41**	.000	.895
	Post-test	45.41	3.60			
	Follow-up	45.76	2.70			

continued on following page

Table 3. Continued

Variable	Test	Mean	*SD*	*F*	Sig.	ηp^2
Communication	Pre-test	22.62	3.21	318.63**	.000	.906
	Post-test	35.68	3.01			
	Follow-up	36.85	1.91			
Emotional Management	Pre-test	25.82	3.09	522.89**	.000	.941
	Post-test	42.97	1.98			
	Follow-up	39.91	2.79			
Decision Making	Pre-test	29.85	3.12	579.37**	.000	.946
	Post-test	48.59	2.10			
	Follow-up	43.82	2.29			

***P*=<.01, **P*=<.05

Table 4. Friedman Test of pre-, post, and follow-up assessments on problem-solving and interpersonal relationship skills

Variable	Test	Median	*SD*	Mean rank	x^2	*P*
Problem-Solving	Pre-test	25	2.23	1.03	54.71**	.000
	Post-test	40	3.67	2.74		
	Follow-up	37	2.43	2.24		
Inter Personal Relationship	Pre-test	32	3.31	1.01	58.68**	.000
	Post-test	49	4.09	2.82		
	Follow-up	44	2.57	2.16		

***p*=<.01, **p*=<.05

Tables 3 and 4 present the outcomes of the life skills training intervention across six psychosocial domains self-awareness, communication, emotional management, decision-making, problem-solving, and interpersonal relationship skills measured at pre-intervention, post-intervention, and follow-up assessments among Paniya tribal adolescent girls.

Repeated measures ANOVA results (Table 3) indicate statistically significant improvements across four life skills domains that met normality assumptions. *Self-awareness* scores increased substantially from pre-test (M = 29.88, SD = 3.40) to post-test (M = 45.41, SD = 3.60) and were sustained at follow-up (M = 45.76, SD = 2.70), $F(2, 66) = 281.41$ $p < .001$, $\eta p^2 = .895$, with a large effect size ($\eta p^2 = .895$). Similarly, *communication skills* demonstrated significant gains across assessment points, increasing from pre-test (M = 22.62, SD = 3.01) to post-test (M = 35.68,

SD = 1.91) and follow-up (M = 36.85, SD = 3.09), $F(2, 66) = 318.63$, $p < .001$, $\eta p^2 = .906$

Significant improvements were also observed in *emotional management*, with mean scores rising from pre-test (M = 25.82, SD = 3.09) to post-test (M = 42.97, SD = 1.98) and remaining elevated at follow-up (M = 39.91, SD = 2.79), $F = 522.89$, $p < .001$, $\eta p^2 = .941$. *Decision-making skills* showed the strongest intervention effect, increasing from pre-test (M = 29.85, SD = 3.12) to post-test (M = 48.59, SD = 2.10), with sustained gains at follow-up (M = 43.82, SD = 2.29), $F = 579.37$, $p < .001$, $\eta p^2 = .946$. These results indicate robust and statistically significant improvements with large effect sizes across all four domains.

For variables that violated normality assumptions, the Friedman test was employed (Table 4). Results revealed significant differences across assessment points for *problem-solving skills*, with median scores increasing from pre-test (Median = 25, Mean Rank = 1.03) to post-test (Median = 40, Mean Rank = 2.74), and remaining elevated at follow-up (Median = 37, Mean Rank = 2.24), $\chi^2(2, N = 34) = 54.71$, $p < .001$ Similarly, *interpersonal relationship skills* showed significant improvement, with median scores increasing from pre-test (Median = 32, Mean Rank = 1.01) to post-test (Median = 49, Mean Rank = 2.82), and sustained at follow-up (Median = 44, Mean Rank = 2.16), $\chi^2(2) = 58.68$, $p < .001$.

Overall, the results demonstrate statistically significant improvements across all six life skills domains following the intervention. Accordingly, the null hypothesis of no difference across assessment points is rejected. These findings suggest that the life skills training program was effective in enhancing psychosocial competencies among Paniya tribal adolescent girls across immediate and short-term follow-up periods.

Structural Determinants of Tribal Adolescent Health

Adolescent health among the Paniya community must be situated within historically embedded structural inequalities shaped by land dispossession, caste stratification, and the legacy of bonded labor. The loss of land and economic autonomy disrupted traditional livelihood systems and entrenched intergenerational poverty, reinforcing dependence on insecure daily wage labor. Such economic precarity constrains educational continuity and narrows future aspirations for adolescents. Persistent caste-based stigma and subtle forms of discrimination within schools further influence identity formation, self-esteem, and social belonging. Although welfare policies exist, uneven implementation and institutional fragmentation limit meaningful access to sustained support. For adolescent girls, gendered labor expectations and restricted mobility intensify these constraints. Together, these intersecting structural forces create cumulative vulnerability, emphasizing that psychosocial challenges are rooted in systemic inequities rather than individual inadequacy.

Cultural Adaptation and Community Engagement

Cultural adaptation was prioritized in designing the intervention. Informal consultations with hostel staff and community-linked educators informed selection of life skill domains relevant to participants' lived realities. The curriculum was translated into Malayalam, and examples were localized to reflect hostel life, family responsibilities, and peer interactions. Sessions were dialogic, encouraging participants to connect skills with their own experiences.

However, tribal elders were not formally involved in curriculum co-design, and no formal pilot study was conducted. While expert validation and iterative adjustments strengthened relevance, deeper community participation remains a limitation and an important direction for future implementation.

Methodological Transparency and Limitations

This study used a single-group pre-test–post-test design due to ethical constraints, as withholding a potentially beneficial intervention from a vulnerable cohort was considered inappropriate. However, the absence of a control group limits causal inference and introduces threats to internal validity. Large effect sizes indicate meaningful change, though interpretation must remain cautious. Intervention fidelity was supported through standardized session plans and attendance monitoring, yet facilitator bias cannot be fully excluded. Hawthorne effects and social desirability bias in self-report measures may also have influenced outcomes. Future randomized or quasi-experimental designs would strengthen causal conclusions.

Health Economics Implications

From a health economics perspective, life skills training can be viewed as a preventive public health investment. Strengthening psychosocial competencies during adolescence may reduce future mental health burdens, school dropout, and maladaptive coping, thereby lowering long-term service costs. Delivered in group formats within existing hostel and school structures, LST is relatively low-cost and potentially scalable.

Enhancing emotional regulation and decision-making also supports educational retention and employability, contributing to human capital development. Although no formal cost-effectiveness analysis was conducted, integrating LST within tribal welfare and education systems positions it as a cost-sensitive component of broader health reform.

Healthcare Marketing Perspective

Implementing life skills programs in marginalized tribal settings requires culturally sensitive health communication. From a healthcare marketing perspective, LST functions as community-based behavior change communication aimed at building trust and participation. Programs should be framed as empowerment-oriented supports rather than corrective interventions.

Localized examples, linguistic adaptation, and participatory dialogue enhance acceptance and credibility, especially where institutional distrust exists. Clear and consistent messaging across schools and welfare systems helps position psychosocial skill-building as integral to adolescent development. Culturally grounded communication strategies are therefore central to program uptake, sustainability, and long-term impact.

Leadership and Governance

Scaling life skills training in tribal contexts requires leadership at institutional and policy levels. Hostel and school administrators play a key role by allocating time, space, and consistent support for psychosocial programs. Their commitment to holistic adolescent development determines whether such interventions become embedded or remain temporary initiatives.

At the policy level, coordination across tribal welfare, education, and public health departments is essential. Integrating life skills education with adolescent health and school retention strategies enhances sustainability. Strong leadership grounded in collaboration, accountability, and preventive mental health advocacy ensures that LST becomes part of long-term systemic reform rather than an isolated pilot effort.

DISCUSSION

The present study demonstrated statistically and practically significant improvements across six life skill domains among Paniya tribal adolescent girls following a culturally adapted intervention. Gains in self-awareness, communication, emotional regulation, decision-making, problem-solving, and interpersonal relationships were sustained at follow-up, suggesting that structured, participatory life skills training can enhance psychosocial functioning in the short to medium term.

Interpreted through a social learning framework, the use of role-play, peer interaction, and guided reflection likely facilitated observational learning, behavioral rehearsal, and reinforcement, thereby strengthening self-efficacy and confidence. From a developmental perspective, improvements in self-awareness and decision-making align with identity consolidation processes central to adolescence. The magnitude of observed effect sizes further indicates that these changes represent substantive psychosocial shifts rather than marginal score variations. The findings also reflect elements of psychological empowerment, evidenced by enhanced confidence and perceived agency within participants' immediate social contexts.

These outcomes illustrate how psychosocial skill-building functions as a proximal developmental mechanism within structurally constrained environments, reinforcing the dynamic interplay between individual agency and systemic conditions outlined in the ecological framework.

Although consistent with prior research on life skills interventions in marginalized settings, the results must be interpreted within enduring structural realities, including poverty, caste-based marginalization, gendered constraints, and uneven welfare implementation. Life skills training cannot independently dismantle systemic inequities; however, it can strengthen adolescents' adaptive capacities, enabling more effective navigation of constrained opportunities.

Overall, culturally responsive life skills programs represent meaningful preventive components of adolescent health and education strategies, particularly when embedded within institutional and policy reforms aimed at advancing equity, inclusion, and long-term social development.

STRUCTURAL AND POLICY CONTEXT

The psychosocial improvements documented in this study must be interpreted within the broader structural conditions shaping the lives of Paniya tribal adolescents. Intergenerational poverty, educational exclusion, gender-based disadvantage, fragmented governance, and uneven implementation of tribal welfare policies continue to limit developmental opportunities. While life skills training cannot dismantle these systemic inequities, it can strengthen internal capacities such as resilience, emotional regulation, decision-making, and social competence that support adolescents in navigating constrained environments more effectively.

Sustainable empowerment, however, depends on coordinated governance across education, health, and tribal welfare systems. In many tribal regions, limited psychosocial services, weak institutional integration, and inconsistent monitoring reduce the impact of otherwise well-intentioned programs. Life skills interventions therefore function most effectively as complementary components within broader service ecosystems, addressing psychosocial determinants often overlooked in access-driven policies.

Accordingly, life skills training should be embedded within multi-level support frameworks rather than implemented as isolated initiatives. Alignment with inclusive education systems, gender-responsive policies, and community-based services enhances both sustainability and impact. Parallel investments in structural reform remain essential to ensure that strengthened psychosocial competencies translate into meaningful, long-term opportunities for marginalized tribal adolescents.

RECOMMENDATIONS AND SOLUTIONS

The findings of this study indicate that culturally adapted life skills training (LST) can enhance psychosocial competencies among marginalized Paniya tribal adolescent girls. However, to ensure that these benefits extend beyond a time-bound intervention and contribute to sustainable adolescent health outcomes, life skills initiatives must be embedded within broader educational, community, and policy frameworks. The following recommendations outline priority actions across institutional, community, and systems levels.

Institutional integration within education systems is a critical first step. Life skills education should be embedded within the formal and co-curricular structures of schools serving tribal populations, rather than delivered as isolated or short-term programs. Government and aided residential schools and hostels in tribal regions should allocate structured time for experiential life skills learning, aligned with developmental needs and local contexts. Integrating life skills pedagogy into pre-service and in-service teacher education would further ensure consistent and scalable delivery, supporting the shift toward holistic, learner-centered education envisioned in national education reforms.

Community-based delivery mechanisms are essential to extend the reach and continuity of life skills training beyond school settings. Establishing locally grounded platforms such as community resource centers or adolescent clubs in collaboration with NGOs and local self-governments can provide safe, sustained spaces for mentorship, peer learning, and psychosocial support. These platforms should incorporate culturally resonant methods, including storytelling and group-based activities, to enhance relevance and participation. Community involvement is central to building trust, ownership, and long-term sustainability.

Capacity building of educators and frontline facilitators is another key priority. Teachers, hostel staff, and social workers require training not only in life skills content but also in participatory, culturally responsive facilitation methods. Continuous professional development focused on adolescent psychology, trauma sensitivity, and inclusive pedagogy can strengthen intervention quality and ethical engagement. Such capacity building should emphasize mentorship roles, enabling facilitators to model the psychosocial competencies they aim to foster.

Given the compounded vulnerabilities faced by tribal adolescent girls, *gender-sensitive policy alignment* is essential. Life skills initiatives should be integrated into existing adolescent and gender-focused programs, with explicit attention to issues such as early marriage, educational discontinuation, reproductive health, and decision-making autonomy. Gender-responsive approaches supported by female facilitators and community role models can enhance relevance and empower girls to navigate social constraints more effectively.

Parental and family engagement is also crucial for reinforcing intervention outcomes. Awareness programs and community dialogues can help parents understand the value of life skills education and its role in adolescent well-being. Involving families as partners can reduce resistance, strengthen support structures, and foster an enabling home environment for adolescents' psychosocial development.

Finally, *integration with health and social services* is necessary to ensure holistic impact. Life skills programs should be linked with adolescent health services, mental health support, and social welfare initiatives to address intersecting educational, health, and livelihood needs. Multi-sectoral coordination among education, health, and tribal welfare departments can enhance continuity of care and support adolescents beyond the intervention period.

In sum, the study supports a *multi-level, context-sensitive strategy* for adolescent empowerment that situates life skills training within institutional systems, community structures, and policy frameworks. While LST alone cannot address structural inequities, its integration within broader support systems can strengthen resilience, psychosocial well-being, and developmental opportunities for tribal adolescents. These recommendations offer a pragmatic roadmap for translating intervention-level gains into sustainable, equity-oriented adolescent health and education practices.

FUTURE RESEARCH DIRECTIONS

While the present study provides evidence for the short-term effectiveness of life skills training (LST) among Paniya tribal adolescent girls, further research is necessary to deepen understanding of its long-term impact, contextual adaptability, and structural relevance. Several priority directions emerge for advancing scholarship and practice in this area.

First, *longitudinal research designs* are essential to assess the sustainability of life skills outcomes over time. Although this study included a follow-up assessment, longer-term tracking across adolescence and early adulthood would clarify whether gains in psychosocial competencies translate into enduring outcomes such as improved educational retention, delayed early marriage, enhanced decision-making autonomy, and greater social participation. Longitudinal evidence is particularly important for informing policy investments aimed at intergenerational mobility and adolescent health equity.

Second, *cross-cultural and cross-tribal validation* of the intervention model is needed to assess its scalability and contextual robustness. Replicating the program among other tribal communities across diverse geographical and cultural settings would allow comparative analysis of how social norms, linguistic contexts, and structural conditions influence intervention effectiveness. Such studies would contribute to the development of adaptable, culturally responsive frameworks for tribal adolescent empowerment at regional and national levels.

Third, future studies should adopt *gender-inclusive and intersectional approaches*. While the present research focused on adolescent girls due to their heightened vulnerability, including boys and examining gendered differences in psychosocial development would provide a more comprehensive understanding of adolescent well-being within tribal communities. Attention to intersecting factors such as disability, migration, and household composition would further strengthen analytical depth.

Fourth, expanding the *range of life skills domains* examined in future interventions would enhance conceptual completeness. In addition to the six core skills addressed in this study, future programs could incorporate competencies such as critical thinking, creative thinking, empathy, and stress management, as outlined in WHO frameworks. Examining how these additional domains interact with resilience, civic engagement, and mental health would extend the explanatory power of life skills research.

Fifth, *mixed-methods and participatory research designs* should be prioritized to capture both measurable outcomes and lived experiences of empowerment. Integrating qualitative methods such as interviews, focus groups, and participatory action research would provide deeper insight into identity formation, confidence, and perceived agency that quantitative measures alone may not fully capture. Such approaches also align with ethical and empowerment-oriented research practices in indigenous contexts.

Finally, future research should explore *responsible integration of digital and hybrid delivery models* for life skills education. As digital access expands in rural and tribal areas, studies can examine the feasibility, acceptability, and equity implications of mobile-based or blended learning interventions. However, this line of inquiry must critically assess digital divides to avoid reinforcing existing inequalities.

In sum, future research should move beyond short-term efficacy toward *sustainability, inclusivity, and structural relevance*. By combining longitudinal designs, cross-cultural validation, intersectional analysis, methodological pluralism, and cautious technological innovation, scholars can contribute to the development of evidence-based, culturally grounded, and scalable life skills interventions that support meaningful and lasting empowerment among tribal adolescents.

IMPLICATIONS

The findings of this study indicate that culturally adapted life skills training (LST) can enhance social, emotional, and cognitive competencies among marginalized Paniya tribal adolescent girls. These results have several implications for research, practice, and policy. First, the intervention model developed in this study can serve as a practical reference framework for educators, school social workers, counselors, and community practitioners working with tribal adolescents. Its structured, participatory design demonstrates how psychosocial skill-building can be implemented within residential schools and hostel settings.

Second, the study underscores the relevance of integrating life skills education into tribal education and adolescent health initiatives. Government agencies and non-governmental organizations may draw on this evidence to inform the design of preventive and promotive programs aimed at improving adolescent well-being, resilience, and educational engagement. The findings also suggest that life skills training can complement existing welfare schemes by addressing psychosocial dimensions often overlooked in access-driven interventions.

Third, the results highlight the importance of family and community engagement. Sensitizing parents and community stakeholders to the value of life skills education may strengthen supportive environments for adolescents' educational and career development. Although life skills training alone cannot ensure social inclusion, it can function as an enabling mechanism that supports adolescents' capacity to engage more effectively with educational and social systems.

Statistical Rigor, Reliability, and Ethical Considerations

For domains analyzed using repeated measures ANOVA, Bonferroni-adjusted pairwise comparisons were conducted to examine differences between assessment points. These comparisons confirmed statistically significant differences between pre- and post-test scores, as well as between pre- and follow-up scores ($p < .001$) across relevant domains. Mean differences were further examined using 95% confidence intervals, none of which crossed zero, reinforcing the stability and precision of the observed changes beyond statistical significance. For example, the mean difference was 15.53, with a 95% confidence interval ranging from 13.42 to 17.64, indicating a substantial and reliably estimated improvement across assessment points.

Because a reduced, domain-specific version of the Life Skills Assessment Scale (LSAS) was utilized, the internal consistency of the adapted instrument was reassessed for the present sample. Cronbach's alpha for the overall adapted scale exceeded the recommended threshold of .70, indicating satisfactory internal consistency and coherent measurement of the intended psychosocial constructs. Domain-specific reliability coefficients likewise met acceptable standards ($\alpha \geq .70$) across the six targeted life skills domains. These findings support the psychometric adequacy of the modified LSAS for assessing life skills among Paniya tribal adolescent girls in the present study.

Ethical clearance for the study was obtained from the Christ (Deemed to be University), Institutional Ethics Committee prior to data collection. Formal permission was secured from relevant government authorities and hostel administration. Written informed consent was obtained from parents or legal guardians, and assent was obtained from all adolescent participants. Participation was voluntary, confidentiality was maintained, and participants were informed of their right to withdraw at any stage without penalty.

LIMITATIONS AND FUTURE RESEARCH

Several limitations of the present study warrant consideration. First, the single-group pre-test–post-test design without a control group limits causal inference. Although statistically significant improvements were observed, changes cannot be attributed exclusively to the intervention in the absence of comparative analysis. Future research employing randomized controlled or quasi-experimental designs would strengthen causal interpretation.

Second, the relatively small sample size and use of convenience sampling from a single tribal residential hostel restrict generalizability and may limit statistical power and precision of effect size estimates. While large observed effect sizes suggest meaningful intervention impact, replication with larger and more diverse samples across multiple tribal communities is necessary to enhance external validity.

Third, the intervention focused on six life skills domains identified through a needs assessment. Although contextually appropriate, future studies could incorporate a broader range of WHO-defined life skills to examine their combined and differential contributions to adolescent development.

Fourth, the follow-up period was limited to short-term assessment. Longitudinal research, including periodic booster sessions, is required to evaluate the sustainability of psychosocial gains and their translation into educational, health, and social outcomes.

Finally, the exclusive focus on adolescent girls reflects gendered vulnerabilities within the Paniya community but limits understanding of gender-differentiated effects. Future studies should adopt gender-inclusive and intersectional designs to examine variation across genders and social subgroups.

Despite these limitations, the study provides valuable empirical evidence on culturally adapted life skills interventions within a highly marginalized tribal context and offers a foundation for more rigorous and scalable future research.

CONCLUSION

This study examined the effectiveness of a culturally adapted life skills training (LST) intervention among Paniya tribal adolescent girls in Wayanad, Kerala, and found statistically significant improvements across six psychosocial domains: self-awareness, communication, emotional management, decision-making, problem-solving, and interpersonal relationships. These findings suggest that structured life skills interventions can enhance psychosocial competence and short-term well-being among adolescents living in conditions of social and educational marginalization.

Importantly, the results indicate that life skills training functions as a *supportive psychosocial intervention*, strengthening internal capacities such as resilience, emotional regulation, and social competence. Rather than operating as a substitute for structural change, LST appears to complement broader educational and health initiatives by addressing social and emotional determinants that influence adolescent development. In this sense, life skills education represents a preventive and promotive approach that links adolescent health, education, and community-based support.

The study also underscores the importance of *cultural adaptation and participatory delivery* when implementing psychosocial interventions within indigenous and tribal contexts. While the findings are encouraging, they should be interpreted in light of the study's design limitations, including the absence of a control group and the focus on a single community. Consequently, conclusions are indicative rather than causal.

Overall, the chapter contributes empirical evidence to a limited body of research on life skills interventions among tribal adolescent girls in India. It highlights the potential value of integrating culturally responsive life skills training within adolescent health and education frameworks, while emphasizing the need for longitudinal, comparative, and intersectional research to assess sustainability, scalability, and broader social impact. Such efforts are essential for advancing equity-oriented strategies that support the holistic development and well-being of marginalized adolescents.

REFERENCES

Asha, C. M. (2020). Education of tribal communities in Kerala. *International Journal of Social Science and Economic Research, 6*, 1390-1399. . 2020. v05i06.001DOI: <ALIGNMENT.qj></ALIGNMENT>10.46609/IJSSER

Bhaskaran, A. A. Child and adolescent psychiatry (2023). *In Revision Guide for MRCPsych Paper B* (pp. 133-152). Routledge. https://www.taylorfrancis.com/chapters/edit/10.4324/9781003376163-6/child-adolescent-psychiatry-arun-arujun-bhaskaran

Census. (2011). Government of India, Census report

Fearon, P., Shmueli-Goetz, Y., Viding, E., Fonagy, P., & Plomin, R. (2014). Genetic and environmental influences on adolescent attachment. *Journal of Child Psychology and Psychiatry, and Allied Disciplines, 55*(9), 1033–1041. DOI: 10.1111/jcpp.12171 PMID: 24256475

Graber, J. A., & Petersen, A. C. (2017). Cognitive changes at adolescence: Biological perspectives. In Baron-Cohen, S., Tager-Flusberg, H., & Lombardo, M. V. (Eds.), *Brain maturation and cognitive development* (pp. 253–280). Guilford Press. DOI: 10.4324/9781315082028-10

Hankin, B. L. (2006). Adolescent depression: Description, causes, and interventions. *Epilepsy & Behavior, 8*(1), 102–114. DOI: 10.1016/j.yebeh.2005.10.012 PMID: 16356779

Joy, J., & Srihari, M. (2014). A Case study on the school dropout Scheduled Tribal students of Wayanad District, Kerala. *Research Journal of Educational Sciences*, ISSN,2321, 0508

Mahanta, P., Deuri, S. P., & Sobhana, H. (2021). Importance of Life Skills Education

Ministry of Tribal Affairs, Government of India. (2013), *Annual Report*. https://tribal.nic.in/downloads/Statistics/AnnualReport/AR2013-14.pdf

Mohindra, K. S., Narayana, D., Harikrishnadas, C., Anushreedha, S., & Haddad, S. (2010). Paniya Voices: A Participatory Poverty and Health Assessment among a marginalized South Indian tribal population. *BMC Public Health, 10*(1), 149. Advance online publication. DOI: 10.1186/1471-2458-10-149 PMID: 20307290

Pao, M., & Bosk, A. (2011). Anxiety in medically ill children/adolescents. *Depression and Anxiety, 28*(1), 40–49. DOI: 10.1002/da.20727 PMID: 20721908

Rahna, K. A., & Nithya, R. (2022). Psycho-social Issues Faced by Tribal Adolescents. IAHRW. *International Journal of Social Sciences Review*, *10*(3), 379–381.

Rockhill, C., Kodish, I., DiBattisto, C., Macias, M., Varley, C., & Ryan, S. (2010). Anxiety disorders in children and adolescents. *Current Problems in Pediatric and Adolescent Health Care*, *40*(4), 66–99. DOI: 10.1016/j.cppeds.2010.02.002 PMID: 20381781

Saranya, T. S., Deb, S., Paul, D., & Deb, S. (2022). Untold and Painful Stories of Survival: The Life of Adolescent Girls of the Paniya Tribes of Kerala, India. In *Child Safety, Welfare and Well-being: Issues and Challenges* (pp. 185-194). Singapore: Springer Singapore. https://link.springer.com/chapter/10.1007/978-981-16-9820-0_11

Saravanakumar, A. R., & Devi, K. P. (2020). Realising life through life skills: An adolescents' perspective. *Journal of Critical Reviews*, *7*(18), 1277–1282. https://www.researchgate.net/profile/Dr-saravanakumar-2/publication/342834193

Seema, G. B., & Kumar, G. V. (2018). Impact of social skills training on self-esteem among male and female adolescent students. *Indian Journal of Positive Psychology*, *9*(1), 147–151. DOI: 10.15614/ijpp.v9i01.11761

Shearer, C., Goss, H. R., Boddy, L. M., Knowles, Z. R., Durden-Myers, E. J., & Foweather, L. (2021). Assessments related to the physical, affective and cognitive domains of physical literacy amongst children aged 7–11.9 years: A systematic review. *Sports Medicine - Open*, *7*(1), 1–40. DOI: 10.1186/s40798-021-00324-8 PMID: 34046703

Shijina, A. V. (2020). Role of Mobile technology in assisting decentralization process among Paniya tribes in Wayanad, Kerala. *Antrocom: Online Journal of Anthropology, 16*(2).

State Council of Educational Research and Training (SCERT). (2016). *A study on problems and challenges of tribal adolescents in Kerala*. SCERT.

Subasree, R., Nair, A. R., & Ranjan, R. (2014). The Life Skills Assessment Scale: The construction and validation of a new comprehensive scale for measuring Life Skills. *Journal of the Humanities and Social Sciences*, *19*(1), 50–58. DOI: 10.9790/0837-19195058

Tavares, D., Freire, T., & Faria, S. (2020). Internal and external factors underlying variations in adolescents' daily optimal experiences. *Journal of Research on Adolescence*, *30*(1), 266–284. DOI: 10.1111/jora.12522 PMID: 31246377

UNICEF. (2005). Life skills-Based Education in South Asia, A Regional Overview Prepared For: The South Asia Life Skills-Based Education Forum. *Paris: The United Nations Children's Fund (UNICEF).*

UNICEF. (2017). *Improving work outcomes for young people: What role for skills? Evidence review* (March 17, 004_edited_002). Retrieved from https://www.unicef.org/india/media/2571/file/Comprehensive-lifeskills-framework.pdf

World Health Organ World Health Organization. (2003). *Skills for Health Skills-Based Health Education Including Life Skills: An Important Component of a Child-Friendly/Health-Promoting School. Geneva: World Health Organ World Health Organization. (1997).* Life Skills Education in Schools.

World Health Organization. (1994). *Life skills education for children and adolescents in schools. Pt. 3, Training workshops for the development and implementation of life skills programmes (No. WHO/MNH/PSF/93.7 B. Rev. 1).* World Health Organization.

KEY TERMS AND DEFINITIONS

Adolescent Health: Adolescent health refers to the physical, mental, emotional, and social well-being of individuals aged 10–19 years. It encompasses not only the absence of disease but also the development of life skills, healthy behaviors, and social competencies that enable adolescents to lead productive and balanced lives.

Cognitive Development: Cognitive development is the process through which individuals acquire and refine mental abilities such as thinking, reasoning, problem-solving, memory, and decision-making. During adolescence, it plays a vital role in shaping critical thinking, creativity, and self-regulation necessary for informed choices and adaptive functioning.

Empowerment: Empowerment is the process of enabling individuals or groups to gain control over their lives, develop self-confidence, and make independent decisions. In this context, it refers to enhancing tribal adolescent girls' capacity to overcome social, cultural, and economic barriers through awareness, education, and self-efficacy.

Healthcare Reform: Healthcare reform refers to systemic changes in health policy and delivery that aim to improve access, quality, and equity in health services. Here, it implies integrating psychosocial and educational interventions like life skills training into public health strategies to promote holistic adolescent well-being. Positioning psychosocial life skills training within preventive public health architecture aligns with emerging models of decentralized, community-based health reform. Early psychosocial investment reduces long-term service burden and supports equity-driven human capital development.

Intervention: An intervention is a structured program or action designed to bring about positive behavioral, emotional, or cognitive change in individuals or communities. The life skills training program served as an intervention targeting social competence, emotional management, and problem-solving among tribal adolescents.

Life Skills Training: Life skills training involves experiential learning programs that equip individuals with essential psychosocial abilities such as communication, empathy, decision-making, and stress management. These skills enable adolescents to cope effectively with daily challenges and improve their overall quality of life.

Resilience: Resilience is the ability to adapt positively and recover from adversity, stress, or trauma. Among tribal adolescents, resilience reflects their capacity to manage socio-economic challenges, emotional distress, and cultural marginalization through learned coping strategies and self-awareness.

Tribal Communities: Tribal communities are indigenous population groups characterized by unique cultural, linguistic, and social traditions, often residing in geographically isolated or rural regions. In India, these communities, such as the Paniya tribe, frequently face marginalization and require targeted interventions to promote education, health, and empowerment.

Chapter 4
Eating Disorders in Higher Education:
Psychosocial Risks, Digital Influences, and Leadership Challenges for Health Reform in Morocco

Mohamed Belomaria
Instituts Supérieurs des Professions Infirmières et Techniques de Santé, Morocco

Yassine Mouniane
http://orcid.org/0000-0002-6037-5301
Faculty of Sciences, Ibn Tofail University, Kenitra, Morocco

Mohamed Rektouti
http://orcid.org/0009-0004-5560-4925
Faculty of Sciences, Ibn Tofail University, Kenitra, Morocco

Brahim El Ouardi
http://orcid.org/0009-0000-4559-6141
Faculty of Sciences, Ibn Tofail University, Kenitra, Morocco

Mohammed Ouhssine
Faculty of Sciences, Ibn Tofail University, Kenitra, Morocco

Driss Hmouni
http://orcid.org/0000-0001-7598-6204
Faculty of Sciences, Ibn Tofail University, Kenitra, Morocco

Farid Elkhlifi
Faculty of Sciences, Ibn Tofail University, Kenitra, Morocco

Nabil Ait Ouaaziz
Faculty of Sciences, Ibn Tofail University, Kenitra, Morocco

Wafaa Benkayba
http://orcid.org/0000-0001-5196-1678
Laboratory of Chemistry Analytical and Bromatology, Faculty of Medicine and Pharmacy, University Mohammed V, Rabat, Morocco

Soukaina Njili
Faculty of Sciences, Ibn Tofail University, Kenitra, Morocco

DOI: 10.4018/979-8-2600-0939-0.ch004

Nada Belmejdoub
Faculty of Sciences, Ibn Tofail University, Kenitra, Morocco

Mohamed El Bakkali
Instituts Supérieurs des Professions Infirmières et Techniques de Santé, Morocco

ABSTRACT

This chapter explores eating disorders among students in Moroccan higher education as a growing public health concern linked to healthcare reform, digital transformation, and leadership in health policy. Based on a cross-sectional study at the Higher Institute of Nursing and Health Techniques (ISPITS) of Kenitra, a synthetic Eating Disorder Risk Score (EDRS) was validated, revealing social pressure and body dissatisfaction as key predictors, with academic stress as a mediating factor. The chapter discusses the economic burden of untreated disorders—productivity loss, absenteeism, and academic dropout—and highlights the need for preventive, cost-effective strategies. It advocates for integrating mental health and nutrition into national health reform through innovative "phygital" approaches that combine digital awareness, institutional counseling, and social marketing. Finally, it underscores the importance of academic leadership in advancing inclusive, evidence-based, and sustainable student health reform in the digital age.

INTRODUCTION

To begin with, it is necessary to keep in mind that eating disorders are now a genuine public health issue that is increasing, particularly with our young adults (Davey et al., 2023; Schmidt et al., 2025). Anorexia nervosa is one of the principal eating disorders that is getting the most attention, as it is a serious, complicated, and enduring disorder, in both physical and psychological aspects, social aspects as well (Zanella & Lee, 2022). Anorexia nervosa is characterized by extreme voluntary restriction of food intake, fear of gaining weight, and a distorted perception of one's body image (Garcia-Burgos et al., 2023; Czubaj et al., 2025). In its most severe forms, this eating disorder could lead to significant medical complications, or ultimately death. Students - especially those studying for paramedical training, to become tomorrow's nurses and healthcare technicians - appear especially vulnerable, even though they are educated in health and nutrition and should be, therefore, in a more informed position to understand the challenges of a moderated diet (Berk et al., 2023; Althagafi et al., 2025). A combination of academic workload, clinical placements to complete schoolwork, and the increasing face of role models imposed upon them by consumer society and social media, could easily contribute to an unhealthy relationship with food and weight, and potentially the development of lifelong disorders involving anorexia.

This issue must be a priority in nursing and healthcare training programs (McLeod et al., 2021). Ensuring it is known (identified), understanding the factors influencing its development (to identify factors), and evaluating the students' knowledge and attitudes regarding eating disorders are all information that would allow for the design of targeted prevention efforts. The purpose of this final year project is investigate the issues of eating disorders (more specifically, anorexia nervosa), amongst students at the Higher Institute of Nursing and Health Technicians. We will endeavor to assess the risk factors and eating behaviors of these students, as well as their levels of awareness of this type of disorder. The intent is not only to highlight this reality, but to contribute to improved prevention and education in our near future areas of professional practice. Although eating disorders (EDs) are increasingly recognized as a problem for students, early identification and assistance for individuals at risk is limited by numerous barriers. Firstly, ED presentations are often trivialized, or go underreported, or mistaken for eating habits that are "normal" within a university setting with much lifestyle variability and social pressure. Furthermore, without any validated screening tools for students, health professionals and schools are restricted in their ability to target prevention strategies. Also, the literature indicates multifaceted risk factors, such as social pressure connected to appearance, body dissatisfaction, and stress, the prevalence and consequences of risk factors are still unknown in the local and/or French-speaking student populations. In this context, a synthetic score that is easy to use and psychometrically indicators of risky eating habits, as well as investigate the proportionally associated social and psychological factors, seems important. This is all part of a broader mandate to bolster prevention and provide appropriate care for EDs at the university level, which is a public health matter that continues to be poorly focused on.

The DSM-5 includes specific or unspecified eating disorders, which incorporate atypical forms of the main EDs. Eating disorders affect almost 10% of the general population, with atypical eating disorders increasing that number to almost 20% (Harrop et al., 2021). Of these melting pot individuals, anorexia nervosa is noteworthy due to its deleterious nature and high mortality rate, with more recent advancements in modern medicine and related health sciences helping to diminish its presence which is still presently a major public health issue due to social, economic, and medical impacts (Feng et al., 2023). These ED classifications assist health care professionals with indicators for understanding and attending to their patients who are affected to grave purposes in attempts to reduce and care for complications and associated health related quality of life (Fleury et al., 2023). Anorexia nervosa is one of the most serious and prevalent eating disorders across adolescents in particular. Indeed, is presents clinically with extreme weight loss, an intense fear of gaining weight despite being underweight, and a distorted body image (Birgegård et al., 2023). In women, it is also associated with amenorrhea. Anorexia nervosa affects adolescents almost exclusively, where the prevalence is estimated to be between 0.2% and 1.3%. Although the somatic complications resulting from anorexia nervosa are serious, they can be reversed best through multidisciplinary care that focuses on re-nutrition and psychological care. Globally, anorexia nervosa is on the rise. In the United States, a retrospective study studying 469 adolescent girls residing in large cities, revealed an incidence of 104 per 100,000 person-years (Kerns et al., 2022).

In Morocco, a study with a sample of 506 medical students in Casablanca, where it was indicated that 25.09% of them were at risk of eating disorders with a SCOFF. The factors associated with increased risk are age, the level of education, and high levels of anxiety and depression (Attouche et al., 2021). The survey results provide a level of insight into the psychological pressures placed on health science professionals, in particular, the stress experienced as it relates to their education or training. Given these worrisome measures, and our intent to complete study in anorexia nervosa in adolescents is, in part, personally and academically driven frustration. As nursing students ourselves managing the demands and pressures of a program, we are aware of the impact stressors and description have upon mental health, and even develop into eating disorders. In addition, anorexia nervosa is a topic often not deemed a priority for study, especially in specific nations such as Kenitra do not have much depth of exploration. This type of study will address a gap in studies on understanding about this disorder and provide a voice for young youth about experiencing a mental health disorder.

HEALTH REFORM AND STUDENT POPULATIONS: WHY EATING DISORDERS MATTER

Eating Disorders as an Emerging Public Health Challenge

In the 21st century, where health systems globally are striving to push to view health and mental health as holistic, the growing incidence of disordered eating (DE) among students is a notable public health concern, and the global epidemiological findings showed that close to 5%-10% of young adults have disordered eating behaviors, while other behaviors that are subclinical such as restrictive dieting, binge eating, and distorted body image are present in the data in one in five students (Ghazzawi et al., 2023). Like many other low and middle-income countries, Morocco is experiencing dietary change, exposure to globalized ideals of beauty, and rapid digitization that equally heighten vulnerability in its university population (Bouhoudan et al., 2024). Health students, including nursing students and medical students, are an interesting paradox as they have been trained to advocate for health and wellness, but have to endure academic and psychosocial stressors that could compromise their own health behaviors (Salamonson ct al., 2009). Eating disorders are public health problems because of their mental health element and chronic effects on a person's physical and social health. Anorexia nervosa, one of the deadliest psychiatric illnesses, has a 5-10% average mortality rate, in addition to the physical toll it takes on long-term survivors - malnourished, hormonal issues, gastrointestinal issues, and fragile bones. An individual with an eating disorder creates distress and burden to the healthcare system, their family, and society as a whole (Meczekalski et al., 2013).

Economic and Societal Burden of Eating Disorders

With respect to direct medical costs, hospitalization, psychotherapy, nutritional counselling and medications are a few examples of the high cost factor associated with these conditions (Iuga & McGuire, 2014). In studies from higher-income countries, the annual average cost per person per year is estimated to be between USD 5,000 and USD 20,000 depending on the level of severity and chronicity; however, indirect costs related to lost productivity, attendance at school, dropping out of school, and life-long impairment, are likely to exceed the direct medical costs (Rashdan & Brodszky, 2020 ; Butt et al., 2022). For developing nations like Morocco, where student health services are still under-resourced, mental health systems are largely non-existent, and health professionals can be rare, the economic implications are even more complex. The absence of early identification and intervention processes frequently results in later diagnosis and higher costs of treatment, and the economic cost of untreated eating disorders extends beyond health systems, as educational success and future productivity are also affected.

While it is difficult to find comparable data for the Maghreb, based on estimated prevalence rates, we could likely find the economic costs to the population at universities in North Africa to be a few million dollars in annual lost productivity and healthcare costs. Additionally, the social cost of eating disorders can have costs that are not visible: stigma, family turmoil, and loss of social cohesion. Students and future students who are suffering from disordered eating generally experience cognitive deficits due to malnutrition—reduced concentration, poor memory, and ineffective decision-making processes— which compromise academic success and future career development. Thus, untreated and poorly managed eating disorders simultaneously fuel social exclusion and economic inefficiency, which is inconsistent with health systems ideals of equity and sustainability.

Role of Health Reform in Addressing Mental and Nutritional Health

Mental health is recognized as one of the leading influences on educational achievement and work readiness. The issue of disordered eating at the university level supports human capital development and aligns with Sustainable Development Goals (SDG 3: Good Health and Well-Being, and SDG 4: Quality Education) (Onyeaka et al., 2024). Therefore, a reformed health care system must integrate holistic care that includes physical, nutritional, and psychological well-being. This may include the establishment of phygital prevention models (integrating digital resources such as self-assessment apps, online awareness campaigns, and virtual counseling with in-person care in student health centers). Phygital models have had some success in a limited number of nations (Canada, France and Australia) when universities worked with the national health care agency to promote early detection and destigmatization (Del Vecchio et al., 2023). In Morocco, integrating phygital models as part of the national reform strategy could represent an important opportunity to fill a gap in access to care. For example, university health units could be testing sites for digital health initiatives in the form of chatbots to screen for mental health, teleconsult with students on a confidential basis, or peer-initiated social media campaigns aimed at at-risk students. Although small-scale, these initiatives can be inexpensive and scalable to be effective ways to improve public health impact by stopping mild symptoms from devolving into chronic mental health conditions.

Intersection of Economics, Prevention, and Leadership

The World Health Organization (WHO) estimates that every dollar spent on preventive mental health programs yields a conservative four to one return on productivity and health care savings (Le et al., 2021). The introduction of low-cost digital screening tools to universities could significantly inhibit the long-term burdens of eating disorders. Beyond this, including ED management as part of national insurance schemes or a public health package would suggest the political will to provide mental health with an equal priority to physical health (Torous et al., 2021). Prevention: Eating disorders can be prevented when identified early. Public health communication and “social marketing” campaigns can change harmful and destructive social norms about body image and food. Prevention involves understanding both digital systems, as well as local culture. For example, while the same media in the West will emphasize thinness, in North African cultures, there is a hybrid impact of traditional cultural valorization of robustness and the globalized idea of thinness. Thus, health reformers must develop prevention messages that respond to and are sensitive to the culture, using influencers, educators, and community leaders to promote healthy body diversity and resistance to the digital pressure.

Leadership: No reform is fully successful without leadership. At the institutional level, universities and schools of nursing should take leadership roles in advocating for health literacy, incorporating body image education and mental health awareness in their curricula (Willis et al., 2014). At the national level, health ministries must take leadership in creating intersectoral partnerships that link education, youth, and digital policy. At the societal level, leadership has to come from student communities to empower youth to co-create the messages and interventions that speak to them.

Mental Health and National Reform: A Shift from Curative to Preventive Paradigms

Many national health systems, including Morocco's, have a history of focusing on treatment rather than prevention. Eating disorders show us again the shortfalls of this model: once clinical symptoms are visible, the cost of treatment is high, and prognosis is poor.

Reform must therefore promote a preventive paradigm—detecting psychological distress and disordered eating behaviors before they crystallize into full-fledged disorders. This involves multiple layers of intervention:

- **Policy Level:** Inclusion of mental health and eating disorder prevention in national public health plans.
- **Institutional Level:** Establishment of student mental health observatories, integrating data collection and early warning systems.
- **Community Level:** Training peer mentors to recognize early signs and refer students to appropriate services.
- **Digital Level:** Deploying AI-based monitoring systems to identify risk behaviors on social media platforms (e.g., pro-anorexia hashtags, excessive diet app usage), while ensuring privacy and ethics.

Such systemic prevention aligns with the broader objectives of health reform—to enhance quality, equity, and efficiency. It also embodies the economics of compassion, where investing in mental health is both a moral and a pragmatic imperative.

Building a Reform-Oriented Framework for Student Health

The case study in Morocco exemplifies the necessity to develop frameworks which give a more comprehensive understanding of student health when considering initiatives for change in student health. In constructing bridges, the disconnect between health ministries, education ministries, and universities administration creates a system with no connected pathways to be responsive to collaborative systems for change, like eating disorders, while still being apprised of those issues that are less amenable. There's an indication that reform is needed, for intersectoral governance and evidence-informed policy. Recent data that has now been reviewed from Kenitra also provides evidence that such work can take place in Schools where that evidence can be displayed in terms of the use of the validated psychometric scores for early identification, as well as the recognition of vulnerabilities of psychosocial risk factor variables and statistical modelling through independent variables which quantify social pressures for our relationships with body dissatisfaction. The indications formed in the data directs directly at national level discourses and decisions around interventions, while also providing assistance for decision making for the next year with resource allocation in mind.

In addition, this reform is not only biomedical; it is also systemic and cultural, specifically in the health communications approaches which will begin to shift the language of eating disorders from individualized nutrient deficiencies to the systemic function of societal expectations. Working with marketing professionals and behaviour scientists opens up collective possibilities for greater reach for your messaging encore again... instead of only promoting a campaign around one idea "balanced living" or "body diversity", we would connect ideas to greater national wellness plans that support and not stigmatize nutrition, mental health, and digital competencies. At the end of the day, student populations are a leverage point for reform with health systems or organizations - your future health workers, educators, and leaders. Investing in steps today to protect the mental health and nutritional health of students could act as precursory ripple agents of change in health systems tomorrow.

CASE STUDY: ISPITS KENITRA (MOROCCO)

Study Context and Objectives

The current case study took place at the Higher Institute of Nursing and Health Techniques (ISPITS) of Kenitra, Morocco to complement a larger study exploring the determinants of eating disorders (EDs) among students studying in health fields. The students are a priority population within the national health framework as they serve as both recipients of health care and future providers of health care. When we think about their wellbeing as it relates to ED diagnoses and treatment, we consider effects beyond the individual. The wellbeing of this student population affects the quality and empathy of future health providers and the stability of the health care workforce.

The research was driven by three main issues. First, increased visibility of body image dissatisfaction and eating disorders among young Moroccan women, created by Western hegemony and online connectedness. Second, the absence of validated screening instruments for eating disorders in local settings, especially university-age students. Third, the limited inclusion of assessment for mental and nutritional health in student healthcare services despite beginning international agreement on early detection.

Hence, the specific objectives of the study were:

- To develop and validate a synthetic score for screening disordered eating behaviors among ISPITS students.
- To estimate the prevalence of eating disorder risk in this population.
- To identify the psychosocial and academic factors associated with high ED risk, including the potential role of academic stress, social pressure, and body dissatisfaction.

Methodology

This study used a cross-sectional descriptive and analytical approach with a period of four months, from March to June 2024. The target population was composed of all students at the Higher Institute of Nursing and Health Techniques (ISPITS) of Kenitra, and they represented varied levels of academic training and different health disciplines such as nursing, midwifery, laboratory sciences and health administration. Of the eligible population, 154 students, from all health disciplines, agreed to participate (voluntarily) in this study upon providing (signed) informed consent. All participants were assured their participation would be anonymous and confidential, allowing freedom and in turn validity of responses.

In order to be eligible for the study, participants had to be a student in a health-related program, between the ages of 18 and 30 years, and agree to participate. The exclusion criteria were developed to ensure internal validity and included being pregnant, having a documented metabolic and/or psychiatric disorder, and inconsistent or incomplete responses to the questionnaires. The criteria provided a homogeneous sample regarding health status and academic setting and allowed for valid representation of the psychological and behavioral precursors of eating disorders in future health professionals. Data were collected through a structured self-administered questionnaire, developed specifically for the research study. Prior to its use, the questionnaire was pre-tested with a small pilot group in order to assess appropriateness, clarity, and content validity. The final questionnaire consisted of six sections in total, with the first section containing socio-demographic and academic information (age, gender, level of study, area of study, and socioeconomic status). The second section included eating behaviors such as eating on a diet, frequency of eating meals, snacking habits, and eating in response to emotion. The third component evaluated body image and satisfaction through comparing perceived body size with preferred body size (e.g. perceived body size 1.75 and preferred body size 1.5), as well as measuring satisfaction with weight and shape. The fourth component measured social pressures and media exposure, both of which are becoming increasingly relevant to disordered eating among young adults. This subsystem reported media use frequency (primarily social media), and whether users engaged in comparison behaviors with peers and influencers, and perceived societal expectations of body ideals. The fifth component included psychological indicators, as measures of stress, mood changes, and self-esteem might all act as mediators between environmental pressures and behavior, or behavioral consequences.

Second, construct validity was evaluated utilizing Principal Component Analysis (PCA), that indicated a single factor with eigenvalue over 1, accounting for 33.2% of total variance. This indicates unidimensionality of the EDRS and supports a coherent interpretation of a measure of a single underlying construct - risk of disordered eating behavior. Third, convergent validity was identified by exploring the correlation between the EDRS and external variables that are theoretically expected to relate to eating disorders such as body dissatisfaction and perceived social pressure. Both significant correlations were both statistically meaningful and positive ($r = 0.48$ and $r = 0.52$ respectively, $p < 0.001$) indicating that students who had a higher score on the EDRS also experienced significantly greater feelings of dissatisfaction with body-image and increased feelings of perceived social pressure. These correlations provided further evidence of the theoretical validity and empirical strength of the new assessment. Based on these results, the EDRS was retained as a screening tool that had demonstrated reliability, validity, and ease of use for screening students with levels of risk for eating disorders in a college setting. Throughout the entirety of the study, ethical considerations were maintained. The study protocol was reviewed and approved by ISPITS Kenitra's Institutional Review Board (IRB). Students were informed of the study purpose, anonymity, and voluntary nature before completing the questionnaire. All procedures for data collection ensured that respondents were anonymous and no personal identifiers were present in the data prior to analysis. The study followed the ethical principles outlined by the Declaration of Helsinki. If students were identified at risk for an eating disorder based on their EDRS score, they were referred for support to on-campus counseling and psychological support services, which was done in a private and timely manner. This ethical measure demonstrated the researchers' sense of obligation to translate academic inquiry into meaningful, practical, and tangible formats for use in mental health and early intervention.

Main Results

The sample consisted of 154 students enrolled in health-related programs at the Higher Institute of Nursing and Health Techniques (ISPITS) of Kenitra (Table 1). The mean age of participants was 21.6 ± 2.1 years. The majority were women (85.7%, n = 132), while men represented 14.3% (n = 22) of the sample (Table 1). Regarding academic level, 38.3% (n = 59) were first-year students, 35.1% (n = 54) were second-year students, and 26.6% (n = 41) were third-year students. Half of the participants (50%, n = 77) reported living away from their families during their training, while the remaining 50% (n = 77) lived with their families. Overall, these characteristics provide a clear overview of the demographic and academic profile of students at ISPITS Kenitra and offer contextual insight into the psychosocial environment in which eating behaviors may develop. The distribution of the Eating Disorder Risk Score (EDRS) revealed a notable level of vulnerability to disordered eating behaviors within this population. Specifically, 43.5% of students were classified as low risk (score 0–1), 39.6% as moderate risk (score 2–3), and 16.9% as high risk (score 4–5). Thus, more than half of the participants (56.5%) exhibited at least a moderate level of risk. Although these findings do not indicate clinical diagnoses, they suggest the presence of behavioral and psychological factors associated with increased vulnerability to eating disorders. While comparable prevalence rates have been reported in international student populations, the results are particularly relevant in the Moroccan higher education context, where systematic mental health screening remains limited. These findings underscore the need for early identification and preventive strategies to support the wellbeing of future healthcare professionals.

Table 1. Frequency distribution of explanatory variables

Variable	Categories	Frequency
Age	18 years	39
	19 years	39
	20 years or older	76
Gender	Female	132
	Male	22

continued on following page

Table 1. Continued

Variable	Categories	Frequency
Year of study	First year	59
	Second year	54
	Third year	41
Housing situation	Living with family	77
	Living away from family	77
Frequency of thinking about food	Sometimes	20
	Rarely	63
	Often	44
	All the time	27
Has followed a diet	Yes	52
	No	102
Age at first diet	Under 15	8
	15–18	20
	18 or older	24
	No	102
Abstains from eating despite hunger	Yes (1)	99
	No (0)	55
Skips meals	Yes (1)	66
	No (0)	88
Frequency of weight measurement	Never	78
	Once a month or less	59
	Once a week	17
Feeling of guilt after eating	Never	70
	Rarely	45
	Often	26
	Always	13
Eats in secret	Yes	52
	No	102
Self-induced vomiting	Yes	29
	No	125
Prolonged fasting	Yes	65
	No	89
Perceived social pressure about appearance	High	57
	None	97

continued on following page

Table 1. Continued

Variable	Categories	Frequency
Binge eating episodes	Yes	58
	No	96
Body dissatisfaction	Yes	73
	No	81
Discrepancy between perceived and desired body image	Yes	52
	No	102
Mood influenced by body image	Yes	88
	No	66
Satisfied with current weight	Yes	81
	No	73
Has discussed concerns about eating	Yes	98
	No	56
Trusted person to talk about eating habits	Friend	44
	Family member	58
	Health professional	18
	No one	34
Interested in eating disorder workshops	Yes	113
	No	41
Able to recognize signs of eating disorders	Yes	99
	No	55
Has met someone with an eating disorder	Yes	58
	No	96
Feels comfortable with patients with eating disorders	Yes	60
	No	94
Feels image pressure during training	Yes	72
	No	82
Has observed signs of eating disorders among peers	Yes	110
	No	44
Stress affects eating behavior	Yes	129
	No	25
Interested in mental health awareness	Yes	128
	No	26
Workload affects eating habits	Yes	136
	No	18

Variable	Categories	Frequency
Avoids meals due to fear of judgment	Yes	65
	No	89

Qualitative responses obtained through open-ended questions provided deeper insight into students' lived experiences and attitudes toward food and body image. Several participants described engaging in restrictive eating before examinations as a way to "feel in control," suggesting that food regulation may function as a coping strategy in response to academic stress. Some students reported avoiding group meals due to anxiety about how their peers might perceive their eating choices or body shape. Social comparison emerged as a recurring theme. Many participants acknowledged comparing themselves to classmates and to individuals portrayed on social media, particularly influencers. These comparison behaviors were frequently associated with dissatisfaction and self-criticism. Feelings of guilt after consuming foods perceived as "off-limits" were also commonly reported. Such episodes were often followed by fasting or increased dietary restriction the following day, reflecting compensatory patterns consistent with disordered eating behaviors. Overall, these qualitative findings enrich the quantitative results by highlighting the emotional and cognitive processes underlying eating behaviors. They illustrate how academic stress, social comparison, and internalized appearance ideals—amplified by digital media exposure—may contribute to guilt, anxiety, and self-regulatory practices aligned with disordered eating risk.

Factors Associated with Eating Disorder Risk

The investigation of possible determinants of disordered eating identified several factors that were significantly associated with an increased EDRS score. In the bi-variate analysis, twelve factors had statistically significant correlations with greater risk ($p < 0.05$). The strongest associations were found for (1) repetitive dieting ($p < 0.001$), (2) body dissatisfaction ($p < 0.001$), or (3) perceived social pressure ($p < 0.001$) variables. Other relevant factors associated with increased EDRS scores included higher academic stress ($p = 0.02$), low self-esteem ($p = 0.04$), frequent social media use ($p = 0.01$), and comparative body image behaviours ($p = 0.02$). Gender, socioeconomic status, and living arrangements had weaker, but relevant, associations, suggesting that psychological and social predictors are stronger than demographic or contextual predictors. In order to identify the most powerful risk factors, a multivariate logistic regression performed all of the significant factors identified in the bivariate analysis. This analysis determined that two factors were independent predictors of having a high EDRS score (greater than 3). The first was perceived social pressure, which increased the odds of a high-risk score by nearly three times (Odds Ratio = 2.87; 95% CI [1.43–5.68]; $p < 0.01$). The second was body dissatisfaction, which had a particularly strong effect (Odds Ratio = 3.11; 95% CI [1.66–6.02]; $p < 0.001$). Although academic stress was not significant in the final model, it remains clear that the effect on vulnerability is mediated by emotional stability and body perception. Overall, these findings further suggest psychosocial factors, relative to demographic or academic factors, are more likely to create risk for disordered eating. For eating disorders are ultimately complex psychological and social constructs rooted in cultural ideals and value, the regulation of emotions and coping, and increasing exposure to social media.

The Role of Academic Stress

Although academic stress was not identified as a separate predictor of eating disorder risk in regression equations, it became evident as a relevant contextual factor in the lives of ISPITS students. From the qualitative findings, we discovered that students often engage with large workloads, long training hours and the pressure to excel academically, which can position them in states of chronic fatigue, anxiety, and emotional distress. In this context of pressure, food and body regulation often became a mechanism for coping with stress. A few students described decreasing food intake during exam periods to either feel disciplined or in control of their bodies. Others reported alternating between periods of overeating and fasting as a way to manage stress and emotional tension.

Although the quantitative results did not point to a direct role of academic stress in terms of disordered eating or eating disorder risks, indirect processes cannot be ignored. Stress may lead to decreased self-confidence, increased emotionality and a distortion of control, contributing to the perpetuation of harmful eating behaviors. International studies have described a vicious cycle of stress and body image dissatisfaction contributing to disordered eating and the need for universities to focus on developing stress and mental health services. Thus, non-academic psychosocial stressors in academic contexts are important protective factors for eating disorders in higher education, especially health-professions programs, where academic stress is likely maximized, and perceptions of expectations for oneself appear greatly inflated.

Interpretation and Discussion

The ISPITS Kenitra study offers valuable information about the psychosocial factors that shape eating habits among upcoming healthcare professionals. By providing a brief and valid measurement—the Eating Disorder Risk Score (EDRS)—the study demonstrates a practical and culturally relevant assessment tool for everyday screening in Moroccan universities. A notable increase in risk behaviors that justified sustained institutional attention and preventive health initiatives. The notion that social pressure and body dissatisfaction are the primary predictors of problematic eating is not only in line with the international literature, but also resonates with the sociocultural context of Morocco. As Morocco encounters a sociocultural transition, the country is torn between their traditional values of modesty, hospitality, and family, and the Western ideals of thinness and beauty that continues to be perpetuated through social media. The notion of social duality, in conjunction with the omnipresence of social media, breeds an internalised anxiety of appearance and increased value to being validated by peers. In this regard, eating disorders are not only a psychological response to stressors, but social behaviour that is learned in the pursuit to conform and gain self-worth within a digital landscape. It suggests that we need to pull interventions at two levels simultaneously. On an individual level, we need to improve emotional resilience, improve body image, and provide students adaptive coping strategies. Institutional and systemic changes need to be made to include mental health education, digital literacy, and critical media literacy at the level of post-secondary education. Addressing eating disorders would not only improve health, but also overall well-being and academic success moving forward.

Implications for Health Reform

Institutions of higher education in Morocco should develop a program, using a validated instrument such as the EDRS, to institutionalize screening for student mental health conditions at each institution of higher education as part of the regular medical check-in and regular counseling programs. The early detection of students at risk for mental illness is the first step in preventing the escalation of their condition into a clinical disorder, as well as decreasing the long term costs of treatment if students seek timely help. Second, the universities together with any student health authority should develop digital educational campaigns regarding body image, social comparison, and stress management. These also should be culturally appropriate and student-focused with students leading positive, inclusive messages about self-acceptance and balanced eating/adopting a healthy approach to eating via social media. Third, training of Academic leaders, faculty and health professionals in mental health literacy training materials is sorely needed to foster a culture of support in the campus environment. Evidently, educators play a big role in cueing into early signs of distress in students, encourage understanding and intervention to decrease stigma, and also encourage help-seeking behavior.

The ISPITS Kenitra case illustrates the interconnection between individual, institutional, and systemic aspects of health reform, educational policy, and digital culture. It demonstrates how countries in the global south can leverage research based in local contexts to develop reform that is sensitive to context while simultaneously protecting students' health and academic productivity. Moreover, it shows higher education institutions can act as promising laboratories for radical, contextualized mental health reform in the digital age. The ISPITS Kenitra case study has shown how the phenomenon of eating disorders among students is not just a discrete psychological condition, but is symptomatic of broader systemic stressors at the levels of educational, social, and cultural structures. The successful validation of a simple, reliable, culturally appropriate screening tool represents a meaningful starting point for moving the field toward evidence-based intervention and deeper reform. In particular, the study results reveal the cumulative impacts of social pressure, body dissatisfaction, and academic pressure on maladaptive eating behaviours and mental distress among students.

DIGITAL AND PHYGITAL DIMENSIONS

As a result, digital environments have a dual impact, providing important health information as well as communities supporting healthy living and balanced lifestyles on the one hand, while entrenching social comparison and modeling of unrealistic bodies and pressures to conform to online representations of beauty and success. In particular, our qualitative findings from the ISPITS Kenitra case study demonstrated that a number of students experiencing these digital phenomenon learned to internalize these referents. Consequently, make frequent comparisons between themselves and their peers in their everyday life, as well as influencers they follow. These comparisons led to feelings of disappointment and guilt, and even restriction of certain behaviors. Digital algorithms, which support and encourage thinness, contributed to the increase in body anxiety by creating an environment where validation is sought through the number of "likes", as well as through recognition in society.

A "phygital" approach to health reform is one that includes several complimentary actions. Universities could develop digital, health "hubs" as a campus-based resource of access to online counseling, self-assessment tools, and evidence-based nutrition information. Social media influencers, trained in health communication, could be a strong ambassador for body positivity campaigns. While campus based, these digital approaches can be backed up with in-person mental health services, student wellness clubs, and seminar series on media literacy and resilience naming these strategies as "ecological" to reinforce each other's effectiveness. The creating synergies between virtual outreach and institutional presence creates continuity between the student's online and offline life, representing today's psychological fragmentation, an effect of the digital era.

ECONOMICS OF EATING DISORDERS IN HIGHER EDUCATION

The financial ramifications of eating disorders do not only apply to individuals; they ultimately carry a cost to education systems, health systems, and loss of productivity on a broader scale (Striegel Weissman & Rosselli, 2017). At the post-secondary education level, where students will soon become the future workforce, eating disorders carry both actionable cost, and indirect costs (Halabieh et al., 2022). Actually - or direct costs - easily accounted for include, but are not limited to, either doctor visits, mental health visits, hospitalization, and follow-up appointments for nutritional rehabilitation, which is estimated internationally to be anywhere from $5,000 - $20,000 a year per person based on the severity of disorder (Lam et al., 2019). Indirect costs, however, are often the lesser perceived, and sometimes carry the greatest impact. Students with an eating disorder tend to demonstrate higher absenteeism rates, lower academic success rates, and ultimately, sometimes never return to school again (Ling et al., 2017). This generated waste can be devastating when we think of time and money invested regarding education. We can examine the educational outcome based on the presumption that students do not graduate on time, and either take longer to enter the workforce or never return to work, and have reduced productivity for the rest of their life. Moreover, we see engagement that is related to chronic stress and malnourishment to be correlated with lower engagement levels as well as lower levels of creativity. Lastly, the impact of being highly engaged in creativity within the educational setting is especially important for students entering in to healthcare profession roles (Morrison-Koechl et al., 2021).

The low-cost intervention options to get large populations at a low-cost (digital awareness campaigns, online-self-referral assessment tools, and peer-led topical discussions) is attractive. Also, the implication of validated instruments, such as the Eating Disorder Risk Score (EDRS) that was designed and presented in this study, allows to better identify and utilize resources to support the groups that are at the greatest risk (Bulik et al., 2021). To further entrench this economic rationale, no national reform agenda would be complete without a cost-benefit analysis for preventive programs as it relates to the notion of investment in mental health for sustainable development. Just as vaccination programs can rationalize cost by herding effects associated with vaccination policy, preventive mental health initiatives can be established by community-wide return to functionality, wellness, and job readiness for our emerging young citizens. And finally, if Morocco were to develop digital health economics frameworks that embed prevention in the reform policy process, it could create a more rational model in thinking of prevention as an investment into human capital rather than an expense.

MARKETING AND SOCIAL PERCEPTION

The social marketing contribution toward changing social attitudes around health and body image is critical for anything to truly occur as a change. Eating disorders are not only medical experiences; they are social constructions that happen through sharing and adopting cultural narratives, the images that we consume in mediated marketing space, and the consequent ways we interact with our societies (Ando et al., 2021; Papageorgiou et al., 2022). Individuals curate and selectively share images of themselves or their families, curated based on the hope of positively inserting them into the narrative around social acceptance. The public health system, if intending to appropriately respond to that, will almost certainly need to incorporate elements of social marketing that are above and beyond the traditional commercialism model of commodification of goods or services as a primary trade off to a more socially neutral process. Social marketing can both exploit all pre-discussed audience segmentation strategies while using branding and behavior change communication to change attitudes, lifestyles and practices toward health (Wei et al., 2025).

They are mini-versions of larger societies and are able to quickly create and spread social norms. A reimagined messaging initiative could involve using visual messaging campaigns showcasing a range of body types, promoting health messaging through student centers, or creating interactive content online with student partners. Incorporating humor, authenticity, and peer endorsement as a part of a campaign could add to respectability and interest. Funding to begin to develop partnerships with post-secondary influencers would also extend reach. For instance, in Morocco, local influencers could be involved in sharing their experiences of living healthy and balanced lives and coming to their own self-acceptance polyomino can help fight against healthy living being framed primarily as how you appear. To successfully reach their target audience messaging campaigns must inspire an emotional connection in the messaging - meaning that they induce feelings of empathy and identification, not guilt and fear.

Policy-wise, social marketing in health reform models helps render prevention efforts audience-aware. Rather than running a campaign that conveys a prescriptive message, a campaign should create a dialogue that allows people to privilege a re-conceptualizing of their understanding of food, health, and identity so that we can prevent eating disorders and will experience a culture of well-being informed from a place of diversity, compassionate concern, and authenticity (Hung, 2022). While there is a changing dialogue around body image and nutrition within postsecondary institutions, health reformers should create points of disruption of the economical and cultural system that perpetuate body dissatisfaction. This exemplifies marketing as connection point between public health objectives and societal change, building consciousness to create sustainable behaviour changes (Goswami & Cherrier, 2025).

In the context of contemporary health system transformation, healthcare marketing should no longer be viewed merely as a promotional or managerial function, but rather as a strategic instrument for value creation and behavioral influence. With the rapid expansion of digitalization, artificial intelligence, and immersive technologies, marketing in healthcare is increasingly positioned at the core of prevention, patient engagement, and system integration. Modern approaches emphasize the creation of interconnected ecosystems that link patients, providers, insurers, and regulators within a unified framework oriented toward proactive and preventive health. Within this perspective, marketing operates as a mechanism of social influence capable of reshaping norms, perceptions, and health-related behaviors. Applied to the issue of eating disorders among students, this approach suggests that carefully designed social marketing strategies—particularly those leveraging digital platforms—can contribute to transforming body image narratives, reducing stigma, and promoting healthier relationships with food and self-perception. Integrating such strategic marketing principles into health reform initiatives therefore represents a culturally sensitive and forward-looking pathway toward sustainable mental health promotion in higher education settings (Djakeli, 2024).

LEADERSHIP AND GOVERNANCE IN HEALTH REFORM

The topic of health reform is more than a technical issue, it is a leadership issue (Reich et al., 2016). The reform that is needed in our health care system requires vision, coordination and the courage to have difficult conversations around mental health stigma, social equity, etc (Patel et al., 2023). In higher education, the expected leadership capacity of presidents, deans, and program directors is significant and frames institutional engagement with student well-being (Thomas et al., 2024). These academic institutional leaders are the first point of influence (Ruan et al., 2024). Their commitment to elevating mental health as a substantial public policy issue related to the institutional context, not as an afterthought or perhaps a consideration in relation to student well-being is the embodiment of what it means to lead inside of a true compassion, inclusiveness innovation framework (Liu et al., 2017). Leaders that prioritize evidence-informed programs of practices like the EDRS, would demonstrate that mental health is a significant measure of educational quality and success for students (Ter Beek et al., 2022; Silva Didier et al., 2025).

The governance framework will allow for mental health promotion to be shared among sectors, rather than being a single sector initiative (Marais & Petersen, 2015). Local actors, such as municipal governments and non-state organizations, are integral to this process because they can provide services within the context of communities and mobilize services when working with students to facilitate access to counseling, and can be part of funding campaigns related to awareness and earmarked benefits. A decentralized governance structure will create a framework for flexibility and responsiveness to diversity among student populations (Bano, 2019). The phygital age requires leadership to similarly evolve and accept different ways to engage (Del Vecchio et al., 2023). The previous, traditional, vertical, top-down leadership approaches aren't good enough in a world with instant and two-way engagement. Leaders are required to blend the positional authority in-person, in a physical space, with their influence online for hybrid uses of engagement with students. University leaders who engage students directly in a digital manner can reduce stigma against their institution as they help to humanize the institution and model positive and healthy behaviors. In the end, health reform governance should reflect those very values we espouse: transparency across the institution, inclusion of those impacted by the governance plan, and accountability to the values espoused. So leadership becomes not just the governance of institutions; it is mobilizing organizations towards collective action. Or, in other words, leaders act as agents of cultural change for instances of eating disorders and mental health to turn universities into cultures of care, innovation, and social responsibility.

DISCUSSION AND POLICY IMPLICATIONS

The findings of the study of ISPITS Kenitra and their relevance in a larger context of health reform have important ramifications for national and international policy. First, the rate of disordered eating behaviors among health students in Morocco is comparable to studies from countries, such as France, Tunisia, and Canada with several similar risk factors (academic stress, body dissatisfaction, media). However, Morocco is distinct from the aforementioned countries, in that there are no large-scale institutional support systems in place and there are few mental health services available to Moroccan students in universities, reinforcing the urgency for reform.

Information from comparable initiatives supports the idea that coordinated national student mental health initiatives can offset some of the impact of eating disorders in the university setting. For example, French school-reform initiatives have resulted in improved and preventive mental health access through a greater focus on mental health as part of national educational reforms (e.g., improved preventive counseling/tele-psychology, etc.). Tunisia campus-based mental health units, which are designed for early detection through peer education, would have a similar cause and effect. The Canadian "Mental Health Commission" has developed an online support system that spends millions of dollars annually exploring greater access to youth eating disorder research. Morocco can explore these pathway examples for strategic coordinated youth health policy processes that might be facilitated through the expansion of digital health, youth, and inter-sectoral considerations. At a policy level, we suggest several action steps. First, mental and nutritional health should be specific and strategic priorities on Morocco's national health reform agenda. This will require funding to establish university health observatories that can provide longitudinal monitoring of student well-being, risk trends, and intervention treatments. Second, state of the art digital health platforms such as tele-consultation processes, self-assessment, and AI-assisted risk detection in health services should be integrated into existing and new campus and university health services. Digital health platforms can serve to improve accessibility and confidentiality for students particularly in advance of their first visit to a live in-person counseling service.

Additionally, a reform agenda needs to incorporate training and capacity-building for academic and health practitioners on early recognition and intervention of eating disorders. Universities, ministries and digital providers could collaborate to develop and deliver certification programs on "Digital Mental Health and Preventive Care." Finally, public communication campaigns should be designed to frame student wellness and mental health as a national investment in human capital and highlight the connection between mental and psychological health to productivity and education quality. In conclusion, eating disorders, as the context for national health reform, requires multi-level health system reform strategies that encompass economics, communications, leadership and technology. When these strategies are synergized within a coherent phygital model (combining physical and digital models), Morocco—and similar countries—can become leaders in establishing a new health governance frame: one that values prevention as highly as treatment, digital care as much as in-person care, and leadership as highly as management. This vision can shift the concern of student health from a marginal issue to a central focus of modern accessibility, inclusivity, and sustainable health system reform.

CONCLUSION

This chapter has examined the interconnections among eating disorders, student well-being, and a growing health reform agenda in a digital context. The illustration of ISPITS Kenitra has shown that eating disorders in students are not standalone psychological disorders, but manifestations of social, academic and cultural pressures. The confirmation of the Eating Disorder Risk Score (EDRS) is a valid and evidenced-based tool that can be used for the early identification and prevention of eating disorders in higher education. The findings illustrate that eating disorder risk has the strongest predictors of social pressure and dissatisfaction with one's body, which are augmented by the pervasive nature of the digital media environment. Although academic stress is not an independent predictor of risk, it contributes to vulnerability by undermining self-esteem and contributes to maladaptive coping mechanisms. The findings recommend consideration of both psychosocial determinants and structural change and reform in education and health frameworks. Thinking Economically, preventing eating disorders is not only a moral issue, it represents an economic valuation. The justification for the inclusion of preventive mental health measures in national reform will be based on considering both direct and indirect costs involved for the treatment of unresolved eating disorders - medical care, educational failure, and time lost from work. Social marketing and phygital strategies will be necessary to facilitate alteration of public perception towards body positivity, and engage the gap between online alternatives and solidarity to organizational change with mental health institutions. In the end, sustainable health reform relies heavily on creative health leadership and inclusion governance investments that establish mental and nutritional health as a commitment to national development. By partnering with universities, ministry officials, and digital innovators, Morocco has an opportunity to develop a progressive model of student health reform based on prevention, youth empowerment, and digital transformation that honour human care without compromising compassion. In conclusion, the ISPITS Kenitra experience, as we ask - who is the client? and - Does is matter? - proves that beginning the journey toward resilient, and equitable, healthcare models must begin with a deeper understanding of the realities of the students. Responding to student realities, however, must be evidence-based, phygital and economically sound - to ensure that there is a standard of commitment to care and a foundation of a modern health reform that is person-centred and equity-focused.

DECLARATION ON THE USE OF ARTIFICIAL INTELLIGENCE TOOLS

The authors used ChatGPT, a generative artificial intelligence tool developed by OpenAI, exclusively for language editing, grammatical correction, and improvement of clarity and academic expression. The tool was not used for data generation, data analysis, interpretation of results, methodological design, or formulation of scientific conclusions. All research content, analysis, interpretations, and conclusions presented in this chapter are the sole responsibility of the authors.

REFERENCES

Althagafi, M. H., Al-Asiri, K. S. K., Almahanna, M. A., Al-Otapi, M. D., Aseri, A. A., Al-Sulami, M. A., Al-Harbi, Y. S., & Al-Mutairi, N. M. S. (2025). A descriptive study of the future qualification level of paramedics in health education programs in Saudi universities. *The Review of Diabetic Studies; RDS*, *21*(S9), 1154–1162. DOI: 10.70082/3q3x9v41

Ando, K., Giorgianni, F. E., Danthinne, E. S., & Rodgers, R. F. (2021). Beauty ideals, social media, and body positivity: A qualitative investigation of influences on body image among young women in Japan. *Body Image*, *38*, 358–369. DOI: 10.1016/j.bodyim.2021.05.001 PMID: 34120098

Attouche, N., Hafdi, S., Somali, R., Battas, O., & Agoub, M. (2021). Factors associated with the risk of developing eating disorders among medical students in Casablanca, Morocco. *The Pan African Medical Journal*, *39*, 270. PMID: 34707771

Bano, M. (2019). Partnerships and the Good-Governance Agenda: Improving Service Delivery Through State–NGO Collaborations. *Voluntas*, *30*(6), 1270–1283. DOI: 10.1007/s11266-017-9937-y

Berk, M., Köhler-Forsberg, O., Turner, M., Penninx, B. W. J. H., Wrobel, A., Firth, J., Loughman, A., Reavley, N. J., McGrath, J. J., Momen, N. C., Plana-Ripoll, O., O'Neil, A., Siskind, D., Williams, L. J., Carvalho, A. F., Schmaal, L., Walker, A. J., Dean, O., Walder, K., & Marx, W. (2023). Comorbidity between major depressive disorder and physical diseases: A comprehensive review of epidemiology, mechanisms and management. *World Psychiatry; Official Journal of the World Psychiatric Association (WPA)*, *22*(3), 366–387. DOI: 10.1002/wps.21110 PMID: 37713568

Birgegård, A., Forsén Mantilla, E., Breithaupt, L. E., Borg, S., Sanzari, C. M., Padalecki, S., Hedlund, E., & Bulik, C. M. (2023). Proposal for increasing diagnostic clarity in research and clinical practice by renaming and reframing atypical anorexia nervosa as "Restrictive Eating Disorder" (RED). *Eating Behaviors, 50,* 101750. DOI: 10.1016/j.eatbeh.2023.101750 PMID: 37263139

Bouhoudan, A., Zian, Z., Khaddor, M., & Mourabit, N. (2024). The impact of societal changes and COVID-19 pandemic on Moroccan food habits: A Mediterranean perspective. *Discover Food, 4*(1), 154. Advance online publication. DOI: 10.1007/s44187-024-00237-x

Bulik, C. M., Thornton, L. M., Parker, R., Kennedy, H., Baker, J. H., MacDermod, C., Guintivano, J., Cleland, L., Miller, A. L., Harper, L., Larsen, J. T., Yilmaz, Z., Grove, J., Sullivan, P. F., Petersen, L. V., Jordan, J., Kennedy, M. A., & Martin, N. G. (2021). The Eating Disorders Genetics Initiative (EDGI): Study protocol. *BMC Psychiatry, 21*(1), 234. DOI: 10.1186/s12888-021-03212-3 PMID: 33947359

Butt, M. D., Ong, S. C., Wahab, M. U., Rasool, M. F., Saleem, F., Hashmi, A., Sajjad, A., Chaudhry, F. A., & Babar, Z. U. D. (2022). Cost of illness analysis of type 2 diabetes mellitus: The findings from a lower-middle income country. *International Journal of Environmental Research and Public Health, 19*(19), 12611. DOI: 10.3390/ijerph191912611 PMID: 36231911

Czubaj, N., Szymańska, M., Nowak, B., & Grajek, M. (2025). The impact of social media on body image perception in young people. *Nutrients, 17*(9), 1455. DOI: 10.3390/nu17091455 PMID: 40362764

Davey, E., Allen, K., Bennett, S. D., Bryant-Waugh, R., Clarke, T., Cooper, Z., Dixon-Ward, K., Dudley, J., Eisler, I., Griffiths, J., Hill, A. J., Micali, N., Murphy, R., Picek, I., Rea, R., Schmidt, U., Simic, M., Tchanturia, K., Traviss-Turner, G., & Shafran, R. (2023). Improving programme-led and focused interventions for eating disorders: An experts' consensus statement—A UK perspective. *European Eating Disorders Review, 31*(5), 577–595. DOI: 10.1002/erv.2981 PMID: 37218053

Del Vecchio, P., Secundo, G., & Garzoni, A. (2023). Phygital technologies and environments for breakthrough innovation in customers' and citizens' journey. A critical literature review and future agenda. *Technological Forecasting and Social Change, 189*, 122342. DOI: 10.1016/j.techfore.2023.122342

Djakeli, K. (2024). Healthcare marketing, meaning, historical development, applications, and current status. In Djakeli, K. (Ed.), *Modern Healthcare Marketing in the Digital Era* (pp. 1–25). IGI Global Scientific Publishing., DOI: 10.4018/979-8-3693-0679-6.ch001

Feng, B., Harms, J., Chen, E., Gao, P., Xu, P., & He, Y. (2023). Current discoveries and future implications of eating disorders. *International Journal of Environmental Research and Public Health, 20*(14), 6325. DOI: 10.3390/ijerph20146325 PMID: 37510558

Fleury, M.-J., Cao, Z., Grenier, G., & Ferland, F. (2023). Profiles of quality of life among patients using emergency departments for mental health reasons. *Health and Quality of Life Outcomes*, *21*(1), 116. DOI: 10.1186/s12955-023-02200-3 PMID: 37880748

Garcia-Burgos, D., Wilhelm, P., Vögele, C., & Munsch, S. (2023). Food restriction in anorexia nervosa in the light of modern learning theory: A narrative review. *Behavioral Sciences (Basel, Switzerland)*, *13*(2), 96. DOI: 10.3390/bs13020096 PMID: 36829325

Ghazzawi, H. A., Nimer, L. S., Sweidan, D. H., Alhaj, O. A., Abulawi, D., Amawi, A. T., Levine, M. P., & Jahrami, H. (2023). The global prevalence of screen-based disordered eating and associated risk factors among high school students: Systematic review, meta-analysis, and meta-regression. *Journal of Eating Disorders*, *11*(1), 128. Advance online publication. DOI: 10.1186/s40337-023-00849-1 PMID: 37537604

Goswami, P., & Cherrier, H. (2025). Intimate neoliberal violence and ungrievable meno bodies. *Journal of Marketing Management*, *41*(3-4), 293–311. DOI: 10.1080/0267257X.2025.2470830

Halabieh, H., Hawkins, S., Bernstein, A. E., Lewkowict, S., Unaldi Kamel, B., Fleming, L., & Levitin, D. (2022). The future of higher education: Identifying current educational problems and proposed solutions. *Education Sciences*, *12*(12), 888. DOI: 10.3390/educsci12120888

Harrop, E. N., Mensinger, J. L., Moore, M., & Lindhorst, T. (2021). Restrictive eating disorders in higher weight persons: A systematic review of atypical anorexia nervosa prevalence and consecutive admission literature. *International Journal of Eating Disorders*, *54*(8), 1328–1357. DOI: 10.1002/eat.23519 PMID: 33864277

Hung, J. (2022). Policy development on upskilling/reskilling older population care staff in China. *International Journal of Environmental Research and Public Health*, *19*(15), 9440. DOI: 10.3390/ijerph19159440 PMID: 35954791

Iuga, A. O., & McGuire, M. J. (2014). Adherence and health care costs. *Risk Management and Healthcare Policy*, *7*, 35–44. DOI: 10.2147/RMHP.S19801 PMID: 24591853

Kerns, J., Itriyeva, K., & Fisher, M. (2022). Etiology and management of amenorrhea in adolescent and young adult women. *Current Problems in Pediatric and Adolescent Health Care*, *52*(5), 101184. DOI: 10.1016/j.cppeds.2022.101184 PMID: 35525789

Lam, P. C., John, D. A., Galfalvy, H., Kunzel, C., & Lewis-Fernández, R. (2019). Oral health–related quality of life among publicly insured mental health service outpatients with serious mental illness. *Psychiatric Services (Washington, D.C.)*, *70*(12), 1101–1109. DOI: 10.1176/appi.ps.201900111 PMID: 31522632

Le, L. K. D., Esturas, A. C., Mihalopoulos, C., Chiotelis, O., Bucholc, J., Chatterton, M. L., & Engel, L. (2021). Cost-effectiveness evidence of mental health prevention and promotion interventions: A systematic review of economic evaluations. *PLoS Medicine*, *18*(5), e1003606. DOI: 10.1371/journal.pmed.1003606 PMID: 33974641

Ling, Y.-L., Rascati, K. L., & Pawaskar, M. (2017). Direct and indirect costs among patients with binge-eating disorder in the United States. *International Journal of Eating Disorders*, *50*(5), 523–532. DOI: 10.1002/eat.22631 PMID: 27862132

Liu, N. H., Daumit, G. L., Dua, T., Aquila, R., Charlson, F., Cuijpers, P., Druss, B., Dudek, K., Freeman, M., Fujii, C., Gaebel, W., Hegerl, U., Levav, I., Munk Laursen, T., Ma, H., Maj, M., Elena Medina-Mora, M., Nordentoft, M., Prabhakaran, D., & Saxena, S. (2017). Excess mortality in persons with severe mental disorders: A multilevel intervention framework and priorities for clinical practice, policy and research agendas. *World Psychiatry; Official Journal of the World Psychiatric Association (WPA)*, *16*(1), 30–40. DOI: 10.1002/wps.20384 PMID: 28127922

Marais, D. L., & Petersen, I. (2015). Health system governance to support integrated mental health care in South Africa: Challenges and opportunities. *International Journal of Mental Health Systems*, *9*(1), 14. DOI: 10.1186/s13033-015-0004-z PMID: 25806085

McLeod, C., Jokwiro, Y., Gong, Y., Irvine, S., & Edvardsson, K. (2021). Undergraduate nursing student and preceptors' experiences of clinical placement through an innovative clinical school supervision model. *Nurse Education in Practice*, *51*, 102986. DOI: 10.1016/j.nepr.2021.102986 PMID: 33621926

Meczekalski, B., Podfigurna-Stopa, A., & Katulski, K. (2013). Long-term consequences of anorexia nervosa. *Maturitas*, *75*(3), 215–220. DOI: 10.1016/j.maturitas.2013.04.014 PMID: 23706279

Morrison-Koechl, J., Wu, S. A., Slaughter, S. E., Lengyel, C. O., Carrier, N., & Keller, H. H. (2021). Hungry for more: Low resident social engagement is indirectly associated with poor energy intake and mealtime experience in long-term care homes. *Appetite*, *159*, 105044. DOI: 10.1016/j.appet.2020.105044 PMID: 33227384

Onyeaka, H., Ejiohuo, O., Taiwo, O. R., Nnaji, N. D., Odeyemi, O. A., Duan, K., Nwaiwu, O., & Odeyemi, O. (2024). The intersection of food security and mental health in the pursuit of Sustainable Development Goals. *Nutrients*, *16*(13), 2036. DOI: 10.3390/nu16132036 PMID: 38999784

Papageorgiou, A., Fisher, C., & Cross, D. (2022). "Why don't I look like her?" How adolescent girls view social media and its connection to body image. *BMC Women's Health*, *22*(1), 261. DOI: 10.1186/s12905-022-01845-4 PMID: 35761231

Patel, V., Saxena, S., Lund, C., Kohrt, B., Kieling, C., Sunkel, C., Kola, L., Chang, O., Charlson, F., O'Neill, K., & Herrman, H. (2023). Transforming mental health systems globally: Principles and policy recommendations. *Lancet*, *402*(10402), 656–666. DOI: 10.1016/S0140-6736(23)00918-2 PMID: 37597892

Rashdan, O., & Brodszky, V. (2020). Productivity loss in patients with chronic diseases: A pooled economic analysis of Hungarian cost-of-illness studies. *Value in Health Regional Issues*, *22*, 75–82. DOI: 10.1016/j.vhri.2020.07.572 PMID: 32798838

Reich, M. R., Javadi, D., & Ghaffar, A. (2016). Introduction to the Special Issue on "Effective Leadership for Health Systems". *Health Systems and Reform*, *2*(3), 171–175. DOI: 10.1080/23288604.2016.1223978 PMID: 31514592

Ruan, J., Cai, Y., & Stensaker, B. (2024). University managers or institutional leaders? An exploration of top-level leadership in Chinese universities. *Higher Education*, *87*(3), 703–719. DOI: 10.1007/s10734-023-01031-x PMID: 37362758

Salamonson, Y., Everett, B., Koch, J., Wilson, I., & Davidson, P. M. (2009). Learning strategies of first year nursing and medical students: A comparative study. *International Journal of Nursing Studies*, *46*(12), 1541–1547. DOI: 10.1016/j.ijnurstu.2009.05.010 PMID: 19541308

Schmidt, U. H., Claudino, A., Fernández-Aranda, F., Giel, K. E., Griffiths, J., Hay, P. J., Kim, Y.-R., Marshall, J., Micali, N., Monteleone, A. M., Nakazato, M., Steinglass, J., Wade, T. D., Wonderlich, S., Zipfel, S., Allen, K. L., & Sharpe, H. (2025). The current clinical approach to feeding and eating disorders aimed to increase personalization of management. *World Psychiatry; Official Journal of the World Psychiatric Association (WPA)*, *24*(1), 4–31. DOI: 10.1002/wps.21263 PMID: 39810680

Silva Didier, L., Schildkamp, K., Visscher, A. J., & Bosker, R. J. (2025). Factors influencing the implementation of a teacher professional development program to improve teaching quality. *Frontiers in Education*, *10*, 1546448. DOI: 10.3389/feduc.2025.1546448

Striegel Weissman, R., & Rosselli, F. (2017). Reducing the burden of suffering from eating disorders: Unmet treatment needs, cost of illness, and the quest for cost-effectiveness. *Behaviour Research and Therapy*, *88*, 49–64. DOI: 10.1016/j.brat.2016.09.006 PMID: 28110676

Ter Beek, M., Wopereis, I., & Schildkamp, K. (2022). Don't Wait, Innovate! Preparing Students and Lecturers in Higher Education for the Future Labor Market. *Education Sciences*, *12*(9), 620. DOI: 10.3390/educsci12090620

Thomas, L. R., Ripp, J. A., & Duncan, J. G. (2024). Graduate medical education well-being directors in the United States: Who are they, and what does the role entail? *BMC Medical Education*, *24*(1), 254. DOI: 10.1186/s12909-024-05243-2 PMID: 38459448

Torous, J., Bucci, S., Bell, I. H., Kessing, L. V., Faurholt-Jepsen, M., Whelan, P., Carvalho, A. F., Keshavan, M., Linardon, J., & Firth, J. (2021). The growing field of digital psychiatry: Current evidence and the future of apps, social media, chatbots, and virtual reality. *World Psychiatry; Official Journal of the World Psychiatric Association (WPA)*, *20*(3), 318–335. DOI: 10.1002/wps.20883 PMID: 34505369

Wei, W., Zhang, L., Ying, T., & Zheng, Y. (2025). Pet influencer marketing appeal in hotel booking: Exploring the power of message appeal and boundary conditions. *International Journal of Hospitality Management*, *126*, 104094. DOI: 10.1016/j.ijhm.2025.104094

Willis, C. D., Saul, J. E., Bitz, J., Pompu, K., Best, A., & Jackson, B. (2014). Improving organizational capacity to address health literacy in public health: A rapid realist review. *Public Health*, *128*(6), 515–524. DOI: 10.1016/j.puhe.2014.01.014 PMID: 24923994

Zanella, E., & Lee, E. (2022). Integrative review on psychological and social risk and prevention factors of eating disorders including anorexia nervosa and bulimia nervosa: Seven major theories. *Heliyon*, *8*(11), e11422. DOI: 10.1016/j.heliyon.2022.e11422 PMID: 36406673

Chapter 5
National Phygital Model for GDM Care:
Bridging Traditional Practice With Digital Technologies for Precision Health

R. Priyanka
http://orcid.org/0009-0006-1623-8496
SASTRA University, India

A. Sumathi
http://orcid.org/0000-0003-4700-5573
Department of CSE, SRC, SASTRA University, India

S. Meganathan
http://orcid.org/0000-0003-4570-8259
SASTRA University, India

ABSTRACT

National health system reform is paramount to the creation of fairer and more efficient systems that meet contemporary clinical needs and advance population health in the long term. From a maternal health perspective, gestational diabetes mellitus (GDM) pinpoints the necessity of national health reform. The global prevalence of GDM has significantly risen because of maternal age, overweight, lifestyle, and genetics. GDM management was uncoordinated with variable diagnosis pathways, a lack of knowledge about GDM among women and providers, and limited follow-up post-delivery. National healthcare reform on GDM is moving away from a decreased focus on pregnancy complications to a life-course prevention strategy for chronic disease prevention by changing maternal health at the public health level. When

DOI: 10.4018/979-8-2600-0939-0.ch005

GDM care is reformulated through an integrated phygital national framework, there will be significant improvements to maternal and child health which will also further support the national goal of reducing the intergenerational burden of non-communicable diseases.

INTRODUCTION

The increase in the number of women diagnosed with gestational diabetes mellitus (GDM) shows the growing recognition of the relationships between a woman's genetic inclination toward diabetes, lifestyle modifications, and the impact of these factors on the population's health both socially and economically. GDM now has the added clinical importance of indicating significant capacity to cause long-term metabolic abnormalities, whereas it used to be thought of as only a pregnancy-related condition. Women With GDM have a significantly higher chance of developing type 2 diabetes (T2DM), cardiovascular illnesses, and eventually developing the metabolic syndrome as they age. Children born to mothers who had GDM also face increased chances of having obesity and developing insulin resistance and cardiometabolic disorders due to their mother's abnormally elevated blood sugar levels while pregnant. Such high blood sugar levels present a challenge for mothers and infants and, therefore, provide an opportunity for an increased focus on GDM for the purpose of developing policies that would reduce the number of people affected by these disorders in upcoming generations. Traditional approaches for managing gestational diabetes mellitus (GDM) typically include the following: All GDM patients should go through either an On-Site Testing (OST) or an Oral Glucose Tolerance Test (OGTT) to confirm diagnosis and gather data for treatment and tracking purposes. For those women who may have developed GDM but have not yet presented with symptoms, the best way for them to be assessed is through the OGTT (which requires follow-up care). In addition, GDM patients should participate in regular follow-up appointments and monitor their glucose levels through self-testing and periodic visits during the postpartum (post-birth) timeframe. Despite these recommendations, the current clinical model for reporting diabetes is limited to measuring blood glucose levels without consideration of the mother's overall metabolic health. The current clinical model for diagnosing GDM has major limitations, which include: delayed diagnosis leading to increased risk of poor maternal and neonatal health outcomes, fragmented access to care from multiple providers, inadequate education of patients about their diabetes treatment options and poor access to diabetes specialists, an increasing number of patients who do not have adequate access to diabetes care (especially in rural areas), and the almost complete lack of postpartum follow-up care after giving birth to a baby who has been diagnosed with GDM. These barriers are compounded in resource-poor and geographically isolated settings where there are limited laboratory resources and specialist availability as well as insufficient infrastructure for ongoing health care monitoring. The current digital transformation of healthcare within the context of phygital healthcare, where traditional clinical care is integrated with new digital healthcare technologies, including Internet of Things (IoT)-enabled sensors, telemedicine, artificial intelligence (AI), cloud computing, and mobile health applications targeted at patients, has created new solutions that can help overcome these challenges. Phygital healthcare does not replace traditional clinical care services; however, it enhances and augments traditional clinical care by providing real-time, continuous, and individualized maternal/child healthcare delivery and ensuring that they remain scalable into the future Combining Artificial Intelligence and Machine Learning allows the proposed solution to process large amounts of glucose and lifestyle data to detect GDM at an earlier time, to categorize the different biologically relevant subtypes of GDM, anticipate GDM-related complications and develop patient-centered treatments. In addition, telehealth services, artificial intelligence chatbots and automated notification systems empower women by providing support, reminders and oversight of practice to reduce the need for multiple visits to hospitals as an alternative method of care. The combined movement to phygital (physical/digital) maternal health will support the goals of national health reform and improve access, universal access and value-based care in addition to establishing the groundwork for Digital Public Health Infrastructure. Countries that are currently implementing changes to their health systems are recognizing the importance of GDM, as it occupies the intersection of maternal health, NCD prevention, strengthening primary health care and supporting informed planning of health services using data. Furthermore, phygital GDM (Gestational Diabetes Mellitus) Pathways allow for creating nationwide registers of population status, as well as real-time analysis of data and resource optimization on the national level. While the creation of a Phygital GDM Monitoring and Prediction Model requires technological advancement, creating this path toward Predictive, Preventive, Social and Precision Maternal Health Care Models is a huge step in the evolution of Maternal Metabolic Health Care Models. Therefore, GDM can be viewed both as a clinical condition and also as a way to evolve our National Health Care Systems in the digital age.

Global and National Epidemiology

The increasing incidence rates of gestational diabetes mellitus (GDM) worldwide are primarily due to the increase in obesity among pregnant women, increasing maternal ages, and the increase in lifestyle-related metabolic diseases. Worldwide, an estimated 1 in 6 pregnancies has hyperglycemia; about 85% - 90% of those cases are diagnosed as GDM. There are significant differences in prevalence rates based on the various diagnostic criteria used, the populations studied, and the level of health care available. In higher income countries, the increase in GDM diagnosis can be attributed to more women being screened for their pregnancy and living in a growing urban population. Additionally, urbanization, reductions in physical activity, and changes in diet have contributed to the increase in GDM observed in lower and middle-income countries. South America, the Middle East, and South Asia are regions of the world that have the highest prevalence rates of GDM, with India being an important contributor to those numbers due to its relatively high degree of baseline insulin resistance and population genetic predisposition to GDM. There are many reasons for GDM being developed in pregnant women, including geographical locations within particular countries (where all have GDM) as different neighborhoods can have higher or lower socio-economic income levels and education levels. There may also be differences in the level of public awareness of GDM and availability of information on GDM, whether it is through newspapers or radio.

Maternal and Neonatal Complications

Gestational diabetes is a significant health threat to women who are pregnant and their developing children. The increased likelihood of women who had gestational diabetes giving birth to children with complications from gestational diabetes such as preeclampsia, gestational hypertension, polyhydramnios (too much fluid around the baby), and increased likelihood of cesarean sections due to large babies or prolonged delivery has been established by the medical community. Complications of gestational diabetes for mothers include increased rates of prolonged labor, hemorrhage after birth, and the use of surgical deliveries to give birth. The reason for the increase in insulin produced by the fetal pancreas is that there is an increase in glucose passing from the mother to the fetus as a result of the mother being hyperglycemic, .In addition to the above complications for mothers who have gestational diabetes, there are many other complications that the infant experiences as a result of the mother's uncontrolled hyperglycemia. Some of the complications of the newborn infant include the following: low blood sugar or hypoglycemic episodes, respiratory distress syndrome, high bilirubin levels (hyperbilirubinemia), higher numbers of admissions to neonate intensive care units, and higher rates of stillbirth and perinatal mortality directly related to the mother's uncontrolled hyperglycemia. The maternal-fetal glucose gradient facilitates the transfer of glucose from the mother to the fetus, resulting in increased levels of glucose in the mother and increased levels of insulin produced by the fetal pancreas, resulting in excessive fetal weight gain and poor metabolic stability following delivery.

Gestational Diabetes Mellitus (GDM) has been shown to impact women's long-term health, especially postpartum and on future generations, making it an urgent and significant public health concern, as opposed to just another pregnancy-related health issue. Women diagnosed with GDM significantly increase their chances of developing Type 2 Diabetes Mellitus (T2DM), metabolic syndrome, and cardiovascular disease within 5-10 years after giving birth, mostly due to a lack of ongoing follow-up care and lifestyle changes after having their baby. It has also been shown that children exposed to intrauterine hyperglycemia are at an increased risk of childhood obesity, reduced glucose tolerance, insulin resistance, and having metabolic disorders at an early age; thus, demonstrating how the intrauterine environment affects the lifelong metabolic programming of children. Moreover, healthcare systems that do not have high rates of postpartum screenings, do not have any digital follow-up services in place after delivery, also place mothers at greater risk due to additional barriers, including their socio-economic status, that prevent them from receiving continued health care after delivery. The large volume of studies presented in this review point to an immediate need for coordinated, continual care for mothers through increased use of technology and early identification, ongoing supervision, extended support and reduced long-term risks to mothers.

Intergenerational Impact and Long-term Cardiometabolic Risks

Gestational Diabetes Mellitus (GDM) has a variety of consequences on maternal and infant health, both directly and indirectly. Maternal health complications caused by GDM can affect both the mother's health throughout the course of her life and the health development of the child from infancy to adulthood. Mothers who had GDM have a significantly increased chance of developing Type 2 Diabetes Mellitus later in life in comparison to those without a history of GDM.Estimates indicate that mothers who have experienced GDM have a 7-10 times greater risk of progressing to T2DM than mothers who do not have a history of GDM. In addition, mothers with GDM have a higher tendency for the development of metabolic syndrome or have increased blood pressure (hypertension), increased triglyceride (dyslipidemia), increased risk of cardiovascular disease (CVD) and related disorders—their risk essentially stems from the genetic conditions derived from chronic maternal metabolic disorders associated with pregnancy. The offspring of mothers who experienced diabetes during gestation have greater potential to develop childhood obesity, insulin resistance, glucose intolerance, and early-onset cardiometabolic diseases mellitus as a result of changes in fetal metabolic programming from maternal hyperglycemia. This process is termed fetal programming, and it is critical to understand DOHaD to comprehend how the intrauterine environment influences future health and disease development. While there is considerable evidence indicating the long-term risk of GDM on the health of both mother and child, modern healthcare systems typically do not provide continued integrated population support to ameliorate the effects associated with the long-term prevalence of GDM. A significant portion of women throughout the world have low postpartum follow-up rates (high percentage of women do not repeat a glucose test and/or receive counseling following delivery) and thus are missing critical windows of opportunity for early detection and prevention of T2DM. Overall, systematic deficiencies in the conventional facility-based paradigm of maternal health indicate that traditional ways of thinking are not responsive to the chronic and intergenerational impact of GDM.

Epidemiology and Public Health Relevance

From 17%-29% of all pregnancies in India are complicated by gestational diabetes mellitus, a much higher percentage than is reported for many other countries. There are a variety of reasons for the elevated incidence of gestational diabetes mellitus in India, including increased maternal age, changing lifestyles, obesity and decreased physical activity levels resulting in increased insulin resistance, and many women inadequately receiving antenatal care. As the incidence continues to increase, the relevance of gestational diabetes mellitus as a public health issue has grown substantially in India. For women who develop GDM, there is an increased lifetime risk of developing type 2 diabetes mellitus between 7% and 10% compared to women who do not develop gestational diabetes mellitus. In addition, infants born to mothers who have elevated blood glucose levels during pregnancy are at a higher risk for developing obesity, insulin resistance, and cardiovascular and metabolic disorders than those whose mothers do not have elevated blood glucose. The growing occurrence of gestational diabetes mellitus (GDM) suggests that GDM will soon become a common early warning sign of intergenerational health problems; however, more than 50% of women diagnosed with GDM do not come back for follow-up diabetes screening, leaving an opportunity for greater implementation of early intervention. The growing prevalence of gestational diabetes will create greater costs for the healthcare system, including higher numbers of prenatal visits, an increase in the number of cesarean births, the higher incidence of neonatal complications, and the higher long-term care costs associated with T2DM in women. The lack of adequate diagnostic capacity, reduced access to specialty care providers, and inadequate digital technology to support the management of GDM in rural areas of India continue to create barriers to managing this condition, necessitating that GDM become a focus of continued national healthcare reform initiatives around maternal health, as well as for expanding access to prenatal care and establishing links between primary healthcare and digital health resources. The increasing incidence of Gestational Diabetes Mellitus (GDM) in India is indicative of the longer-term, serious systemic deficits within India's maternal healthcare delivery infrastructures and highlights the urgent need for both the modernisation and coordination of the service delivery from within, among the various delivery systems. While there are various service providers and programmes, i.e. National Health Mission (NHM), Reproductive and Child Health (RCH) Programme. Due to a continued reliance on overburdened public laboratories, a limited supply of glucose testing meters and the lack of consistency in adherence to national guidelines, many facility-based health providers do not have adequate screening or diagnostic services available for diagnosing GDM. Because of these issues, the time it takes to make a diagnosis is extended, and there is often a lost opportunity to provide preventive care for women who are at risk for developing GDM. Moreover, the shortage of medical specialists (endocrinologists and obstetricians) and trained community-based health workers is a significant factor contributing to the inequities that exist between women living in both rural and urban areas. The problems that arise from deficiencies in these systems highlight the urgent necessity to develop new models of care that provide continuous monitoring of women versus simply providing episodic care through office visits. A model that incorporates both physical and digital care (phygital) as well as IoT-enabled monitoring and AI-facilitated risk stratification creates a tremendous opportunity to enhance the maternal health infrastructure and to prevent preventable complications.

RELATED WORK

Lu and Huang (2022), research studies showing that incorporating these new technologies into nursing systems significantly improves patient adherence, dietary compliance, and short-term metabolic control and leads to better immediate pregnancy outcomes. However, these studies had limitations in terms of follow-up times and are unable to comment on the long-term impact of these technologies. Concurrently conducted studies using telemedicine interventions (e.g., Rigla et al.'s Mobi Guide Pilot Study in 2018 and Varnfield et al.'s Mother platform) found significantly higher rates of patient acceptance of telehealth interventions, greater frequency of glucose checks and improved communication between patients and providers, all without increasing the clinical burden on patients and providers, demonstrating that there is a viable option for real-time decision support and feedback as part of routine GDM management. Expanded evidence bases will continue to support telehealth interventions as they have the potential to reduce rates of fetal overgrowth in rural areas (Tancredi et al., 2024).

Lu et al. (2022), developed a new stack of Long Short-term Memory Networks (LSTMs) applied to time series glucose levels to predict future glucose levels and trends with high levels of accuracy comparable to that of CGMs. Using these analyses, individuals can use cost-effective self-monitoring options for continuous diabetes risk detection. Similarly, there are multi-sensor mother-to-be platforms (IMFHMS-ODL, with Nandini and Rahimunnisa in 2025) and IoT telehealth platforms enabled by medical algorithms trained on a decision tree to assist providers in identifying the early stages of abnormal fetal development. Papri et al. (2025) developed prototypes of IoT technologies specifically for pregnancy and employing sustainable wearable systems.

Gaps in Traditional GDM Care

Harrison et al. (2021) state that traditional approaches to managing GDM typically result in delays regarding both the screening and diagnosis of pregnant women with GDM. This clearly limits the opportunity for early interventions to help manage GDM successfully. As well, according to Moses et al. (2017), traditional management of GDM leads to a slow process for adjusting treatment as the frequency of in-person visits are much lower compared to how many times it needs to be done; therefore, this means that the management of GDM does not occur as quickly as possible, resulting in poor control of glycemia. Finally, as stated by Sakai et al (2019) observe that patients' adherence to SMBG (self-monitored blood glucose) is poor. The burden of manual logging, inconsistency in feedback, and low health literacy make it difficult for patients to monitor their blood glucose. Combined, these findings demonstrate that traditional management lacks timeliness, continuity, and patient engagement.

Digital Interventions for Remote Monitoring

Research conducted by Griauzde and colleagues (2020) indicates a positive correlation with increased adherence to SMBG for those who have glucose monitoring apps and receive automated reminders compared to the traditional method of using paper based logs. Telemedicine also allows patients to engage in regular visits without physically visiting a clinician while maintaining stable blood glucose levels; thus, Dalfra et al. (2014) support this finding. According to Miremberg and associates (2018), the mobile enabled daily glucose transmissions lead to quicker therapeutic modifications as well as superior fasting glucose levels when compared with traditional methods of care. As a whole, these studies point towards the benefits of improved monitoring through remote access for GDM management by increasing the frequency and accuracy of reporting as well as providing patients to be more responsive to their health needs.

Behavioural Support and Patient Engagement

The study performed by Hirst et al. (2015) demonstrated that the utilization of educational modules through smartphones was beneficial in providing patients with knowledge regarding exercise and nutrition and enabling the patients to manage their own health more effectively. Kaufman et al. (2020) showed that the addition of personalized digital prompts increased adherence to the monitoring of blood glucose and dieting. In contrast, Kim et al. (2019) demonstrated that when the content of a digital tool is not culturally reflective of the user, engagement with the tool decreases. The overall results from these studies indicate that digital support tools are most successful when they provide the user with personalized recommendations, allow for interaction between the user and their provider via the digital tool, and are relevant based upon the context in which the user resides.

Hybrid ("Phygital") Models Combining Digital and In-Person Care

Peacock and co-authors claim that Hybrid Care Models decrease the workload of clinicians and improve the ability of clinicians to provide oversight of high-risk women. Cheung et al., 2018 showed increased patient satisfaction as well as timely adjustments in insulin dosing when using a combination of telehealth along with onsite assessments. D'Souza et al., 2022 highlight how hybrid models provide care based on risk, with stable patients mostly managed through electronic means and unstable/complex patients receiving highest priority for clinic-based care. Overall, all of these studies reveal how hybrid care models overcome limitations related to the either complete digital or complete in-person delivery of care.

TRADITIONAL CARE AND LIMITATIONS

Traditionally, GDM was managed using a facility-dependent model ("clinic-centric") that involved face-to-face appointments, laboratory tests and procedures, and in-person third-party monitoring by health care providers and family members, among other practices. While this framework has provided critical medical support to help ensure the safety of both the mother and her developing fetus, the growing prevalence of logistics problems (delays), behaviour problems (non-compliance), socio-economic issues (limited access), and systemic failures (barriers to access) has limited this model's ability to successfully treat GDM. The increasing global number of GDM cases illustrates these limitations and sheds light on the gaps in access to care, continuity, and individualised care that have historically characterised the management of GDM. Historically, GDM has been categorised into three areas: (1) Screening and Diagnosis; (2) Clinical Management; and (3) Postpartum Follow-up. In some cases, these three areas are based on established medical protocols, but in reality each area is essentially reliant on the woman being available, on time, and in person to follow established medical protocols. Additionally, aside from the excessive amount of time that can elapse between delivery and the initiation of postpartum care, these areas of GDM management rely on manual, time-consuming processes (e.g., appointment scheduling) and delayed responses to medical provider communication within the health care system. In addition to the complexities resulting from these characteristics, the GDM management model is reactive rather than proactive and is unable to accommodate the evolving needs of today's mothers in their journey toward optimal maternal health. Additionally, the traditional clinic-centric model of care is less compatible with the changing health and social-behavioural environments and needs of the pregnant woman. Particularly in low- to middle-income settings, where health systems are already facing enormous challenges, pregnant women often have to make multiple visits to a health care facility to obtain glucose screening, receive nutritional counselling, or make adjustments to their treatment. Coupled with financial barriers to care and social barriers, such as long travel times, limited transportation options, family obligations, or lack of family support, the burden of multiple appointments can be overwhelming for pregnant women. Also, long delays in getting results back from the lab, interruptions in supply, and differences in test results and diagnoses prevent the quick decisions needed by the physician in the office setting. There is no clear communication between the doctor who is providing primary care, the physician in the specialty area that provides currently available care, or the hospital-based physician who provides specialty care in a local area. This lack of communication leads to multiple tests being ordered; conflicting recommendations being given to patients; and missing the opportunity for timely interventions to be performed. The high incidence of manual record keeping in many parts of the world increases the risk of inaccurate data and lost records of antenatal care, which limits the ability to track patterns of maternal risk and contribute to developing a plan of care that will enable them to receive personalised services. Collectively, these inefficiencies result in disrupted continuity of care, reduced responsiveness and decreased equity of care for women with gestational diabetes mellitus, which creates an urgent need to develop more integrated, technology-enabled and patient-centred care models that can provide for real-time monitoring of gestational diabetes mellitus.

Screening and Diagnosis

Traditionally, screening for gestational diabetes mellitus (GDM) is the responsibility of healthcare providers during pregnancy weeks 24 through 28 through a variety of means including; the Oral Glucose Tolerance Test (OGTT) and Fasting Plasma Glucose Test (FPGT). While the OGTT and FPGT are both widely in use today and validated by scientific evidence, these tests also present many challenges to pregnant women. The OGTT requires a person to fast, travel early in the morning for an appointment, endure a long wait time, and have blood taken multiple times over several hours. For pregnant mothers who work outside the home, live in rural areas, or have trouble accessing reliable transportation, these conditions create serious challenges when obtaining GDM screenings. Those living in areas where healthcare access is limited often have to delay or miss their GDM screenings due to these challenges. Adding to the issue of access to GDM screenings and the follow-up care required for GDM patients are the significant differences that exist around the world and even within regions of the same country regarding GDM screening protocols. The difference in cut-off points that are used to determine whether a woman has Gestational Diabetes Mellitus (GDM), the testing method(s) utilized to diagnose the disease and the difference in screening practices between selective screening versus universal screening, have resulted in significant differences in how GDM is diagnosed and treated across the globe. In places with limited resources, selective screening methods are often used which fail to identify up to 50% of women with GDM resulting in a delayed diagnosis of GDM and the initiation of necessary medical intervention until complications occur. Relying on laboratory-based methods to diagnose conditions results in extended delays between the time that samples are obtained, processed, and treated, especially in areas with no adequate digital reporting system. Consequently, conventional diagnostic approaches frequently ascertain the presence of gestational diabetes mellitus only after the individual has experienced substantial metabolic disturbances attributable to the condition itself.

Clinical Management

The traditional way of treating gestational diabetes mellitus (GDM) is by using a combination of medical nutrition therapy (MNT), physical exercise, self-monitoring blood-sugar levels (SMBG), and medication when indicated. All procedures will generally occur through direct patient consultation with obstetricians, endocrinologists, nutritionists, and diabetes educators. Although this management method is considered effective in theory, it assumes that patients will participate regularly and have easy access to a health care facility along with adequate patient understanding—only a small percentage of patients do. Nutritional Counseling, which is very important in the treatment of GDM, is usually provided in one session instead of continuing contact with the patient about food choices; this reduces the effectiveness of this management method long-term. Women attempting to make dietary changes for GDM often have barriers such as cultural food customs, available funds, and low health literacy. Similarly, exercise recommendations are often vague and not individualized and most women have difficulty adhering to them without continuous reinforcement. Patients must perform multiple finger-stick tests every day to monitor their blood sugar levels, and they must then input these results manually. As a result, blood sugar levels are only reviewed at pre-scheduled appointments. This leaves extended periods without physician oversight. If patients document their results incorrectly or do not communicate them properly, this will lead to mistakes by physicians when interpreting the results. Also, because of the pain associated with repeated pricking of the fingers, many patients do not comply with self-monitoring of their glucose levels. In addition, patients must manage insulin in conditions where access to insulin is limited and the costs associated with insuring insulin is prohibitive.

BRIDGING GAPS IN TRADITIONAL GDM MANAGEMENT THROUGH A PHYGITAL CARE FRAMEWORK

Traditional GDM care is limited by delayed diagnosis, infrequent in-person reviews, poor adherence to glucose monitoring and fragmented coordination between obstetricians, diabetologists and community workers. The proposed phygital model directly addresses these gaps through remote glucose tracking and automated alerts, digital education and nudges, virtual multidisciplinary consultations and targeted in-clinic follow ups supported by risk stratification data.

Proposed Phygital GDM Care Model

We intend to implement a hybrid ecosystem to manage Gestational Diabetes Mellitus (GDM) using many different advanced technologies in a phygital manner. Using non-invasive physiological sensors, IoT-based devices, cloud computing and artificial intelligence to analyze our collected data combined with telemedicine for monitoring our patients we will create a Continuous & Predictive System (CPS) for improving maternal metabolic health management. Our framework's main component will be the use of non-invasive glucose monitoring technologies (compared to current blood glucose monitors) such as Optical Spectroscopy and Bio-impedance Sensing that provide continuous information on glycaemic changes without the need for blood draws (phlebotomy). In addition, our devices will connect with mobile apps via low-energy Bluetooth and through Edge Computing to operate in areas without traditional telecommunication service. The data collected from the wearable devices will be securely stored and forwarded to our cloud-based digital health platform, which meets and exceeds all of the National Interoperability Framework guidelines developed by the Health Level Seven (HL7) and Fast Healthcare Interoperability Resources (FHIR).

This framework uses AI/ML algorithms to produce risk classification scores, identify GDM, estimate future glucose levels and alert the physician when the patient's data indicates a potential adverse event. These alerts and reports will be provided to physicians through a dashboard that provides real-time access to glucose readings and trends for each individual patient. In addition, these reports will support physicians when making care decisions, enabling them to intervene quickly through either face-to-face visit or telehealth through this framework, patients will receive automated messages, meal plans, and personalized recommendations, while physicians will receive immediate identification of risk factors to make necessary changes to their treatment method. In order to ensure the successful implementation of this innovative technology-based healthcare delivery model, it will be necessary to develop a systematic approach within a tiered structure of operation. The first step in developing this systematic approach is to identify the necessary clinical and technological components to be included in the framework; this should be done collaboratively between the various stakeholders, i.e., physicians, endocrinologists, medical staff, data analysts, biomedical engineers and public health policy makers.

A user-centered mobile application and clinical dashboards that alert providers when their patients' glucose levels move outside the normal range should be part of the technology platform. Additionally, there should also be offline capabilities available for patients who live in rural areas where internet access is unavailable. The artificial intelligence model and machine learning models should be developed and empirically validated using a multisite database to improve the generalizability of results. Whenever possible, these artificial intelligence and machine learning models that are developed should utilize federated learning models in order to protect patient privacy/confidentiality. The first phase of the project should begin with pilot testing in tertiary care institutions, district hospitals, and primary care clinics to determine the need for further refinements to enhance usability and integration into the current clinical workflow while providing continuous education for staff and comprehensive support to patients. All components of the implementation of this model on the National level should be aligned with existing national digital health initiatives, with the required allocation of government-sponsored technology resources, and with ongoing technical support. There are important ethical and operational considerations when creating a remote Diabetes Management Program including securing an informed consent for each participant, ensuring the confidentiality of patients' medical records, looking for potential algorithm biases and security issues around patients' health records (e.g. protecting them with encryption and allowing only authorized individuals access through a role based access model). Additionally, it is vital to improve both patients' and healthcare providers' general level of digital literacy; provide linguistic resources in multiple languages; improve access to affordable equipment and/or subsidize the costs of acquiring equipment for patients who have low incomes; increase the strength of rural health systems; and lastly to assess the long term success of this program based on clinical outcomes; patient adoption rates; predictive accuracy; cost/benefit ratios; levels of satisfaction experienced by patients; and the reduction of maternal and neonatal morbidity and mortality rates. The ultimate goal of the Phygital GDM model is to create a maternal health system that is predictive, preventive, personalised and precise in order to reduce the incidence of intergenerational Cardiometabolic Disease; enhance the quality of postnatal care in the 12 months following delivery; and close the Gap between Urban and Rural Health Care access concerning Maternal & Neonatal Health Care.

The Phygital Model of Care for Gestational Diabetes Mellitus (GDM) includes a complete and integrated Multi-Layered Digital Ecosystem that allows for a Comprehensive Connected Care experience for a wide variety of services within one central system or organization. A component of the Phygital GDM Care Model's Digital Ecosystem is Non-Invasive Physiological Monitoring (NIPM) via a Smart Wearable Device. The Smart Wearable allows for Continuous Monitoring of Glucose Levels via Continuous Glucose Monitoring (CGM), Heart Rate (HR), Physical Activity (PA) Levels, and Several Other Maternal Health Measures. The information collected by the Smart Wearable Device is transmitted via Bluetooth Low Energy Technology to a Secure Cloud-based Health Management Application. This Application utilises Edge Computing Technology to process and interpret information collected by the Smart Wearable Device on the Patient Mobile Device before the Patient's information is uploaded to the secure Health System/Agency Cloud/Health Information Exchange (HIE) Environment.

Figure 1. Pydigital -GDMCare Model

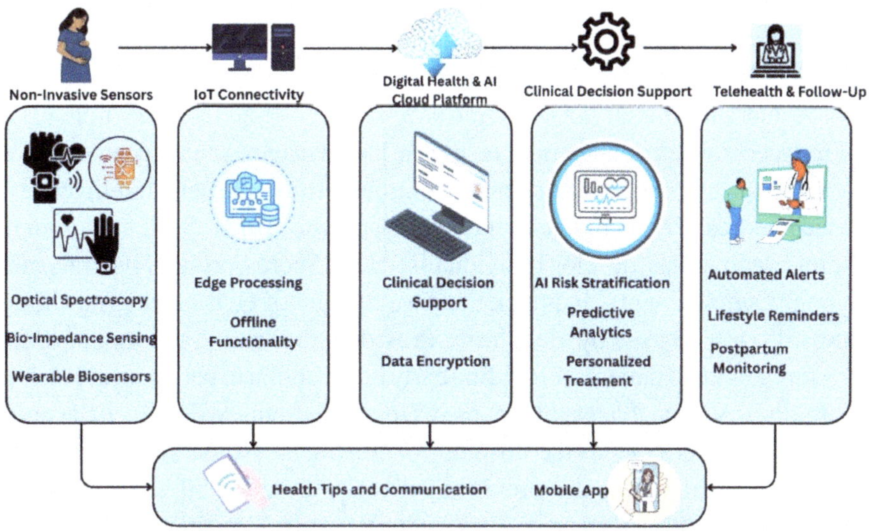

The Safe and Secure Transfer of Patient Information will adhere to National Interoperability Standards (NIS) including #-HL7-FHIR. Consequently, the integration of the Patient's Clinical Data from Electronic Health Record (EHR) and Digital Public Health System (DPHS) is accomplished. An important part of the NIS is addressing the need for a Centralized Repository to House/Store all Electronic Health Records and Additional Electronic Data, including All Tables/Data Sources Related to the Patient, in one central location. This Central Repository provides Patients with Access to their Individual Health Record Data via the Secure Digital Ecosystem that is maintained by their Healthcare Provider at any time. Once the Data has been Segmented, the ML/AI Algorithms will perform a detailed analysis of each segment.

Workflow Overview

The proposed workflow for a Phygital GDM (Gestational Diabetes Mellitus) Care Model connects the patient's continuous care through pregnancy and postpartum with real-time physiological data and clinical decision making, creating an uninterrupted maternal healthcare experience. The workflow for the patient commences with Antenatal Registration where the patient first registers for the Phygital program, is introduced to how to utilise a connected device, and receives access to a Mobile Health Application that serves the patient as the interface to their healthcare provider. Once onboarded, the user will wear a non-invasive wearable glucose monitoring sensor that continuously collects and sends glycaemic and physiological data via Bluetooth Low Energy to the user's smartphone. Since the sensor uses Edge processing capabilities, it can remain operational even when there is no connectivity or if the user resides in a rural location where connectivity may not always be guaranteed, as it can temporarily store the collected data and upload to the cloud for access when connectivity resumes. The glycaemic and physiological data collected by the glucose sensor is sent continuously to an Artificial Intelligence (AI) and Machine Learning (ML) system for analysis. The AI/ML System will identify glycaemic fluctuations, develop Individualised Risk Scores, project Hyperglycaemic or Hypoglycaemic Events, and track the development of GDM subtypes. Clinician Dashboard's will be used by Healthcare Providers to identify and monitor Health Trends for individual patients. Providing early intervention to patients via Telehealth Consultations, Virtual Triage, or Adapted Treatment Plans, will reduce the number of times the Patient goes to the hospital for treatment. At the same time that the application is operating, it also provides patients with alerts, lifestyle suggestions, nudges for behaviour change as well as reminders for taking their medications and for appointments through the app. This process continues beyond the time of birth; through postpartum monitoring and automatic reminders for patients to be screened for diabetes, we will be able to provide long-term follow-up and early identification of progression to Type 2 Diabetes. Thus, combining these processes allows us to provide patients with pre-emptive, individualised and easily accessible Care throughout the continuum of Care, both in Urban and Rural settings, by creating a synchronised Adaptive Continuous Care Environment that encompasses all aspects of clinical and digital health technology for managing Gestational Diabetes.

Technologies used

The suggested Phygital GDM Monitoring and Management Solution will be based on a collaborative and multidimensional technology ecosystem with connected biomedical devices (sensors) for monitoring blood glucose levels, integrated with IoT, 'AI,' cloud computing, and the National Digital Health Infrastructure. Sensors will allow for continuous glucose monitoring using non-invasive methods such as Optical Spectroscopy, Raman Spectroscopy, Photoacoustic Sensing and Bio-Impedance Spectroscopy, eliminating the need for blood sugar finger-stick tests and Glucose Tolerance Testing (OGTT). Access to real-time patient physiological data through wearable devices featuring IoT technology enables transmission of these data to an mHealth application via Bluetooth Low Energy (BLE) and Edge Processing, which is effective even in rural areas that have limited or poor network connections. Wearable device Data is securely transferred to a Cloud Computing platform (AWS, Google Cloud Platform or the National Health Cloud) that adheres to the same Interoperability Standards (HL7 and FHIR) used by all National Health Record (NHR). Remote Health Delivery (Telehealth and Virtual Care) is supported through WebRTC Video Consultation Providers, Automated Alerts linked to Electronic Medical Record Dashboards for Clinicians, and Chatbots for Guidance during Decision Making. Various Big Data Systems (e.g., Hadoop, Spark) are employed for Public Health Analysis and Optimization of Resources in All Levels of Community Care (Community Care, Secondary [Intermediate] Care, and Tertiary Care); thereby creating a Hybrid Intelligent Ecosystem of Scalable, Equitable and Predictable, Preventable and Personalized; Medicaid or National Health Reform model Maternal Care.

Data Integration and Real-Time Monitoring

According to the proposed phygital GDM care model, the approach will integrate and monitor real-time physiological data such as glucose level, activity rate, heart rate, and behaviour of a GDM patient with the help of Artificial Intelligence and Machine Learning (AI/ML) continuously through Continuous Glucose Monitoring (CGM/CGM) Technology and Wearable Technology. This type of integration will allow clinicians to intervene at the earliest opportunity. All information gathered through Non-Invasive Wearable Sensors will be sent via Bluetooth to the patient's mobile app. Once this data is received, it is processed locally (within the patient mobile app), filtered and temporarily stored, and had excessive background noise removed to ensure the quality of the data when sent to areas with limited connectivity. Once the data are gathered from these resources by the mobile app, all data will be securely uploaded to an Electronic Health Record (EHR) System using standard Electronic Health Record Interoperability protocols (e.g. HL7-FHIR). The patient's app will automatically send them updates for automated actions, therapy updates, nutritional recommendations, and alerts for issues that need to be corrected by them immediately. The ability to track the treatment in real-time allows for postpartum follow-up tracking to decrease the chances of missing follow-ups and allows for early identification of Type 2 diabetes risk. The tightly coupled multilateral communication between maternal health providers and the patient ensures that a maternal care plan is continually updated, accountable, and supported by predictive analytics, thereby closing the gap between episodic clinical visits and real-time digital-based health oversight for the maternal health care team.

Integrated Implementation Strategy and Key Considerations

The phygital GDM model is expected to be realised using a complex multi-pronged implementation strategy that involves integrating technology, reshaping operations and aligning with current national health care systems. The implementation process starts with an evaluation of the requirements (clinical and technical) for obstetricians, endocrinologists, biomedicine engineers, artificial intelligence (AI) experts, public health officials, and government representatives, all of whom will play an essential role in developing and implementing the proposed model. Developing the prototype(s) will include integrating wearable sensors, mobile apps, clinician dashboards, real-time alert systems and cloud computing platforms that function where there is limited internet or mobile network connectivity. The training of AI and machine learning (ML) algorithms will require using multiple geographical and regional datasets to ensure they can all be standardised, and federated learning will be used to efficiently maximise the use of raw data while reducing user privacy issues during the development of the model. To determine whether the pilot implementation is likely to be successful, there will need to be a series of pilot trials run at the three levels of tertiary hospitals, district hospitals and primary health centres, to evaluate the following four factors: Usability, Preparedness of Staff for Pilot Implementation, Feasibility in Rural Locations, and Aligning Current Clinical Workflows with Digital Technology. In addition to these evaluations, the ability to scale nationally will depend on the linkages between any digital health initiatives and the Federal Government's provision of device distribution grants and the establishment of long-term maintenance plans for those devices. There are a number of ethical issues that will require careful attention: Informed Consent; Ownership of Data Generated by the Algorithm; Transparency in Algorithmic Processes; and Security Measures to Mitigate Potential Misuse of Algorithms. In addition to these ethical issues, there will also be a number of operational factors that will need to be considered: The Cost of the Device; Providing a Multilingual Software Interface; Training Community Health Workers; Offering Digital Literacy Training to Community Members; and Developing a Robust Technical Support System to Support the Community Health Workers. The parameters used to evaluate the benefits, efficiency, and effectiveness of Artificial Intelligence in Improving the Framework for Maternal Health Delivery Models should include: Clinical Outcomes, Customer Satisfaction, Economic Benefits, and Adoption Rates; and used to support future improvements to the framework for delivering maternal health services through the use of Artificial Intelligence tools and technologies. Ultimately, the successful enactment of Predictive, Preventive, Personalised, and Precision-oriented systems will contribute to the enhancement of maternal health delivery by mitigating complications, advancing Post-Partum Care, broadening access to healthcare for Rural Women, and markedly diminishing Intergenerational Cardiometabolic Risk through the reduction of complications and morbidity.

CHALLENGES AND RISKS IN IMPLEMENTING PHYGITAL NATIONAL HEALTHCARE REFORM FOR GDM CARE

In order to create a phygital hybrid environment for gestational diabetes mellitus (GDM) within all national healthcare systems, there are therefore numerous operational, technical, regulatory, clinical, and socio-ethics considerations to be evaluated comprehensively prior to successfully implementing and providing for equal access. Of major concern is the digital divide, which is defined as the unequal distribution of smartphones, internet access, varied devices and related costs, as well as the limited digital literacy skills of women living in rural and/or socio-economically depressed areas. Women in these environments may not be able to access the digital monitoring options to their full potential. Additionally, differences in women's health literacy levels, cultural views of technology, and reluctance to use wearable devices or participate in remote consultation are all additional barriers to using GDM monitoring alternative options. A key aspect of clinical implementation of any new non-invasive glucose monitoring devices is how accurately and reliably they measure glucose levels; however, non-invasive glucose monitoring devices using optical and/or bio-impedance technology still require additional validation specific to pregnancy before being considered safe and offer similar performance as traditional invasive monitoring devices. The use of inaccurate non-invasive devices can create the risk of a potential misclassification of a woman's GDM status, under- or over-treatment, or poor clinical outcomes. There are significant impediments to successfully implementing non-invasive glucose monitoring devices in clinical practice due to the need to integrate these devices with existing national Digital Health system(s) (e.g., Electronic Medical Records, Clinical Workflows). As Digital Health solutions are being implemented into existing clinical practice only as isolated and fragmented systems, this has resulted in multiple format(s) of Shared Data being available, and a failure to Synchronise Data in Real-Time. The result of this situation has created many difficulties in the area of Clinical Decision-Making and the Coordination of Patient Care. It takes a vast amount of time and effort to successfully integrate Digital Health technology into practice for any clinician, nurse or Community Health Worker who must learn how to change their current Workflow, monitor their patients remotely, and utilise Artificial Intelligence (AI) Decision Support technologies. There are also a number of additional Major Concerns regarding Privacy, Security, and Ethical Issues arising from the use of Internet of Things (IoT), Cloud-Based Data Interchange, AI and Machine Learning to predict Maternal-Infant health outcomes. Moving to a phygital model will require Organizational Change Management, and there will likely be resistance to implementation on the part of some institutions, a slow rate of adaptation to new processes and procedures, and lags behind in policy adjustments. Healthcare models established prior to digital health technology operating with episodic acute care-focused models will be challenged to incorporate new continuous remote monitoring and proactive disease management strategies. In order to properly mitigate these identified risks, implementation will need to include co-designing with: Patients and Frontline Healthcare Workers (i.e., Emergency Medical Technicians), conducting Iterative Pilots, creating defined Governance Models, creating Ethical AI frameworks, and Developing Strong Community Engagement Strategies.

Potential for Phygital Personalization & Precision Medicine in GDM Monitoring

Integrating phygital healthcare frameworks into current methods of managing Gestational Diabetes Mellitus (GDM), has the potential to significantly advance personalization and precision in Maternal health systems through their ability to provide individualized medical interventions. Current treatment protocols for GDM, such as standardized care practices and general dietary or medication guidelines, do not consider the diverse Biological, Metabolic and Psychosocial characteristics of pregnant women and therefore are not adequately suited to meet their needs. The newly implemented "phygital" model combines in-the-moment (real time) physical observation and evaluation, along with Digital Analytics, to develop continuous and individualized assessments and adaptive care methodologies that allow for the provision of proactive and predictive care, versus the traditional practice of episodic and reactive management. With the availability of wearable devices and continuous glucose monitoring technology that utilizes the Internet of Things, detailed real time glycaemic data can be easily captured, allowing for dynamic modification of lifestyle, dietary intake, insulin administration and clinical consultations based on individual biological responses, rather than general norms. Through the establishment of longitudinal datasets, pregnant women will experience greater autonomy, awareness and engagement with their health behaviours due to the increase in information available to their care providers regarding their Glucose metrics, compared to the assessments provided during discrete clinician visits. Integrating phygital healthcare systems into existing methods of the management of Gestational Diabetes Mellitus (GDM) provides an opportunity to greatly improve both personalization and precision within Maternal Health Systems by enabling the development of customized medical treatments. Currently, the adoption of the standardised treatment protocol for GDM, which utilises only generalised dietary guidelines and medication prescriptions, do not consider the differences between pregnant women, including their Biological, Metabolic and Psychosocial differences. As a result, these treatment protocols are not sufficiently supportive of the individualised needs of pregnant women. The recently developed 'Phygital' healthcare support model incorporates both digital analytics and momentary (real-time) observations/assessments to create personalised, continuous assessments and adaptive care models that deliver proactive/predictive care compared to the current episodic/reactive care management model. With the use of wearable devices and continuous glucose monitoring technology that is connected to the IoT, continual real-time glycaemic information can now be collected from a pregnant woman's body, which allows for dynamic adaptations to her lifestyle choices (diet), insulin dosage and clinical consultations, based on individualised biological responses as opposed to standard norms. By enabling remote monitoring of other aspects of wellness—including blood pressure, heart rate variability, weight trends, sleep patterns/durations, activity levels, and nutrition—the integration of these additional data within the National Digital Health Ecosystem provides a means to develop a standardised approach to the collection and storage of health records across multiple sites, allows for the collection and analysis of population-based data, and provides all individuals (including those who may live in remote or rural areas or be economically disadvantaged) with access to advanced health care services via Telehealth and other methods (such as offline data synchronisation and collaboration with Community Health Workers). With this approach, the integration of clinical data with patient-generated health information along with the use of artificial intelligence-based analytics will provide the basis for a feedback loop that supports continuous improvement of therapeutic interventions designed to optimise maternal-fetal health while minimising long-term Cardiometabolic Risks for both mothers and their children. The Phygital Precision Medicine framework conceptualises Gestational Diabetes Mellitus (GDM) as more than simply a medical condition rather, it provides women with a means of reshaping their life course to prevent future chronic diseases (including diabetes and cardiovascular disease) for themselves and their children by providing them with access to integrated, predictive, preventative, personalised, and continuous care. As a platform for monitoring GDM experiences in a Phygital (physical/digital) environment, the Phygital GDM Monitoring Platform is laying the groundwork for the creation of Evidence-Based Public Health Systems that can deftly and effectively respond to the worldwide challenge of Metabolic Disease, particularly in those communities where Metabolic Disease is disproportionately represented compared to elsewhere in the world.

COMPARATIVE INSIGHTS FROM GLOBAL AND INDIAN DIGITAL MATERNAL-HEALTH INNOVATIONS

Global and Indian digital maternal health programs show that impact depends on modality, reach and system integration. South Africa's MomConnect demonstrates large scale SMS enrolment and strong health system linkage, while India's Kilkari and mMitra use voice messaging to overcome literacy barriers and improve maternal knowledge. Provider tools like the Safe Delivery App reliably boost frontline skills. These examples highlight that digital interventions work best when locally adapted and supported by robust monitoring and integration with health services.

Future Directions for Phygital GDM Care

The future development of phygital GDM (Gestational Diabetes Mellitus) management systems will greatly depend on the creation of a mother's health ecosystem that is intelligent, adaptive, and fully interoperable; an ecosystem that can efficiently integrate innovative technologies such as Biosensors, multi-omics precision medicine, Predictive Analytics, and National Digital Health Systems, with their associated infrastructure. Over the next few years, the capabilities and effectiveness of non-invasive glucose monitoring technology will significantly improve. These technologies will transition into Hybrid Multi-Sensor Devices that utilize Optical Technology, Electrical Technologies, and Chemical Technologies to provide the highest degree of Accurate Continuous Glucose Monitoring possible with one device. The user Interface for Continuous Glucose Monitoring will evolve into a simpler interface for both pregnant women, as well as the general population; therefore, non-invasive glucose monitoring should become very common throughout pregnancy. Currently used AI-based Rule-Based Prediction Models will dramatically change to more advanced AI-based Personalized Digital Twin Models for women, whereby each woman will be able to access a digital clone of her Metabolic Profile, to predict her Glycemic Response during periods of Stress, Diet, Sleep, and Medication use. Moreover, the next phase of integrating Genomics, Metabolomics, and the Microbiome with Environmental Exposure Data will allow for earlier identification of individuals at risk for GDM (i.e., Preconception). This means that, moving forward, individuals with an increased chance of developing GDM will be able to employ Life Course Metabolic Prevention Strategies. Third, the new methods of Federated Learning and Privacy Preserving Computing will allow for a continued evolution of better formulated AI models created through the aggregation of data from a variety of populations while also protecting the privacy of the data used. And finally, the development and implementation of sophisticated Telehealth and Virtual Maternity Care Clinics and the growth of Mobile Community Health Programs will allow individuals living in rural and underserved communities access to clinical care in real time. Together these advances will further enhance and change the way that Phygital Maternal Care will be experienced now, and looking forward.

CONCLUSION

The phygital model of care for gestational diabetes mellitus (GDM) integrates traditional clinical practices, continuous monitoring via digital technology, and Artificial Intelligence (AI) into a comprehensive framework to allow for real-time assessment of maternal health. Based on current literature, there is a need for modernization, access to and equity of GDM care for many areas with high rates of GDM but few resources. The phygital model utilizes non-invasive sensor technologies, Internet of Things (IoT) enabled wearable technology, cloud-based electronic medical records, AI predictive analytic capabilities with subtype functionality, and a secure national digital health infrastructure; through these combined systems and services, the phygital model creates a collaborative ecosystem that promotes early detection of problems and proactive health management rather than reactive treatment and disjointed healthcare delivery. To achieve successful implementation of the phygital model, it is essential to develop and implement good data ethics practices, improve digital literacy among healthcare providers, provide access to care for women who live in remote/rural locations, and conduct large-scale validation studies on the effectiveness of this model among diverse populations.The phygital model tackles the many challenges that are present in gestational diabetes mellitus (GDM) screening and GDM management by creating a robust foundation for decreasing long-term metabolic issues for mothers and offsprings, strengthening the growth of the national public health system, and promoting an all-inclusive vision of precision maternal health delivery on a national scale. Incorporated phygital technology in national programs developed for maternal health has transformed the episodic model of managing pregnancy into an ongoing life course approach with the objective of managing both immediate and long-term metabolic risk factors as the pregnancy progresses. Using digital monitoring, Artificial Intelligence (AI) predictive analytic capabilities, and decision support systems, healthcare providers will be able to intervene earlier, apply appropriate treatment protocols and tailor lifestyle counselling to the individual based on their glycemic pattern and biological sub-type distinction. Additionally, the continuous use of digital technologies such as interoperable electronic health records, telemedicine solutions, and federated learning models has provided a significant increase in opportunities to grow and sustain phygital GDM services in many national healthcare systems globally. This transition has further created collaborative opportunities across many different organisations such as clinical teams, data scientists, engineers, policy makers, and community health practitioners, to ensure that innovations are grounded in real-world data and therefore are culturally appropriate.

REFERENCES

Chcung, N. W., Byth, K., Cincotta, R., & Fong, B. (2018). Telehealth combined with in-person care improves satisfaction and glycaemic control in gestational diabetes. *Diabetes Care, 41*(9), 1830–1835.

D'Souza, R., Arbuckle, S., & Koren, G. (2022). Risk-stratified hybrid models for gestational diabetes: Integrating digital monitoring with targeted in-clinic review. *Journal of Obstetrics and Gynaecology Research, 48*(5), 1123–1132.

Dalfra, M. G., Nicolucci, A., Bisson, T., & Lapolla, A. (2014). Telemedicine and pregnancy: Monitoring gestational diabetes mellitus improves outcomes. *Diabetes Technology & Therapeutics, 16*(9), 650–657.

. Griauzde, D., Kullgren, J. T., Liestenfeltz, B., et al. (2020). *A mobile health intervention supporting self-monitoring improves adherence in gestational diabetes.* JMIR mHealth and Health, 8(3), e16195.

Harrison, A. L., Shields, N., Watson, M. J., & Taylor, N. F. (2021). Gestational diabetes mellitus screening and care: A review of challenges and opportunities for improvement. *Diabetes Research and Clinical Practice, 175*, 108789.

Hirst, J. E., Raynes-Greenow, C. H., & Jeffery, H.. (2015). Smartphone education supports improved self-management in gestational diabetes mellitus. *Diabetic Medicine, 32*(8), 1057–1065.

Kaufman, N., Stone, K., & Holland, E. (2020). Digital interventions with personalised feedback improve adherence in gestational diabetes management. *Journal of Medical Internet Research, 22*(4), e15515.

Kim, H., Lee, S., & Lee, M.-H.. (2019). Challenges in sustaining engagement with mobile health apps among women with gestational diabetes. *BMC Pregnancy and Childbirth, 19*, 108.

Lu, L., & Huang, T. (2022). Effects of early nursing monitoring on pregnancy outcomes of pregnant women with gestational diabetes mellitus under the Internet of Things. *Computational and Mathematical Methods in Medicine, 2022*(1), 8535714. DOI: 10.1155/2022/8535714 PMID: 35693264

Miremberg, H., Ben-Ari, T., & Betzer, T.. (2018). The impact of a smartphone-based daily monitoring system on care quality and glycaemic control in gestational diabetes. *American Journal of Obstetrics and Gynecology, 218*(4), 448.e1–448.e7. DOI: 10.1016/j.ajog.2018.01.044 PMID: 29425836

Moses, R. G., Wong, V. C., Lambert, K. A., & Morris, G. J. (2017). The management of gestational diabetes: Evidence gaps and emerging solutions. *The Medical Journal of Australia*, *207*(4), 152–158. PMID: 28814215

Peacock, A. S., Lavery, J. A., & Farrell, C.. (2020). Hybrid telemedicine models reduce clinic burden while maintaining quality of gestational diabetes care. *Obstetrics and Gynecology*, *135*(3), 583–591. PMID: 32028504

Rigla, M., Martínez-Sarriegui, I., García-Sáez, G., Pons, B., & Hernando, M. E. (2018). Gestational diabetes management using smart mobile telemedicine. *Journal of Diabetes Science and Technology*, *12*(2), 260–264. DOI: 10.1177/1932296817704442 PMID: 28420257

Sakai, K., Iwama, N., & Nishigori, H.. (2019). Adherence to self-monitoring of blood glucose in women with gestational diabetes: Barriers and facilitators. *Journal of Diabetes Investigation*, *10*(6), 1608–1617.

Chapter 6
New Technologies and Enduring Challenges in the Healthcare Market

J. Sudarvel
http://orcid.org/0000-0001-6656-1992
Karpagam Academy of Higher Education, India

J. Smruthymol
http://orcid.org/0009-0002-8911-7530
Karpagam Academy of Higher Education, India

R. Velmurugan
http://orcid.org/0000-0002-7925-9757
Karpagam Academy of Higher Education, India

K. Jothi
http://orcid.org/0000-0002-8625-863X
KPR College of Arts, Science, and Research, India

Ravi Thirumalaisamy
http://orcid.org/0000-0002-5954-5940
Modern College of Business and Science, Oman

R. Sankar Ganesh
http://orcid.org/0000-0003-0708-8327
Vel Tech Rangarajan Dr. Sagunthala R&D Institute of Science and Technology, India

ABSTRACT

The health care business is undergoing a high rate and unprecedented change due to the combination of new technologies and the changing societal needs. AI, telemedicine, Internet of Medical Things (IoMT), robotics, and data-driven diagnostics are all transforming the healthcare delivery, monitoring, and administration modalities. These changes in technology have become necessities in addressing increasing needs triggered by aging of the population, increase in chronic diseases, and increase in healthcare spending. However, the challenges remain, such as the lack of workforce, the unequal access to the high-quality care in both the urban and rural areas, and the complexity of the functioning of the modern healthcare struc-

DOI: 10.4018/979-8-2600-0939-0.ch006

tures. Considering that millions of healthcare staff spread across the globe, and the scope of service demands is rapidly expanding, there is an urgency with regard to technology-powered solutions that enable clinical decision-making, improve patient outcomes, and streamline the allocation of resources.

1. INTRODUCTION

The health-care industry around the world is presently experiencing an acute change of structure, which was initiated by the fast-growing technological progress and increasing pressure on affordable, easily available, and high-quality medical services on the part of the population (Burrell, 2023). The recent advances in the digital health such as artificial intelligence, precision medicine, robotics, telehealth, genomic analytics, and the Internet of Medical Things (IoMT) have radically transformed the provision of health-care, creating opportunities to increase the efficiency of its operations, personalized care, and predictive decision-making. This technological outburst is not just a show of zeal; it is an organisational strategy to the systemic weaknesses that have undermined the strength of health-service delivery in the past decades.

One of the most important forces that contribute to such a change is the international demographic migration towards the ageing population. The chronic and degenerative disease rates are directly proportional to the number of older people, putting an unprecedented strain on the state health-care budgets and facilities (Sariyildiz, 2022, p. 10; Singhal et al., 2025). This has forced governments and health-care givers all over the world to embrace the use of technologically advanced care paradigms which enable chronic disease management, cost containment, and the allocation of resources in the most sustainable manner (Singhal et al., 2025).

The rising demand of health services shows that there has always been an inequitable allocation of health services especially between urban and rural areas. The allocation of clinicians and specialised facilities is substantially urbanised, and rural populations are not adequately offered the services of diagnostic processes, emergencies, and preventive health programmes (Hassan et al., 2024, p. 137). These geographic inequalities indicate the need to have remote-care solutions, such as teleconsultation, virtual hospital, mobile health applications, and AI-based diagnostic services implemented to guarantee fair distribution of services regardless of the residential location.

The global labour shortage that is increasing is another structurally inherent problem that faces health-care markets. Even though the health -care staffing market is estimated to expand to about USD 3 billion by 2033, the industry is simultaneously projected to have a shortage of 10 million employees by 2030, with a disproportionate effect on low- and low-income countries (Sinha, 2024, p. 2). This shortage endangers both operational performance and patient safety and continuity of care. Thus, health systems are considering the possibilities of automation, digital workforce optimisation, remote medical expertise and simulation-based training to reduce workforce shortage and improve performance.

Combined, these socioeconomic and demographic changes reveal that the use of the new technologies has ceased to be a fashionable decision and it has become a need to maintain the health-care markets. The emerging technologies provide solutions to overcome service bottlenecks, increase diagnostic accuracy, broaden access, minimize clinical errors, patient experience, and public-health preparedness. With health-care systems attempting this difficult shift their ability to strategically adopt technological solutions will have a significant impact on the future competitiveness, sustainability and social worth.

2. THE EVOLVING LANDSCAPE OF HEALTHCARE TECHNOLOGY

The modern environment of the healthcare sector is rapidly changing into a technological-focused paradigm, where advanced computing infrastructure and smart devices are becoming primary tools of diagnostic, treatment, and management guidelines. Artificial intelligence (AI), the Internet of Things (IoT), blockchain, and quantum computing technologies contribute to this change as they can be used to automate, support decision making in real-time, and to administer data safely in both non-clinical and clinical environments (Mahendrakar, 2025, p.2005).

In particular, quantum computing has become one of the disruptive capabilities, providing calculating capabilities outperforming the traditional system. It has potentials to simulate molecular interactions to speed up drug discovery and to decompose large genomic data to further personalized medicine (Sinha, 2024, p. 12). At the same time, diagnostic information technologies based on machine learning are capable of providing medical knowledge at low costs to rural and resource-limited populations, hence eliminating the geographic and socioeconomic differences in access to healthcare (Khan et al., 2023, p. 5; Vats, 2024). These technologies coming together are an indicator of a shift to a more active, more data-driven and fairer healthcare ecosystem.

2.1 Digital Health Innovations

The basis of the modern patient-centred care models is online health technologies. The widespread use of wearable gadgets, remote health strategies, and AI-driven web-based health applications has also changed the health surveillance and administration of individuals on daily operations (Adelson et al., 2003, p. 2). These sensors constantly record physiological and behavioural information, therefore, making it possible to notice health anomalies early enough and provide the necessary clinical attention, at the same time representatives do not have to visit a physical hospital and it reduces the load on health care facilities (Singhal et al., 2025). In 2023 alone, more than 500 million wearable gadgets were shipped across the world, and they mostly included smartwatches and fitness trackers (Adelson et al., 2003, p. 2). The adoption by consumers is also strong due to the growing curiosity of wellness, high rates of sensor accuracy improvement, straightforward health apps, and overall interoperability between smartphones and cloud systems. The area of digital health is not limited to wearables; the digital health finds its expression in the field of telemedicine which has become the main tool in the quest to improve the access to care, especially in rural and geographically isolated areas. Teleconsultations, online clinics, and mobile health services give patients an opportunity to access specialist knowledge without the limitations of traveling, which reduces structural inequalities in healthcare delivery (Ahmed et al., 2025; Zahidi et al., 2024, p. 6). The intersection of these digital innovations aims to make healthcare more democratic, enhances clinical outcomes, and makes it a shift toward sustainable hybrid care models.

2.2 Biotechnology and Pharmaceutical Advancements

The present-day generations of biotechnology and pharmaceutical sciences are passing the period of revolution, where the levels of genetic engineering, molecular therapeutics, and computational drug design developments are astounding. The gene-editing systems, especially CRISPR, have provided new therapeutic opportunities on hereditary diseases that were previously inaccessible. At the same time, mRNA-based vaccines have proven to be extremely versatile and able to be created within a short timeframe in response to newly identified infectious diseases (Mahara et al., 2023, p. 1). Besides, the application of artificial intelligence and machine learning to drug-discovery processes has improved clinical trial design, the prediction of molecular efficacy, as well as lightened the time and financial costs of the traditional pharmaceutical development procedures (Liu et al., 2024, p. 205).

Other than the laboratory-based innovation, biotechnology is also transforming the distribution and accessibility of pharmaceuticals. New directions focus on the localized and decentralized drug production, which increases supply-chain resilience and ensures timely access to drugs in underserved regions (Ogbewele et al., 2024, p. 2456). All these developments are a paradigm shift in therapeutic innovation as well as the logistical models on which healthcare delivery is based.

2.3 Artificial Intelligence and Machine Learning in Healthcare

Artificial intelligence and machine learning technologies have been increasingly integrated into health-care service provision on several levels, as highly complex engines of analysis. These technologies make the diagnostic process more streamlined, strengthen therapeutic planning, support patient monitoring guidelines, and personalized interventions by predictive analytics (Artuso & Guijt, 2020, p. 32). It is unique since AI/ML algorithms combine large data sets in the biomedical sector, providing accurate risk assessment of diseases, comorbidity likelihood, and patient-specific results. Their influence is especially strong in those areas of research where genomics, proteomics, transcriptomics, and metabolomics converge to provide a more detailed picture of tumour biology and guide the accuracy-based therapy of cancer (Ansari et al., 2025, p. 2).

The computer-aided diagnostic procedures have changed radically due to the deep-learning techniques, particularly in the field of radiological imaging. The AI can reduce the cognitive load of clinicians by automatising the process of identifying and classifying salient features in radiographs, CT scans, and MRI sequences due to the absence of human saturation and perceptual errors (Rawat et al., 2023, p. 1232; Shatnabi et al., 2024, p. 100188). New uses are also being created in metabolomics, which will allow complex diseases to be predicted at an early stage, including gastric and oral cancer due to subtle changes in biochemical behavior (which would have been undetectable in traditional clinical practice). The innovations provide a clear understanding of the crucial impact of AI to revolutionize medical care, making it more precise, efficient, and personalized.

3. PERSISTENT CHALLENGES IN HEALTHCARE MARKETS

Digital, computational, and biotechnological technologies are now integrated in the world health care systems, having radically changed the operations of health care systems worldwide, but structural and ethical issues continue to disrupt this transformation. The major concerns include the accuracy of datasets used to train the artificial intelligence (AI) models, interpretability of complex algorithms, and the ethical aspects of making the decisions by the robots in the area of individual medicine and pharmaceutical development (Patria et al., 2024).

These issues highlight the importance of having well-developed regulations and interdisciplinary cooperation between clinicians, computer scientists, policy makers, and bioethicists in order to implement the emerging technologies in a responsible manner (Saini, 2025, p. 553). At the same time, patient confidentiality, data security, and algorithmic fairness are also essential to the development of trust in AI-enhanced healthcare, especially when digital systems gain more control over clinical decisions (Ansari et al., 2025, p. 23). All these concerns assert the necessity of the socio-technical approach to innovation, where technological progress has to be adjusted to the moral protection and fair allocation.

3.1 Access and Equity Disparities

Even though state-of-the-art medical technologies have the potential to improve health outcomes, there is an unequal distribution of this technology all over the world, which only contributes to the perpetuation of historic health inequities. In developing nations, as well as in remote areas, the populations of the countries many times lack access to high-quality health facilities, professional labor force, and sophisticated digital resources, leading to significant differences in mortality and morbidity rates (Dunker, 1998, p. 541). To address these inequities, there is a need to mitigate the inequity by scaling the telehealth services, mobile health clinics, community-based interventions, and digital health literacy programs concurrently to facilitate equitable access.

Moreover, the inequalities in technologies do not simply concern the physical access. Many AI systems have significant computational requirements and a great amount of data prerequisites, which restrict the use of these systems in resource-constrained environments, where cloud computing, server, and secure data storage infrastructure is limited (Wang et al., 2025, p. 13). Besides, the lack of representative data, such as the information on ethnic minorities, the elderly, rural setting, and low-income communities, contributes to the biases in the algorithm and decreased diagnostic accuracy in various clinical settings (Nguyen, 2024, p. 100153). When unchecked, such disparities are likely to further exacerbate the health disparity gap of the world, undermine trust in AI-based diagnostic and treatment procedures, and undermine the inclusiveness of healthcare innovation.

3.2 Cost Containment and Economic Pressures

Although the introduction of new health technologies promises to bring a long and more efficient performance and greater effectiveness in clinical patient results, their high initial costs of implementation pose a significant financial burden on the healthcare providers and governments across the world. The costs related to the acquisition of the newest diagnostic technologies, the implementation of digital architecture, the modernization of informational systems, the introduction of systems that are compatible, and education of medical staffs are constantly increasing (Fahim et al., 2025, p.'1). The fiscal strain is especially high in low and middle income nations where healthcare expenditure is limited and alternative claims on the public service means further limit the spending power.

Besides material expenses, the aging world population together with the growing number of chronic diseases are straining the healthcare system, increasing the demand to find economical care models. This condition highlights the necessity of switching to value-based care, according to which the payment is associated with patient outcomes but not with the volume of services, which will guarantee the sustainability of the financial process, stimulate the development of novel payment models, and optimize the distribution of resources. Without such economic restructuring, the fruits of the technological innovation do run the risk of being left unexplited by the institutions and people needing them the most.

3.3 Regulatory and Ethical Considerations

With the age of sophisticated AI systems entering the healthcare industry, laws and regulations are not keeping up with the technical side of it. Current health policies that were initially oriented to be applied to traditional medical equipment and pharmaceuticals are not well equipped to consider the problems of accountability, validation, and safety in AI-generated diagnoses and treatment suggestions (Arab et al., 2025). This ambiguity poses difficulties to the developers, clinicians, and policymakers, and it calls on agile and adaptable regulation systems that can accommodate the swift technological change and give priority to the safety of patients (A Review of Hybrid AI Approaches for NDVI-Based Detection and Classification of Maize Crop Stress and Diseases, 2024, p. 7).

Among the most topical challenges is associated with the interpretability of AI models. The majority of advanced neural networks are black box systems and make extremely accurate predictions without giving clinicians a clear understanding of the line of thought behind these predictions. In order to introduce responsible medical deployment, interpretability studies are becoming indispensable to assist practitioners comprehend the nature of algorithmic decisions, gauge their performance, and when automation might be necessary (A Review of Hybrid AI Approaches to NDVI-Based Detection and Classification of Maize Crop Stress and Diseases, 2024, p. 8). In difficult diagnostic cases, in particular, subtle or early-stage disease diagnosis, transparency is especially important, as diagnostic errors can be very destructive (Gayap & Akhloufi, 2024, p. 267; Nguyen, 2024, p. 100153). It is thus important to reinforce the governance, transparency, and auditability of AI systems to facilitate ethical deployment and long-term confidence of people in digital healthcare.

4. INTERACTIONS BETWEEN NEW TECHNOLOGIES AND ENDURING CHALLENGES

The merging of new technology in the healthcare sector and old systemic issues has created an environment of dynamic and multifaceted ecosystem that requires constant adjustment. Although the digital and computational innovations hold the promise of reshaping the diagnostics, delivery of treatment, and administrative efficiency, their implementation comes with significant trade-offs. One of the most evident conflicts is a clash between the cost control and technological development as at first, the use of advanced systems always increases the costs of activities, even though these systems promise high-quality patient outcomes and long-term efficiency benefits (DosSantos & Oliveira, 2020, p. 179). In addition, the use of state-of-the-art AI models, which are the best in pattern recognition and predictive accuracy, is often based on computationally intensive architectures, which prevents real-time integration into clinical workflows (Gayap and Akhloufi, 2024, p. 268). This has led to a focused effort to come up with AI solutions which minimise computational needs without affecting accuracy and further improve the aptness of AI systems to clinical decision-making (Gayap & Akhloufi, 2024, p. 268).

In spite of these developments, there are still ongoing issues in the medical fraternity especially with regards to the bias of AI to over-sell and under-deliver real value. As it is observed, human factors, including empathy, communication, collaboration, and emotional support continue to be essential elements of high-quality patient care (Fendrick et al., 2023, p. 15). More so, the fact that large and heterogeneous datasets are required makes the implementation of deep-learning models more challenging, as most existing datasets are not big enough to include the population size and clinical setting required to make unbiased and broadly generalized predictions (Shariif et al., 2023, p. 10). Consequently, the main issue, is not the technical effectiveness of these systems, but the necessity of the equitable, ethical, and socially responsible implementation of such technologies in the healthcare practice.

4.1 Technology's Role in Addressing Access and Equity

Digital health solutions were shown to have a great potential to eliminate the disparity in healthcare access, especially to those who are situated in remote, rural, or socioeconomically disadvantaged settings. Telehealth technologies, mobile apps and telehealth monitoring systems will decrease reliance on physical health care infrastructure and alleviate the logistic pressures of travel expenses, time and resource limitations. These technologies help people with low mobility or limited access to hospitals and specialists to receive quality care within the context of their localities.

The AI-based diagnostic tools also encourage equity by spreading specialised knowledge to underserved areas, delivering high-quality decision support, even those departments without specialist doctors (Udegbe et al., 2024, p. 504). Nonetheless, to make benefits equal it is necessary to consider the digital literacy, availability of the internet, cost-effective, linguistic suitability and cultural sensitivity (Acharya, 2025, p. 7). In the absence of such considerations, the implementation of digital and AI technologies can inadvertently increase instead of mitigating health inequities. Thus, the technological advances should be combined with community education and the development of infrastructures to maximise the achievement of equitable patient outcomes.

4.2 Economic Implications of Technological Adoption

There is a significant potential in long-term efficiency of emerging healthcare technologies, but their initial implementation cost is a critical threshold. The purchase of medical artificial intelligence systems, genomic sequencing systems, and digitally connected diagnostic devices require a lot of capital investment, which can affect the financial stability of healthcare organizations in the short term (Santana et al., 2023, p. 2). In addition to equipment purchase, the use of human resources in this sector, including training of clinicians to operate AI-assisted applications, may also contribute to financial inequalities between healthcare systems globally (McLean, 2023, p. 736).

Lots of Electronic Health Record (EHR) architectures in many health systems are fragmented, which adds extra burdens to them by making their interoperability more difficult to achieve to ensure the use of the AI smoothly. The discrepancies between the data systems inhibit the real-time access to comprehensive patient data, reducing the quality and validity of AI-assisted diagnostics and care planning (Mitera & Harasimowicz, 2024, p. 250). This, therefore, necessitates the need to ensure that a technology ecosystem is financially sustainable, which requires strategic planning, cost-benefit analysis, and the socioeconomic diversity in order to avoid disproportionate implementation of the technology across geographical areas and institutions.

4.3 Navigating the Regulatory Environment for New Technologies

The fast progress in the digital and artificial intelligence-based healthcare has demonstrated that current regulatory frameworks have many gaps, most of which were originally designed to regulate the work of traditional medical devices and pharmaceuticals but not the work of autonomous computing systems (Husnain et al., 2023, p. 1690). To prevent unethical deployment and safeguard the patients, the regulators need to develop dynamic governance systems, which can be flexible to ongoing technological change, including algorithms validation standards, accountability, and post-deployment monitoring (Wani et al., 2023, p. 107880).

One of the primary regulatory issues relates to the so-called black box phenomenon of many high-performance AI systems that produce results without providing a reason that would be interpretable. Both physicians and patients should be required to trust AI prescriptions and, therefore, to promote the use of trust in AI-assisted clinicians, it is crucial to ensure the transparency and explainability of AI-based solutions (Gayap & Akhloufi, 2024, p. 267). Systematic regulatory interventions and solid data governance protocols, in this turn, will be inevitable to guarantee the safe, scalable, and ethically justified introduction of AI technologies into the healthcare ecosystems.

5. CASE STUDIES AND EXAMPLES

Recent trends in the international healthcare sector suggest that the greatest advantages can be achieved through the combination of the emerging technologies and the strict quality control and continuous evaluation of the healthcare performance. Therefore, the governance system is essential to identify and address the bias of the algorithm and, thus, maintain its ability to work across different backgrounds and groups of patients without favoring a certain segment of the population (Aprajita et al., 2025). Ongoing validation based on real-world evidence is also of first importance, because performance metrics can change with time depending on changes in treatment guidelines and acquisition of new clinical knowledge (A Review of Hybrid AI Approaches to NDVI-Based Detection and Classification of Maize Crop Stress and Diseases, 2024, p. 10; Trzmielak et al., 2024, p. 82). This iterative assessment retains the clinical utility and safety of AI tools, which is a requirement especially in fast-changing fields of medicine (Arab and Moosa, 2025, p. 556).

This is even complicated by the heterogeneity of international regulatory regimes. The healthcare developers and institutions have to align the legal expectations that are at variance in terms of data management, algorithm transparency, and system liability, thus obstructing the general uptake (Aldwean & Tenney, 2024, p. 140). These challenges are compounded by the fact that the continuous need to consider explainability even poses a challenge to clinicians, who are still unwilling to rely on AI systems that act as the black boxes and do not explain why they arrived at such conclusions (Gayap & Akhloufi, 2024, p. 267; Kumar, 2025, p. 2; Wani et al., 2023, p. 107880). As such, to be accepted by the clinicians as a clinical decision-support mechanism, interpretability should be part and parcel of the system architecture, and not an afterthought.

5.1 Telemedicine and Rural Healthcare Access

Telemedicine has become one of the key means of ensuring health equity, especially in remote and rural settings with scarce health care resources. Telemedicine, in turn, provides patients with timely care by enabling safe online consultations, regardless of geographic conditions, thus increasing access to quality care significantly (Havlik, 2024, p. 171). Recurring teleconsultations, allowing individuals with chronic illnesses, such as diabetes and cardiovascular, to regularly monitor their health, early diagnose complications, and continue care, will be possible without requiring people to travel far to distant health centers (Khalifa and Hussein, 2025, p. 15).

In addition to the clinical benefits, telemedicine reduces cost implications of low-income families, eliminating transport, housing, and missed employment costs. This in turn makes it possible to manage diseases that have been long-term especially to those people who have a history of uneven access to medical services.

All of these findings describe that digital health platforms, with the right design to be inclusive and easy to use, have a great potential to reduce deep-rooted healthcare disparities.

5.2 AI in Diagnostic Imaging and Workforce Impact

The concept of artificial intelligence has redefined the scope of diagnostic imaging by acting as a high capacity analytical teammate of radiologists and clinical technologists. Artificial intelligence technology can rapidly scan radiographs, computed tomography images, and magnetic resonance images to detect slight anomalies that otherwise may not be detected during human analysis, thus improving the accuracy of diagnosis and preventing medical errors (Sarkar, 2023, p. 2091). The AI is even more useful in those areas where radiology specialists are limited, and thus, using the technology, local clinics can also provide images interpretations at the expert level without having to employ the help of experts on-site (Gayap & Akhloufi, 2024, p. 237).

Additionally, AI solutions significantly relieve the burden of employees. They are also effective at processing large volumes of imaging data, thus eliminating radiological backlogs and decreasing the patient waiting time to result, hence leading to better treatment outcomes (Chassagnon et al., 2022, p. 1). Implementation of AI therefore not only increases the diagnostic skills of the medical staff, but it also supports overloaded systems that are faced with continuous labour deficit (Balakrishnan et al., 2025, p. 29).

5.3 Drug Development Costs vs. Innovation Benefits

The traditional barriers to pharmaceutical innovation are the cost of research and development, length of discovery process, and high regulatory standards. The AIs pinpointed in the drug discovery systems are changing this face by using biological data to generate potentially promising drug candidates, predicting potential toxicity, and simplifying trial design stages, as quickly as possible (Balakrishnan et al., 2025). Such acceleration also considerably saves on money and time-to-market making life-saving drugs available to patients earlier than in traditional approaches (Zeb et al., 2024).

Artificial intelligence is particularly effective in biomedical innovation acceleration, particularly in the field of oncology. As one example, deep learning solutions have made lung cancer diagnosis and treatment possible in earlier stages when treatment is more effective (Chassagnon et al., 2022, p. 1).

6. FUTURE DIRECTIONS AND POLICY IMPLICATIONS

The next generation of policy efforts should be proactive and uniform to lead to safe, equitable, and scalable integration of artificial intelligence into health systems worldwide as artificial intelligence becomes an indispensable part of the healthcare industry. At the core of this work is the implementation of interoperability models that would allow AI tools to communicate with various electronic health records platforms and clinical information systems without violating patient privacy and continuity of care (Mitera and Harasimowicz, 2024, p. 249; Tippur, 2023, p. 6). In addition to interoperability, reinforcing digital infrastructure to enable federated learning is important since it will allow models to be trained on distributed datasets, which are found in different institutions and will reduce the exposure of sensitive patient information and will increase the volume of datasets (Nguyen, 2024, p. 100154).

The technical and ethical consequences of integrating big size and multi-source clinical data, such as genomics, imaging data sets, and real-world evidence based on wearable devices and remote patient monitoring systems, should also be covered in the future AI strategies (Gu et al., 2022, p. 3). This integration will necessitate sophisticated data governance systems determining the owner rights, giving transparent monitoring, and controlling the ethical reuse of health data in the creation of AI (Santhosh, 2024, p. 1582; Zeb et al., 2024, p. 126).

It is also necessary to create regulatory avenues that will allow keeping up with the fast development of AI. Specialized frameworks like regulatory models of software as a medical device (SaMD) offer a framework that defines how to organize approval processes along with defining the issue of liability in cases where AI determines the medical choice (Spear et al., 2023, p. 2).The end result will be the successful AI implementation in healthcare under the condition of encouraging innovation without jeopardising patient safety, transparency, and social trust..

6.1 Strategies for Equitable Technology Integration

It is important to make sure that the implementation of artificial intelligence will not reinforce the already existing healthcare disparities to make it feasible in the long term. The fair use of technology presupposes the specific properties of investing in digital infrastructure, training activities, and workforce in rural areas and resource-scarce regions to reduce the inequality in institutional preparedness (Nguyen, 2024, p. 100154). Local knowledge and personalisation of the algorithms to the population demographics, culture, and epidemiology can be fostered by creating regional hubs or AI competency centres (Fahim et al., 2025, p. 17).

Through joint ventures, between healthcare providers, state agencies, academic investigators, and even individual technology creators, the implementation of context-specific AI solutions, tailored to the specific needs of underserved communities, may proceed more quickly, instead of failing to address all challenges with generic, one-size-fits-all solutions (Najjar, 2024, p. 19).

This kind of multi-stakeholder, cooperative strategy does not only democratize access to healthcare innovation but it also ensures that AI strengthens equity, inclusiveness, and better clinical outcomes regardless of geography and socioeconomic status.

6.2 Balancing Innovation with Cost-Effectiveness

Artificial intelligence integration has potential in triggering the radically improved healthcare provisions though the policy initiatives should integrate the elements of affordability in the long run to ensure that the applications are universal and sustainable. Strict health-economic evaluations are required to determine that AI interventions provide tangible patient outcomes, operational efficiencies, and resources allocation that are capable of justifying the high costs of deployment and maintenance (Fahim et al., 2025, p. 17).

The international data-governance agreements will be critical in aligning ethical principles, working across international borders to address health data, and prevent the accumulation of technological benefits and capabilities in a set of regions or health systems (Fahim et al., 2025, p. 17). These contracts are especially relevant because the formation of AI depends not only on the large, heterogeneous, and high-quality data but also on the fact that they can be difficult to gather independently by low-income nations (A Review of Hybrid AI Approaches to NDVI-Based Detection and Classification of Maize Crop Stress and Diseases, 2024, p. 7). Lastly, the augmentation of the interpretability of algorithms is a critical aspect of clinical acceptance. Physician confidence, shared decision-making, and reducing institutional concerns about opaque black-box decisions are supported using transparent, human-readable models of AI in sensitive medical settings (Gayap & Akhloufi, 2024, p. 267). By focusing on the ethical design and explainability, policymakers can adjust innovation to human-centred care.

7. ETHICAL FRAMEWORKS FOR EMERGING TECHNOLOGIES

The urgent necessity to develop a thorough set of ethical principles addressing the well-being of patients, their trust in the system, and responsible innovation can be highlighted by the blistering growth of the sphere of artificial intelligence in healthcare. The key ethical aspects, including accountability, privacy, transparency, and fairness, are to be integrated in each step of AI development and implementation to guarantee the compatibility with the values of the population and the standards of professional healthcare provisions (Horgan et al., 2019, p. 151; Jha et al., 2023, p. 12). Along with the fact that the AI tools are often based on large datasets that represent a wide range of people, the protection against the bias of the algorithm becomes essential. Otherwise, bias may unwillingly contribute to structural health disparities, especially when applied to the demographic subgroups under marginalization (Adibi et al., 2025, p. 29).

Thus, ethical standards need to include clear specifications on how bias can be detected, measured, and addressed in the entire lifecycle of AI, including curation of datasets and training of models as well as their use in the clinic. To identify the bias that can be exhibited over time as the disease patterns, clinical procedures, and population trends change, constant algorithm monitoring and regular reevaluation with newly obtained data are essential (Zhang, 2023, p. 245). Modern ethical principles, including those advocated by the European policy of trustworthy AI, prioritize the following principles, including the human agency and control, technical soundness and safety, openness, inclusivity, and societal good, which make sure that AI supplements, as opposed to substituting, clinical decision-making (Hobbs, 2020, p. 57). These values support the importance of having significant human control over AI-based decision-making, considering that medical decisions usually contain certain contextual depth that cannot be explained by computational analysis.

To make these ethical principles operational, the scholars have suggested that the AI systems engaged in instances of fundamental rights, life-changing medical choices, or patient protection be mandated to perform an impact assessment (Hobbs, 2020, p. 57). This evaluation should also include not only algorithmic performance and explainability, but also possible downstream impacts, such as differences in the accuracy of particular demographic subgroups, the risk of harm to patients, and potential medical liability implications. Additionally, ethical frameworks are also supposed to be dynamic and ongoing which makes sense to change with the development of technology so that the implementation of AI in healthcare facilities can be safe, fair and trustworthy.

8. CONCLUSION

Artificial intelligence implementation in the healthcare field is one of the most radical changes in modern medicine, which has provided unprecedented possibilities to improve the accuracy of diagnoses, diversify treatment regimens, and streamline healthcare processes (Goktas' & ' Grzybowski, 2025). However, to harness the capabilities of AI, it would be essential to have a multidisciplinary approach to deal with such underlying issues as medico-legal uncertainty, ethical complexity, regulatory ambiguity, and unequal access to technological solutions (Jeyaraman et al., 2023; Udegbe et al., 2024, p. 506).

In order to facilitate equal distribution of AI benefits, policymakers, researchers, system developers, and clinical practitioners should work together to build strong regulatory mechanisms, enhance transparency, and enable equal distribution of AI benefits to the populations. A pressing focus is related to the issue of explainability in AI decision-making; explicit interpretability is expected to increase the trustworthiness of clinicians in algorithmic recommendations, and patients may not be eager to involve themselves in the AI-assisted intervention (Jha et al., 2023, p. 14 , 2025). Clinical trust, usability, and ethical adoption of new tools in routine care can be supported by empowering healthcare professionals and engaging them in AI co-design processes, empowerment through education, and solving the issues.

In addition to enhancing the transparency of the model, AI governance should focus on long-term post-deployment monitoring to reduce the likelihood of bias drift, data drift, and shift in epidemiological patterns (Chinta et al., 2024, p. 21). Artificial intelligence technologies are also difficult to keep the performance objective fair among various demographics and socioeconomic populations, and this requires constant monitoring and re-tuning. The next stage of AI in healthcare, therefore, cannot be viewed as the logical continuation of algorithmic complexity, but as a combination of technological representation and ethical accountability, clinical skill, and the trustworthiness the society is ready to assign. AI can be the basis of fair, safe, and patient-centred care on a global scale through a careful design, open and decentralized governance, and the joint effort of implementation.

REFERENCES

Acharya, V. (2025). Intelligent Healthcare Ecosystems: Optimizing the Iron Triangle of Healthcare (Access, Cost, Quality). *arXiv (Cornell University)*. https://doi.org// arxiv.2510.03331DOI: 10.48550

Adelson, P. D., Bratton, S. L., Carney, N., Chesnut, R. M., du Coudray, H. E. M., Goldstein, B., Kochanek, P. M., Miller, H. C., Partington, M. D., Selden, N. R., Warden, C. R., & Wright, D. W. (2003). Chapter 1: Introduction. *Pediatric Critical Care Medicine, 4*(SUPPLEMENT), S2–S4. Advance online publication. DOI: 10.1097/01.CCM.0000066600.71233.01 PMID: 12847337

Adibi, A., Xu, C., Ji, Z., Kaur, J., Chen, W., Healey, E., Nuwagira, B., Ye, W., Woollard, G., Xu, M., Cui, H. T., Xi, J., Chang, T., Bikia, V., Zhang, N., Noori, A., Yuan, X., & Hossain, Md. B., Frank, H. A., … Jabbour, S. (2025). Recent Advances, Applications and Open Challenges in Machine Learning for Health: Reflections from Research Roundtables at ML4H 2024 Symposium. *arXiv (Cornell University)*. DOI: 10.48550/arxiv.2502.06693

Ahmed, M. M., Okesanya, O. J., Olaleke, N. O., Adigun, O. A., Adebayo, U. O., Oso, T. A., Eshun, G., & Lucero-Prisno, D. E. (2025). Integrating Digital Health Innovations to Achieve Universal Health Coverage: Promoting Health Outcomes and Quality Through Global Public Health Equity [Review of *Integrating Digital Health Innovations to Achieve Universal Health Coverage: Promoting Health Outcomes and Quality Through Global Public Health Equity*]. *Healthcare, 13*(9), 1060. Multidisciplinary Digital Publishing Institute. DOI: 10.3390/healthcare13091060

Aldwean, A., & Tenney, D. (2024). Artificial Intelligence in Healthcare Sector: A Literature Review of the Adoption Challenges [Review of *Artificial Intelligence in Healthcare Sector: A Literature Review of the Adoption Challenges*]. *Open Journal of Business and Management, 12*(1), 129. Scientific Research Publishing. DOI: 10.4236/ojbm.2024.121009

Ansari, M. M., Kumar, S., Chola, C., Heyat, M. B. B., Akhtar, F., Hayat, M. A. B., Sayeed, E., Parveen, S., Abbasi, R., & Pomary, D. (2025). A Novel Machine and Deep Learning–Based Ensemble Techniques for Automatic Lung Cancer Detection. *BioMed Research International, 2025*(1). DOI: 10.1155/bmri/6666688

Aprajita, K., Capucine, B., Ganash, T., & Jasper, T. (2025). *Responsible, safe, and inclusive AI for sustainable development in health in Southeast Asia*. DOI: 10.53832/ evidence-fund.0006

Arab, R. A. E., & Moosa, O. A. A. (2025). Systematic review of cost effectiveness and budget impact of artificial intelligence in healthcare. *NPJ Digital Medicine*, *8*(1), 548. DOI: 10.1038/s41746-025-01722-y PMID: 40858882

Arab, R. A. E., Moosa, O. A. A., & Sagbakken, M. (2025). Economic, ethical, and regulatory dimensions of artificial intelligence in healthcare: an integrative review [Review of *Economic, ethical, and regulatory dimensions of artificial intelligence in healthcare: an integrative review*]. *Frontiers in Public Health, 13*, 1617138. Frontiers Media. https://doi.org/DOI: 10.3389/fpubh.2025.1617138

Artuso, F., & Guijt, I. (2020). *Global Megatrends: Mapping the forces that affect us all*. DOI: 10.21201/2020.5648

Balakrishnan, K., Velusamy, D., Hinkle, H. E., Li, Z., Ramasamy, K., Khan, H. U., Ramaswamy, S., & Shah, P. (2025). Artificial Intelligence in Rural Healthcare Delivery: Bridging Gaps and Enhancing Equity through Innovation. *arXiv (Cornell University)*. https://doi.org//arxiv.2508.11738DOI: 10.48550

Burrell, D. N. (2023). Dynamic Evaluation Approaches to Telehealth Technologies and Artificial Intelligence (AI) Telemedicine Applications in Healthcare and Biotechnology Organizations. *Merits*, *3*(4), 700–721. DOI: 10.3390/merits3040042

Chassagnon, G., Margerie-Mellon, C. de, Vakalopoulou, M., Marini, R., Hoang-Thi, T.-N., Revel, M., & Soyer, P. (2022). Artificial intelligence in lung cancer: current applications and perspectives [Review of *Artificial intelligence in lung cancer: current applications and perspectives*]. *Japanese Journal of Radiology*. Springer Science+Business Media. DOI: 10.1007/s11604-022-01359-x

Chinta, S. V., Wang, Z., Zhang, X., Viet, T. D., Kashif, A., Smith, M. A., & Zhang, W. (2024). AI-Driven Healthcare: A Survey on Ensuring Fairness and Mitigating Bias. *arXiv (Cornell University)*. https://doi.org//arxiv.2407.19655DOI: 10.48550

DosSantos, P., & de Oliveira, S. B. (2020). A Financial Theory Perspective of the Metrics Employed to Measure Value in the "Value in Healthcare" Methodologies. *Portuguese Journal of Public Health*, *38*(3), 176–186. DOI: 10.1159/000512564

Dunker, A. K. (1998). The pacific symposium on biocomputing. *Journal of Molecular Graphics & Modelling*, *16*(4-6), 267. DOI: 10.1016/S1093-3263(98)80012-0

Fahim, Y. A., Hasani, I. W., Kabba, S., & Ragab, W. M. (2025). Artificial intelligence in healthcare and medicine: clinical applications, therapeutic advances, and future perspectives [Review of *Artificial intelligence in healthcare and medicine: clinical applications, therapeutic advances, and future perspectives*]. *European Journal of Medical Research, 30*(1). BioMed Central. DOI: 10.1186/s40001-025-03196-w

Fendrick, A. M., Bagley, N., & Bonavitacola, J. (2023). Michigan Professors Offer Insights Into What Braidwood Ruling Could Mean for Preventive Screening in Cancer Care. *The American Journal of Managed Care*, *29*(Spec. No. 5), SP353–SP354. Advance online publication. DOI: 10.37765/ajmc.2023.89392 PMID: 37341474

Gayap, H. T., & Akhloufi, M. A. (2024). Deep Machine Learning for Medical Diagnosis, Application to Lung Cancer Detection: A Review [Review of Deep Machine Learning for Medical Diagnosis, Application to Lung Cancer Detection: A Review]. *BioMedInformatics*, *4*(1), 236–284. DOI: 10.3390/biomedinformatics4010015

Gu, C., Dai, C., Shi, X., Wu, Z., & Chen, C. (2022). *1-s2.0-S2452414X22000541-main.pdf.*

Hassan, A., Khan, H., Ali, A., Din, I. U., Sajid, A., Husain, M., Ali, M., Naz, A., & Fakhar, H. (2024). An Enhanced Lung Cancer Identification and Classification Based on Advanced Deep Learning and Convolutional Neural Network. [BBE]. *Bulletin of Business and Economics*, *13*(2), 136–141. DOI: 10.61506/01.00308

Havlik, D. (2024). TELEMEDICINE AND RURAL HEALTHCARE ACCESS: A COMPARATIVE ANALYSIS OF EMERGING TECHNOLOGIES. *Journal of Population Therapeutics and Clinical Pharmacology = Journal de la Thérapeutique des Populations et de la Pharmacologie Clinique*, *169*, 169–179. Advance online publication. DOI: 10.53555/37d41t64

Hobbs, C. (2020). *EUROPE'S DIGITAL SOVEREIGNTY: FROM RULEMAKER TO SUPERPOWER IN THE AGE OF US-CHINA RIVALRY.*

Horgan, D., Romao, M., Morré, S. A., & Kalra, D. (2019). Artificial Intelligence: Power for Civilisation – and for Better Healthcare. *Public Health Genomics*, *22*(5-6), 145–161. DOI: 10.1159/000504785 PMID: 31838476

Husnain, A., Rasool, S., Saeed, A., Gill, A. Y., & Hussain, H. K. (2023). AI'S Healing Touch: Examining Machine Learning's Transformative Effects On Healthcare. *Journal of Wood Science*, *2*(10), 1681–1695. DOI: 10.58344/jws.v2i10.448

Jeyaraman, M., Balaji, S., Jeyaraman, N., & Yadav, S. (2023). Unraveling the Ethical Enigma: Artificial Intelligence in Healthcare [Review of *Unraveling the Ethical Enigma: Artificial Intelligence in Healthcare*]. *Cureus*. Cureus, Inc. DOI: 10.7759/cureus.43262

Jha, D., Durak, G., Sharma, V., Keleş, E., Çiçek, V., Zhang, Z., Srivastava, A., Rauniyar, A., Hagos, D. H., Tomar, N. K., Miller, F. H., Topcu, A. E., Yazidi, A., Håkegård, J. E., & Bağcı, U. (2025). A Conceptual Framework for Applying Ethical Principles of AI to Medical Practice. *Bioengineering (Basel, Switzerland)*, *12*(2), 180. DOI: 10.3390/bioengineering12020180 PMID: 40001699

Jha, D., Rauniyar, A., Srivastava, A., Hagos, D. H., Tomar, N. K., Sharma, V., Keleş, E., Zhang, Z., Demir, U., Topcu, A. E., Yazidi, A., Håakegård, J. E., & Bağcı, U. (2023). A Conceptual Algorithm for Applying Ethical Principles of AI to Medical Practice. *arXiv (Cornell University)*. https://doi.org//arxiv.2304.11530DOI: 10.48550

Khalifa, A., & Hussein, R. (2025). Artificial Intelligence For 6P Medicine: Consolidating AI Needs of Predictive, Preventive, Personalized, Participatory, Precision, and Public Health Trajectories. Research Square *(*Research Square*)*. DOI: 10.21203/rs.3.rs-7402571/v1

Khan, R. H., Miah, J., Nipun, S. A. A., Islam, M., Amin, M. S., & Taluckder, M. S. (2023). Enhancing Lung Cancer Diagnosis with Machine Learning Methods and Systematic Review Synthesis. *2021 7th International Conference on Electrical, Electronics and Information Engineering (ICEEIE)*, 1. DOI: 10.1109/ICEEIE59078.2023.10334739

Kumar, S. (2025). Patient-centered AI. *Frontiers in Digital Health*, *7*, 1638098. Advance online publication. DOI: 10.3389/fdgth.2025.1638098 PMID: 40881731

Liu, B., Zhou, H., Tan, L., Siu, K. T. H., & Guan, X. (2024). Exploring treatment options in cancer: tumor treatment strategies [Review of *Exploring treatment options in cancer: tumor treatment strategies*]. *Signal Transduction and Targeted Therapy, 9*(1), 175. Springer Nature. DOI: 10.1038/s41392-024-01856-7

Mahara, G., Tian, C., Xu, X., & Wang, W. (2023). Revolutionising health care: Exploring the latest advances in medical sciences. *Journal of Global Health*, *13*, 03042. Advance online publication. DOI: 10.7189/jogh.13.03042 PMID: 37539846

Mahendrakar, N. (2025). Adopting Technologies in Medical and Healthcare Systems. *International Journal for Research in Applied Science and Engineering Technology*, *13*(7), 1997–2009. DOI: 10.22214/ijraset.2025.73297

McLean, A. L. (2023, July 14). Towards Precision Medicine in Spinal Surgery: Leveraging AI Technologies. In *Annals of Biomedical Engineering* (Vol. 52, Issue 4, p. 735). Springer Science+Business Media. DOI: 10.1007/s10439-023-03315-w

Mitera, B., & Harasimowicz, K. (2024). Balancing Act: The Dual Impacts of AI and Healthcare Algorithms on Patient Welfare in Telemedicine. *European Research Studies, 243*(2), 243–254. Advance online publication. DOI: 10.35808/ersj/3400

Najjar, R. (2024). Digital Frontiers in Healthcare: Integrating mHealth, AI, and Radiology for Future Medical Diagnostics. In *Biomedical engineering*. DOI: 10.5772/intechopen.114142

Nguyen, M. (2024). A scoping review of deep learning approaches for lung cancer detection using chest radiographs and computed tomography scans [Review of *A scoping review of deep learning approaches for lung cancer detection using chest radiographs and computed tomography scans*]. *Biomedical Engineering Advances, 9*, 100138. Elsevier BV. DOI: 10.1016/j.bea.2024.100138

Ogbewele, E. G., Mbata, A. O., & Nwosu, N. T. (2024). Advancing pharmaceutical care in rural and underserved communities: Strategies for improving global healthcare access. *International Journal of Applied Research in Social Sciences, 6*(10), 2447–2461. DOI: 10.51594/ijarss.v6i10.1641

Patria, D. G., & Ram, B. (2024). AI and Machine Learning in Biotechnology: A Paradigm Shift in Biochemical Innovation. *International Journal of Plant Animal and Environmental Sciences, 14*(4). Advance online publication. DOI: 10.26502/ijpaes.4490166

Rawat, D., Sharma, S., & Bhadula, S. (2023). Deep Learning Techniques in Digital Clinical Diagnostic System for Lung Cancer. *2022 8th International Conference on Advanced Computing and Communication Systems (ICACCS)*, 1232. DOI: 10.1109/ICACCS57279.2023.10113055

SAINI. (2025). Accelerating Drug Discovery: How Agentic AI and Multi-Agent Collaboration Transform BioPharma R&D. *Journal of Information Systems Engineering & Management, 10*(59s), 545–553. DOI: 10.52783/jisem.v10i59s.12898

Santana, G. O., Couto, R. de M., Loureiro, R. M., Silva, B. C. R., Rother, E. T., Paiva, J. P. Q. de, & Correia, L. R. (2023). Economic Evaluations and Equity in the Use of Artificial Intelligence in Imaging Exams for Medical Diagnosis in People With Skin, Neurological, and Pulmonary Diseases: Protocol for a Systematic Review [Review of *Economic Evaluations and Equity in the Use of Artificial Intelligence in Imaging Exams for Medical Diagnosis in People With Skin, Neurological, and Pulmonary Diseases: Protocol for a Systematic Review*]. *JMIR Research Protocols, 12*. JMIR Publications. DOI: 10.2196/48544

Santhosh, C. S. (2024). Revolutionizing Healthcare: The Transformative Power of Artificial Intelligence. *International Journal for Research in Applied Science and Engineering Technology*, *12*(5), 1581–1586. DOI: 10.22214/ijraset.2024.61755

SARIYILDIZ, A. Y. (2022). New Approaches to Healthcare Marketing. *DergiPark (Istanbul University)*. https://dergipark.org.tr/tr/pub/ssd/issue/72835/1143346

Sarkar, A. (2023). The Impact and Potential of Artificial Intelligence in Healthcare: A Critical Review of Current Applications and Future Directions [Review of *The Impact and Potential of Artificial Intelligence in Healthcare: A Critical Review of Current Applications and Future Directions*]. *International Journal for Research in Applied Science and Engineering Technology, 11*(8), 2089. [IJRASET]. *International Journal for Research in Applied Science and Engineering Technology*. Advance online publication. DOI: 10.22214/ijraset.2023.55537

Singhal, V., Shyam, R., Singhal, S., Tiwari, A., & Mangal, D. (2025). Healthcare and cutting-edge technology: Advancements, challenges, and future prospects. [Review of *Healthcare and cutting-edge technology: Advancements, challenges, and future prospects.*]. *PubMed, 196*, 110861. National Institutes of Health. DOI: 10.1016/j.compbiomed.2025.110861

Sinha, R. K. (2024). The role and impact of new technologies on healthcare systems. *Discover Health Systems*, *3*(1), 96. Advance online publication. DOI: 10.1007/s44250-024-00163-w

Spear, J., Ehrenfeld, J. M., & Miller, B. J. (2023, November 17). Applications of Artificial Intelligence in Health Care Delivery. In *Journal of Medical Systems* (Vol. 47, Issue 1). Springer Science+Business Media. DOI: 10.1007/s10916-023-02018-y

Tippur, A. (2023). AI-Powered Precision Oncology: Computational Insights Redefining Therapeutic Landscapes. *DHR Proceedings*. DOI: 10.47488/dhrp.v3iS1.95

Trzmielak, D., Lipka-Matusiak, I., & Oftedal, E. M. (2024). Responsible Innovation in E-Health Care: Empowering Patients with Emerging Technologies. *Marketing of Scientific and Research Organizations*, *52*(2), 68–87. DOI: 10.2478/minib-2024-0010

Udegbe, F. C., Ebulue, O. R., Ebulue, C. C., & Ekesiobi, C. S. (2024). The Role of Artificial Intelligence in Healthcare: A Systematic Review of Applications and Challenges [Review Of *The Role Of Artificial Intelligence In Healthcare: A Systematic Review Of Applications And Challenges*]. *International Medical Science Research Journal, 4*(4), 500. Fair East Publishers. DOI: 10.51594/imsrj.v4i4.1052

Vats, K. (2024). Navigating the Digital Landscape: Embracing Innovation, Addressing Challenges, and Prioritizing Patient-Centric Care. *Cureus*. Advance online publication. DOI: 10.7759/cureus.58352 PMID: 38756283

Wang, J., Haq, A. U., Afzal, N., Khan, S., Alsolai, H., Alanazi, S. M., & Zamani, A. T. (2025). Developing an innovative lung cancer detection model for accurate diagnosis in AI healthcare systems. *Scientific Reports*, *15*(1), 22945. Advance online publication. DOI: 10.1038/s41598-025-03960-2 PMID: 40592932

Wani, N. A., Kumar, R., & Bedi, J. (2023). DeepXplainer: An interpretable deep learning based approach for lung cancer detection using explainable artificial intelligence. *Computer Methods and Programs in Biomedicine*, *243*, 107879. DOI: 10.1016/j.cmpb.2023.107879 PMID: 37897989

Zahidi, K., Obtel, M., & Naji, S. (2024). Healthcare Accessibility: Metrics, Assessment, Policies, and Barriers. In *IntechOpen eBooks*. IntechOpen. DOI: 10.5772/intechopen.1006821

Zeb, S., Fnu, N., Abbasi, N., & Fahad, M. (2024). AI in Healthcare: Revolutionizing Diagnosis and Therapy. *International Journal of Multidisciplinary Sciences and Arts*, *3*(3), 118–128. DOI: 10.47709/ijmdsa.v3i3.4546

Zhang, S. (2023). Artificial Intelligence and Applications in Structural and Material Engineering. *Highlights in Science Engineering and Technology*, *75*, 240–245. DOI: 10.54097/9qknfc57

Chapter 7
Policy for Regulating the Implementation and Use of Artificial Intelligence in Medicine

Revaz Gvelesiani
Ivane Javakhishvili Tbilisi State University, Georgia

Irina Gogorishvili
Ivane Javakhishvili Tbilisi State University, Georgia

ABSTRACT

The advent of artificial intelligence has changed a lot. One of the main advantages of this technology is its ability to process large volumes of data. Machine learning allows you to identify patterns and predictions that are not impossible for humans to make, but require a lot of energy, financial resources, and time. In medicine, artificial intelligence can analyze large volumes of information, including medical images, with high accuracy to support early disease diagnosis. The use of artificial intelligence in healthcare is a rapidly growing, powerful, and promising process. This technology, as a successful tool for implementing healthcare policy, has significant potential to ease the work of all healthcare workers significantly. At the same time, its implementation requires a responsible, ethical, and balanced approach that recognizes that artificial intelligence technology does not replace the human mind, its creativity, or its intuition. By using this technology, people use resources, which is a key component of sustainable development.

DOI: 10.4018/979-8-2600-0939-0.ch007

1. INTRODUCTION

The advent of artificial intelligence has changed many things. One of the main advantages of this technology is its ability to process large volumes of data. Machine learning enables the identification of patterns and the making of predictions that are not impossible for humans, but require significant energy, financial resources, and time. In medicine, artificial intelligence can analyze large volumes of information, including medical images, with high accuracy to support early disease diagnosis. Furthermore, artificial intelligence can accelerate research and assist medical personnel in disease prevention. Artificial intelligence already plays a significant role alongside humans (though not everywhere or always) in forecasting and making innovative medical decisions. The implementation and proper use of this technology open new possibilities in medicine, improving the quality of life and enhancing work efficiency. At the same time, the implementation and use of artificial intelligence is spreading across all spheres of human activity. It is ubiquitous and rapidly integrating into our lives, which is already creating (and will continue to create) several problems and challenges. It is especially important to gain insight into and analyze these issues in small, open economies that face shortages of capital and skilled labor.

One of the most serious ethical concerns is that machine learning algorithms can reflect and amplify existing biases and discrimination inherent in the data on which they are trained. The automation of work processes driven by artificial intelligence could lead to mass unemployment and social instability, necessitating carefully considered public policy. Artificial intelligence is also generating debate in the academic healthcare community. It can be a useful tool for generating projects, exploring ideas, and structuring thoughts, but the results must be imbued with personal reflection. Critical thinking, fact-checking, and introspection remain integral to intellectual work. Currently, artificial intelligence serves as an auxiliary tool: it helps improve style, correct grammar, and find precise wording, but it does not replace the creative process. Artificial intelligence can certainly replace human knowledge, but it will never replace human creative thinking. The widespread use of artificial intelligence is precisely the phygitalization of our lives.

It is currently expected that by the end of 2026, completely new IT technologies will enter the global market. For example, a new generation of scanners has emerged in military operations. They visualize the movement of objects and processes within confined spaces using artificial intelligence. The emergence of new technological products will likely lead to instability in the supply chain for products manufactured with legacy technologies, as well as regional pressures, requiring special attention and preparedness from economic policymakers.

According to a study by Precedence Research, approximately 8 out of 10 companies in the life sciences sector are increasingly implementing and using artificial intelligence. Furthermore, according to the same study, various pharmaceutical and medical device companies are implementing advanced automation to handle approximately 75-85% of their work processes. The use of artificial intelligence in healthcare is a rapidly growing, powerful, and promising process. This technology, as a successful tool for implementing healthcare policy, has significant potential to significantly facilitate the work of all healthcare workers. At the same time, its implementation requires a responsible, ethical, and balanced approach that recognizes that AI technology does not replace human intelligence, creativity, and intuition. By using this technology, people (both medical staff and patients) conserve resources, which is a key component of sustainable development. However, the availability of capital, labor, and natural resources varies significantly across countries (Gigauri & Djakeli, 2021a).

North America, Western Europe, and Australia are the most prepared to implement AI in healthcare. These regions have more developed digital infrastructure, stronger research capacity, and more robust AI policies. Developing regions in many countries across Africa, South America, and Central Asia are less prepared to implement AI and other digital technologies in healthcare, given their current capabilities. This is due to the generally unsatisfactory level of digital infrastructure development, as well as significant challenges in disseminating AI across policy and education. The goal of this work is to identify and characterize highly promising areas of AI systems and policies for implementation in medicine (Mordor Intelligence, 2024).

2. DIRECTIONS OF APPLICATION OF AI IN MEDICINE

The map of the Artificial Intelligence Readiness Index reveals a significant global gap in readiness for its use, which largely corresponds to the existing economic and technological inequality. At the same time, it is worth noting that among the areas of application of generative artificial intelligence in health care, medical visualization currently dominates (IBM, 2025).

The global market for artificial intelligence in medical imaging will grow rapidly, reaching almost 22.97 trillion US dollars by 2034, compared to 2.01 trillion US dollars in 2025. The growth is driven by increased demand for early disease diagnosis and the automation of radiology workflows. The increase in imaging volumes, the growing prevalence of chronic diseases, and the shortage of radiologists are accelerating the adoption of AI in CT, MRI, radiography, and ultrasound diagnostics. AI provides faster, more accurate diagnostics, increases the efficiency of work processes, and reduces clinical workload, positioning itself as the most important technology shaping the future of diagnostic healthcare worldwide (GlobeNewswire, 2026).

The growing demand for early diagnosis of cancer, cardiovascular diseases, neurological disorders, and diseases of the respiratory system — which together account for more than 70% of deaths in the world — continues to stimulate the introduction of AI. At the same time, medical institutions use AI to manage the growing volume of scanning and reduce the global shortage of radiologists, which is 30-40% (Precedence Research, 2025).

The growth in the use of artificial intelligence in the medical imaging industry is also driven by the rising prevalence of chronic diseases, the push for earlier diagnosis, the development of personalized medicine, the need to automate routine medical tasks, and the desire to reduce the burden on radiologists.

Artificial intelligence in medical visualization is the use of computer algorithms to enable efficient and accurate disease diagnosis. AI minimizes scanning time and easily recognizes complex patterns in magnetic resonance imaging (MRI), X-ray images, and computed tomography (CT). Artificial intelligence helps detect diseases early and develop personalized treatment plans for patients. AI in medical visualization offers advantages such as early disease detection, improved planning of surgical interventions, automated image segmentation, and increased accuracy and reduced human error.

Factors affecting the market and economic impact:

- Growth in the volume of diagnostic studies: more than 5 billion studies per year, growth rates of 6–7% per year;
- Automation of working processes: AI reduces the time by 30-50%.
- Economic efficiency: Improved scanner use and reduced repeat scans increase the profitability of medical institutions' investments.
- Cost recovery optimization: higher throughput and improved diagnostic accuracy support results-oriented care delivery models.

The key growth factors are:

- Early diagnosis of diseases. burden of chronic diseases (70% of deaths in the world), automation of work processes, and precision medicine;
- Level of clinical implementation. Image analysis with AI is used in more than 45% of stroke and lung disease visualization processes in developed markets.
- Technological superiority. Deep learning occupies 48% of the market, increasing diagnostic accuracy by 20–30% when processing large volumes of images.
- Explainable Growth AI. The XAI market is growing at approximately 30% per year, driven by regulatory transparency and clinical trial requirements. Mordor Intelligence

3. DEPLOYMENT SPLITTING

Hybrid systems combine on-premises servers and clouds (e.g., Veeam Cloud Connect, VDI), optimizing costs and ensuring data protection compliance. Key services include the Google Cloud Healthcare API, Microsoft Cloud for Healthcare, and telemedicine platforms such as Zoom(Gabelaia et al.,2024)

Hybrid clouds: Used to meet strict regulatory requirements by storing sensitive data locally and less critical data in the public cloud. The Google Cloud Healthcare API provides AI tools for data analysis and improved patient outcomes. The SaaS (software as a service) model eliminates the need for capital investments in on-premises servers. Popular solutions on the market today include MTS Web Services Infrastructure, Cloud4Y, and Oxygen, as well as specialized software such as 3D4Medical (training/diagnostics) and VisualDx (diagnostics) (Wheatley, 2022).

On-premises solutions are the most common. (58%), cloud and hybrid solutions (28%), and edge/embedded solutions (14%).

Edge AI performance improvements reduce image processing latency by 40–60% in emergencies. What is edge AI?

The combined share of CT imaging methods is 37%, MRI 26%, and X-ray and ultrasound 30%. MRI efficiency is improving and increasing. Artificial intelligence reduces MRI scan times by 25–50%, increasing the throughput of clinics and treatment centers.

In oncology research, image analysis accounts for 51% of the market, and segmentation accuracy has improved by more than 90%. Software accounts for 77% of the IT product usage, while AI-enabled hardware accounts for 23%, with hardware growth at approximately 28% per year.

End users are primarily hospitals (65%). Diagnostic imaging centers (22%) and research and academic institutions (13%).

Today, the fastest-growing end user is diagnostic imaging centers, growing at 28.90% annually, undoubtedly driven by the development of outpatient diagnostics.

In 2025, North America led the market (with a 45% share), as evidenced by the highest per capita utilization of diagnostic services. Meanwhile, the Asia-Pacific region is the fastest-growing region from 2026 to 2035, with a CAGR of 30.80%. An aging population and smart hospital initiatives drive this. The Chinese market is growing each year. The healthcare industry accounts for over 35% of growth in the Asia-Pacific region, driven by government policy support for artificial intelligence. Significantly, over the past five years, AI startups in imaging have attracted more than $3 billion in private investment.

Regulatory approvals accelerate adoption. Over 700 AI-based medical imaging algorithms have received approval worldwide from agencies such as the US FDA,

European CE bodies, and China's NMPA. Growing attention to explainable AI (XAI) promotes regulatory transparency, physician trust, and ethical implementation.

Artificial intelligence is moving from decision support to clinical assistant, becoming a key diagnostic infrastructure. AI applications in medical imaging have the following characteristics:

- Lung imaging dominated clinical practice (22% share, 2025);
- Oncology became the fastest-growing segment (30.20% CAGR).
- Deep learning remains a key technology (48% market share, 2025), while explainable AI is gaining momentum (30% CAGR).
- On-premises deployments held the largest share (58% in 2025), but AI development at the network edge and in embedded systems is rapidly accelerating (30.80% CAGR);
- Cloud adoption continues to grow.
- Computed tomography (CT) has a high market share (37%, 2025), while magnetic resonance imaging (MRI) is expected to grow significantly (~30% annually).
- Image analysis is the dominant function (51% market share), enabling automation and increased diagnostic accuracy;
- Software solutions account for the majority of revenue (77% in 2025), with AI-enabled hardware gaining popularity.
- Hospitals remain the primary end users (65% share), while diagnostic imaging centers are expanding the fastest (CAGR of 28.90%). Market Medical Reshapes AI in the Imaging Industry. FIME by Report
- Risks and limitations of generative AI may include the following:
- High initial integration costs;
- Data bias and model generalization issues;
- Compatibility issues with legacy systems;
- Data privacy and cybersecurity risks under HIPAA and GDPR;
- Regulatory framework and compliance landscape.

Regional Leadership (2025). North America accounts for 45% of the market share.

4. PRIVATE INVESTMENTS IN HEALTHCARE AI FOR MEDICAL IMAGING

The following products and companies using them stand out in this area:

Aidoc is an enterprise platform built on AI (iOS) for medical image analysis (CT, X-ray, MRI). It identifies critical indicators, such as strokes and pulmonary embolisms, and alerts medical teams in real time, accelerating diagnosis and treatment.

Viz.ai coordinates medical care using artificial intelligence when immediate intervention from medical staff is required (e.g., in a stroke). The system identifies the disease in images and automatically notifies interdisciplinary teams, reducing diagnosis and treatment time.

Qure.ai develops AI-powered solutions for analyzing and reporting medical images (particularly chest X-rays and head CT scans). This facilitates the early diagnosis and treatment of diseases such as tuberculosis, lung cancer, and stroke. These solutions are highly effective for handling high workloads (Qure.ai, 2025).

Subtle Medical is developing Subtle-ELITE™, an advanced MRI suite combining SubtleHD(MR)™, SubtleSYNTH™, and SubtleALIGN™ to deliver time savings, high image quality, and streamlined workflows. This enables faster MRI and PET scans or reduced radiation doses without compromising image quality (Subtle Medical,2025).

Cleerly is a digital health company that uses artificial intelligence to analyze coronary computed tomography angiography (CCTA) images to quantify plaque and stenosis, helping physicians with personalized treatment planning and early cardiovascular risk assessment.

Inequality in the use of AI technologies poses both challenges and opportunities. On the one hand, it risks exacerbating global inequality, as AI technologies become increasingly important for economic growth and societal development. On the other hand, it opens a clear path for targeted measures and international cooperation to bridge the AI readiness gap. These varying levels of readiness highlight the need for a coordinated global approach to AI development and deployment. By promoting collaboration and knowledge sharing and supporting less prepared regions, the international community can work toward a more equitable distribution of AI opportunities and benefits. The rate at which artificial intelligence is spreading across all areas of our lives is so rapid that without understanding forecasts, it is impossible to explore and evaluate the potential direction and level of AI implementation in healthcare. However, it is safe to say that blockchain technology will be widely adopted (Djakeli, 2024).

By 2030, a promising area for the use of artificial intelligence in medicine will be the combination of artificial intelligence and blockchain technology. By 2030, blockchain could become a fundamental technology for digital medicine. Decentralized solutions can be used across various sectors and tools, enabling deep integration of healthcare with digitalization. Blockchain will no longer be simply a data storage and verification system. It will increasingly be used in conjunction with artificial intelligence, particularly for early diagnosis and disease prognosis. The reliability of blockchain ensures the authenticity of the source data, while artificial intelligence enables its intelligent processing. Together, they form the basis for self-regulating algorithms that can predict disease progression, select a treatment regimen, and adjust it in real time. The exponential growth in demand for computing resources (i.e., digital work) is driven by several new technologies, primarily artificial intelligence (AI). Training and running AI algorithms and models require significant computing resources. Stability.AI, the creator of Stable Diffusion, a text-to-image generator, used 4,000 Nvidia A100 GPUs running in the AWS cloud to train its AI models. This cost them over $50 million per month. Blockchain AI is believed to reduce the resource intensity of AI training and operation (Kassab & Devens, 2022).

To ensure that the formalization of artificial intelligence using blockchain technology proceeds without significant controversy, it is necessary to accelerate the development of an appropriate legislative framework(FIME,2025).

Blockchain, coupled with AI, makes medicine and pharmaceuticals more secure, transparent, and patient-focused. A unified, decentralized system replaces disparate databases with controlled access to data. This ensures:

- Data security. All medical records are encrypted and timestamped. Once entered into the blockchain, data cannot be altered or deleted, protecting against hacker attacks and accidental leaks(FIME,2025).
- Transparency. Any information—from drug production and logistics to data entry in medical records—is recorded on the blockchain. This allows for verification at any time and the identification of errors, storage violations, or counterfeit medications.
- Efficiency. Smart contracts can automate routine processes, such as confirming drug delivery, coordinating access to medical records, and processing insurance payments. This reduces paperwork and eases staff workload.
- Patient trust. Users can access their health information and check at any time who viewed or modified it and when.
- Process unification. Blockchain provides a unified standard of interaction between all industry participants. This eliminates data duplication and accelerates coordination between organizations, even if they are located in different countries.
- Thanks to these capabilities, blockchain lays the foundation for a new, more transparent, reliable, and patient-focused digital healthcare infrastructure.

Along with all the benefits of implementing and using blockchain with AI in medicine, problems no less serious than those in the financial and monetary spheres may arise, and will inevitably arise. The challenges and limitations of using blockchain in healthcare require careful, in-depth study; otherwise, irreparable harm to human health could occur. Despite their potential, blockchain and AI face several obstacles hindering their widespread adoption in healthcare. Key barriers include:

- High implementation costs. Developing and integrating a full-fledged blockchain system requires significant investment. This can amount to millions of dollars for security audits, staff training, and integration with existing medical systems. For public and small clinics, these costs are often prohibitive.
- Regulatory requirements. Legislation such as the General Data Protection Regulation (GDPR) in the EU requires the ability to delete personal information upon user request completely. This contradicts the immutability principle of blockchain and requires the creation of more complex hybrid systems.
- Lack of qualified specialists. Implementing blockchain solutions in healthcare requires teams with a rare combination of skills: an understanding of medical processes, knowledge of data protection legislation, and technical expertise in distributed systems.
- Low level of understanding of the technology. Many small clinics and regional hospitals, especially in developing countries, use outdated technical solutions or even work with paper-based documentation. In such a context, even basic integration of digital systems is a complex task, let alone implementing blockchain. One challenge that should be addressed in legislation in the US and other countries is eliminating the possibility of errors (or "hallucinations") in AI operations. "Hallucinations" arise already during the preliminary model training stage. The system is trained on enormous data sets, so the model is highly likely to forget or confuse information encountered only once. AI companies are trying to improve the technology with the help of human testers. When users interact with GPT models, they evaluate the chatbot's responses, effectively indicating which answers are useful and truthful and which are false. Then, using a technique called Reinforcement Learning from Human Feedback (RLHF), the system analyzes these evaluations over several weeks to better distinguish fact from fiction.
- Furthermore, other approaches enable neural networks to combat "hallucinations" in their responses. Corporations are using them when developing their own LLMs. The most effective approach would be to involve government agencies in solving this problem (Precedende Research,2025)

Overcoming these barriers requires a comprehensive approach: from government support and the creation of adaptive standards to investments in education and the development of internal development departments. Large-scale implementation of blockchain in medicine is only possible when the industry is ready not only technically but also organizationally (Gigauri & Djakeli, 2021b).

To address these issues, it is necessary to develop a regulatory framework for blockchain implementation at various levels, which can only be achieved through coordinated cooperation among governments and international organizations. Well-thought-out policies can simultaneously protect patients' rights and improve the efficiency of the healthcare system(Precedence Research, PrecedenceQ, 2025)

5. HEALTHCARE DATA TOKENIZATION

One key concept will be the tokenization of medical data. The idea is to return full control over personal information to patients, allowing them to grant and revoke access to medical records through secure interfaces. Physicians' work is strictly regulated, and this significantly impacts the design of the medical system interface. Norms, rules, standards, and laws represent a vast number of formalized requirements that must be reflected in the interface and are impossible to influence.

These processes are quite extensive, complex, and nonlinear. It should be noted that we are often dealing with a physician's direct actions when working with a patient or their medical history, as well as with actions related to compliance with all regulations and requirements. In the near future, each hospital and medical center will likely have its own tokens that can be exchanged or liquidated as needed (Precedence Research, Sample Report, AI in the medical imaging market,2025)

5.1. The Role of Regulation of the Blockchain Application with Artificial Intelligence in Healthcare

Regulation plays a crucial role in the implementation of blockchain technologies with artificial intelligence in medicine. Since sensitive personal data is involved, any new system must comply with regulatory requirements. In this context, blockchain faces several legal contradictions (Djakeli, 2025).

Thus, the aforementioned General Data Protection Regulation (GDPR) requires developers to use solutions that store sensitive information off-chain, with only hashes or links added to the blockchain. This approach helps ensure legal compliance, particularly the right to erasure, but increases technical complexity. Overcoming these barriers requires a comprehensive approach: from government support and the creation of adaptive standards to investments in education and the development of internal development departments. Even with growing support from international organizations, blockchain still faces several systemic barriers:

- Privacy and the "right to be forgotten." In a context where patients have the legal right to request the deletion of their data, the immutability of blockchain records becomes a legal obstacle(Djakeli,2025 B).
- Jurisdiction of data storage. The distributed nature of blockchain makes it difficult to determine where the data is actually stored. This gives rise to legal disputes regarding compliance with local laws, especially during cross-border transfers of information.
- Lack of liability standards. In the event of a leak, error, or access breach, it is not always clear who bears legal responsibility: the platform provider, the smart contract developer, or other system participants. This reduces trust between medical institutions and insurance companies.
- Lack of uniform standards. Currently, there is no globally recognized regulatory framework governing the use of blockchain in healthcare.

Successfully addressing these challenges requires creating a regulatory framework for implementing blockchain and AI at various levels. This is possible through coordinated collaboration between developed and developing countries, small states, and international organizations. A well-designed blockchain and AI implementation policy can simultaneously protect patient rights and improve the efficiency of the healthcare system (Stanford Institute for Human-Centered Artificial Intelligence, 2025)

As interest in this technology grows, blockchain is gaining increasing support at the regulatory and research levels. Stellar Market Research predicts that the global market for blockchain solutions in healthcare could reach $230 billion by 2032. A 2021 report from the European Commission notes significant investment in the digitalization of healthcare, including blockchain technologies. The exponential growth in demand for computing resources (i.e., digital workflows) is driven by emerging technologies, primarily artificial intelligence, the Internet of Things (IoT), and the metaverse. Artificial intelligence: training and running AI algorithms and models require significant computing resources.

CONCLUSIONS

By 2030, blockchain will likely cease to be solely a data storage and verification system. It will increasingly be used in conjunction with artificial intelligence, particularly in early diagnosis and disease prognosis. Blockchain's reliability ensures the authenticity of the source data, while AI enables its intelligent processing. Together, they form the foundation for self-tuning algorithms capable of predicting disease progression, selecting a treatment plan, and adjusting it in real time.

The implementation of AI in healthcare creates unique cybersecurity challenges. AI systems require large data sets to train and operate effectively, increasing the risk of large-scale data breaches (Żak et al.,2024).

All of these factors combined will negatively impact initial investments and pose a direct threat to the competitive advantage of innovative healthcare organizations. In 2024, the US Department of Health and Human Services announced the renaming of the Office of the National Coordinator for Health Information Technology (ONC). Moreover, the risk extends beyond intellectual property theft to encompass serious privacy concerns. This is confirmed by incidents in which generative AI models trained on massive datasets inadvertently reveal sensitive information from their training data in response to certain queries. This confirms that the technology is becoming established not as an experiment, but as a new industry standard. At the same time, blockchain is shaping a new paradigm in which security, transparency, and trust become systemic values in healthcare (Gigauri & Djakeli, 2021b).

In the future, this model allows for the monetization of anonymized data: individuals will be able to decide for themselves whether their records are used in research or clinical trials—and receive compensation for doing so. This will not only expand patients' rights but also open new data sources for science and AI training.

REFERENCES:

Djakeli, K. (2024). Healthcare marketing: meaning, historical development, applications, and current status. In *Modern Healthcare Marketing in the Digital Era* (pp. 1–25). IGI Global Scientific Publishing.

Djakeli, K. (2025). A). Phygitalization of Palliative Care and Its Social Marketing. In *Phygital Approaches to Social Marketing* (pp. 267–288). IGI Global Scientific Publishing.

Djakeli, K. (2025 B). Strategic Management for Digital Platform Brands in the Phygital Era. In Brand Creation and Management in the Phygital Era (pp. 499-520). IGI Global Scientific Publishing.

FIME. (2025). *Radiology industry report.* https://www.worldhealthexpo.com/content/dam/esa/emea/worldhealthexpo/events/healthcare/miami/en/2025/pdfs/FIME25-radiology-industry-report.pdf

Gabelaia, I., Djakeli, K., & McElroy, J. W. (2024, September). The power of customer journey mapping with artificial intelligence: a case study method. In International Conference on Reliability and Statistics in Transportation and Communication (pp. 244-257). Cham: Springer Nature Switzerland.

Gigauri, I., & Djakeli, K. (2021a). National health reforms in Georgia during 1994-2021cnd their success. *HOLISTICA–Journal of Business and Public Administration, 12*(2), 102–108. DOI: 10.2478/hjbpa-2021-0017

Gigauri, I., & Djakeli, K. (2021b). Expecting Transformation of Marketing During the Post-Pandemic New Normal: Qualitative Research of Marketing Managers in Georgia. [IJSEM]. *International Journal of Sustainable Economies Management, 10*(2), 1–18. DOI: 10.4018/IJSEM.2021040101

GlobeNewswire. (2026, January 23). *Press release/knowledge base article.* https://www.einpresswire.com/knowledge-base/how-to-get-into-ai-platforms

IBM. (2025). *What is edge AI?* https://www.ibm.com/think/topics/edge-ai

Kassab, S., & Devens, C. (2022). *The exponential demand for comput*ing. Messari. https://messari.io/report/the-exponential-demand-for-compute

Mordor Intelligence. (2024). *Latin America medical imaging software market size & share analysis – Growth trends & forecasts (2024–2029).* https://www.mordorintelligence.com/industry-reports/latin-america-medical-imaging-software-market-industry

Precedence Research. (n.d.). *AI in the medical imaging market.* https://www.precedenceresearch.com/ai-in-medical-imaging-market

Precedence Research. (n.d.). *PrecedenceQ.* https://www.precedenceresearch.com/precedenceq/

Precedence Research. (n.d.). *Sample report: AI in the medical imaging market.* https://www.precedenceresearch.com/sample/2380

Qure.ai. (2025). *Qure.ai FY 2024–25 impact report.* https://www.qure.ai/impact-stories/qure-ai-fy-24-25-impact-report-global-ai-healthcare-innovations

Stanford Institute for Human-Centered Artificial Intelligence. (2025). *AI index report 2025.* https://hai.stanford.edu/ai-index/2025-ai-index-report

Subtle Medical. (n.d.). *Subtle Elite.* https://subtlemedical.com/subtle-elite/

Wheatley, H. (2022). Google Cloud's medical imaging suite to make AI-based diagnosis more accessible. *SiliconANGLE.* https://siliconangle.com/2022/10/04/google-clouds-medical-imaging-suite-make-ai-based-diagnosis-accessible/

Żak, A., Djakeli, K., & Bielińska-Dusza, E. (2024). Cross-Sector Partnerships and Relationship Marketing in Healthcare: The Example of Fairy Tale Therapy in Children's Hospitals in Poland. In Modern Healthcare Marketing in the Digital Era (pp. 164-192). IGI Global Scientific Publishing. REVISED

Chapter 8
Algorithmic Neutrality in Healthcare AI: Critical Perspectives on Bias, Inequality, and the (Re) Production of Health Disparities

Nada Belmejdoub
Faculty of Sciences, Ibn Tofail University, Kenitra, Morocco

Mohamed Rektouti
http://orcid.org/0009-0004-5560-4925
Faculty of Sciences, Ibn Tofail University, Kenitra, Morocco

Wafaa Benkayba
http://orcid.org/0000-0001-5196-1678
Laboratory of Chemistry Analytical and Bromatology, Faculty of Medicine and Pharmacy, University Mohammed V, Rabat, Morocco

Yassine Mouniane
http://orcid.org/0000-0002-6037-5301
Faculty of Sciences, Ibn Tofail University, Kenitra, Morocco

Mohamed Belomaria
Instituts Supérieurs des Professions Infirmières et Techniques de Santé, Morocco

Brahim El Ouardi
http://orcid.org/0009-0000-4559-6141
Faculty of Sciences, Ibn Tofail University, Kenitra, Morocco

Nabil Ait Ouaaziz
Faculty of Sciences, Ibn Tofail University, Kenitra, Morocco

Farid Elkhlifi
Faculty of Sciences, Ibn Tofail University, Kenitra, Morocco

Soukaina Njili
Faculty of Sciences, Ibn Tofail University, Kenitra, Morocco

Driss Hmouni
http://orcid.org/0000-0001-7598-6204
Faculty of Sciences, Ibn Tofail University, Kenitra, Morocco

Abdellatif Bour
Faculty of Sciences, Ibn Tofail University, Kenitra, Morocco

DOI: 10.4018/979-8-2600-0939-0.ch008

Soad Khal-Layoun
http://orcid.org/0009-0004-0783-5841
Faculty of Sciences, Ibn Tofail University, Kenitra, Morocco

Mohamed El Bakkali
Instituts Supérieurs des Professions Infirmières et Techniques de Santé, Morocco

Mohammed Ouhssine
Faculty of Sciences, Ibn Tofail University, Kenitra, Morocco

ABSTRACT

This chapter critically examines the assumption of algorithmic neutrality in healthcare artificial intelligence (AI). Although AI is often promoted as a driver of accuracy, efficiency, and equity, evidence shows that it can reinforce disparities through biases in data, model design, and implementation. Based on a review of biomedical, computational, and policy literature from 2017 to 2025, the chapter highlights how underrepresentation of marginalized populations, limited validation across contexts, opaque algorithms, and weak stakeholder engagement contribute to inequitable outcomes. It argues that technical bias mitigation alone is insufficient without addressing structural inequalities. Emphasis is placed on participatory and justice-oriented frameworks, transparent audits, accountable governance, and inclusive design. Embedding equity and accountability across the AI lifecycle is presented as essential for ensuring digital innovation advances health justice.

INTRODUCTION

The rapid integration of artificial intelligence (AI) into healthcare has sparked extraordinary hope for transformative improvements in diagnosis, clinical decision-making, and resource allocation. Advocates portray AI as a vehicle for "democratizing" healthcare—promising greater accuracy, efficiency, and equity in access to high-quality care. Yet this optimistic narrative stands in sharp contrast to a growing body of critical research, which challenges the presumed neutrality of algorithms and cautions that, rather than eliminating disparities, AI can inadvertently reproduce or even amplify the deep-seated biases and social injustices that persist within health systems (Ali & Nikberg, 2024; Haider et al., 2024; Aquino et al., 2025).

Recent empirical studies and high-profile incidents have illuminated the ways in which AI-enabled tools—designed for diagnosis, triage, and population health management—can encode and perpetuate racial, gender, and socioeconomic inequities. Algorithms trained primarily on data from privileged or majority populations often underperform for marginalized groups, leading to delayed diagnoses or suboptimal care for those already vulnerable to adverse outcomes (Haider et al., 2025). These issues arise not only because of representativeness and provenance of the training data, but also, and perhaps more significantly, because machine learning models are often "black boxes" in terms of their lack of transparency. This opacity makes it even more challenging to audit systems for bias or accountability (Ali & Nikberg, 2024; Singhal et al., 2024).

Despite mounting evidence of these challenges, much of the academic literature continues to frame AI chiefly as a technical solution to clinical problems, with limited attention to the complex social, ethical, and organizational dynamics at stake. As Munk and colleagues point out, peer-reviewed articles focus on presenting algorithms as valuable agents of progress and invariably avoid even considering the risks that those algorithms could generate or exacerbate existing inequities (Munk et al., 2024). The dominance of that discursive framing risks reinforcing the myth that algorithms are neutral and ignore the experiences of patients and practitioners facing the unknown consequences of automated decision-making (Braveman et al., 2017; Aquino et al., 2025).

Recognising these gaps is urgent as health systems globally are having difficulty addressing systemic inequalities in access, quality and outcomes. If we do not examine the impact of AI on health equity, the widespread use of AI could exacerbate and entrench existing patterns of disadvantage, with the potential to support continued injustice in pursuit of better health equity (WHO, 2024). By contrast, a better and grounded understanding of AI's impact in the 'real-world' could inform technologies that are truly inclusive and responsive to the needs of different communities (Mergen et al., 2025).

Within this framework, the current review engages in critical inquiry with the myth of neutrality in healthcare AI. Building on recent scholarship and a multi-level investigation of algorithmic bias and health inequities, we explore the role that prevailing narratives, data practices and implementation efforts play in the (re) production of inequity in digital health. We also discuss prominent and emerging frameworks and practical approaches to auditing, addressing, and eventually overcoming these issues, with the goal of ushering in a more equitable and ethically responsible future for AI in medicine.

BACKGROUND

The document presents Artificial Intelligence (AI) as an omnipresent technology within the healthcare value chain, with global investments projected to exceed $45 billion by 2026. While AI promises to "democratize" healthcare by improving diagnostics and efficiency, a sharp contrast exists between this optimistic narrative and empirical reality. Research indicates that algorithms, far from being neutral, can reproduce or amplify deep-seated prejudices and social injustices. For instance, diagnostic or triage tools can encode racial, gender, or socioeconomic inequalities, particularly when models are trained on data from privileged populations.

THEORETICAL FRAMEWORK

The theoretical framework of the document is built around challenging the "myth of AI neutrality" in healthcare. It draws upon:

- The Critique of Technological Solutionism: The tendency to view AI as a panacea capable of erasing human error without considering complex socio-technical realities.
- Technological Optimism Bias: The fact that academic literature often prioritizes technical "successes" at the expense of analyzing failures or unintended real-world consequences.
- The "Black Box" Concept: The opacity of machine learning models which makes it difficult to audit for bias or establish accountability.

CONCEPTUAL FRAMEWORK

The conceptual framework is based on several key definitions and a multidimensional analysis of equity in digital health:

- Artificial Intelligence and Machine Learning: Computational systems that learn from large datasets to perform diagnostic or predictive tasks.
- Algorithmic Bias: Systematic errors that create unfair outcomes by privileging one group over another.
- Health Equity: The absence of avoidable and unjust differences among populations.
- Stakeholder Engagement and Contextual Validation: The involvement of patients and clinicians at all stages, and the testing of models in real-world environments to ensure reliability and justice.

The document also proposes a typology of biases (sampling, measurement, labeling, deployment, historical, and aggregation) to structure the analysis of AI failures.

METHODOLOGY

This review adheres to best practices for comprehensive literature synthesis in health sciences, emphasizing transparency and methodological rigor. The search strategy encompassed leading biomedical and interdisciplinary databases—including PubMed, Scopus, Web of Science, and Embase—as well as specialized repositories such as arXiv and SSRN to capture relevant preprints and policy papers. Searches were conducted using a combination of controlled vocabulary (e.g., MeSH terms) and free-text keywords: "artificial intelligence," "machine learning," "algorithmic bias," "health equity," "disparities," "ethics," "regulation," "validation," and domain-specific terms such as "clinical decision support," "medical imaging," and "real-world evidence." Boolean operators and filters for publication type (reviews, empirical studies, policy documents) and date range (2017–2025) were systematically applied to ensure breadth and relevance.

Titles and abstracts were independently screened for eligibility. Full texts were then reviewed based on predefined inclusion criteria: (i) explicit focus on AI or machine learning in healthcare, (ii) direct discussion of bias, equity, fairness, or social determinants, and (iii) presentation of empirical findings, methodological frameworks, or regulatory perspectives. Studies were excluded if they fell outside the healthcare domain, lacked clinical or ethical relevance, or provided insufficient methodological detail. Duplicate articles and redundant preprints were excluded after cross-verification.

To enhance comprehensiveness, backward and forward citation tracking was performed, ensuring inclusion of influential and foundational works. All sources were classified by methodological approach (systematic review, empirical research, qualitative study, conceptual paper, or policy document), geographical focus, and main thematic contribution. Key documents from authoritative organizations—including the World Health Organization, U.S. Food and Drug Administration, European Commission, and relevant professional societies—were systematically reviewed to integrate regulatory and normative perspectives.

The study selection process was structured according to the Preferred Reporting Items for Systematic Reviews and Meta-Analyses (PRISMA) guidelines. Figure 1 summarizes the identification, screening, and inclusion of articles for this review.

Figure 1. PRISMA Flow Diagram for Study Selection

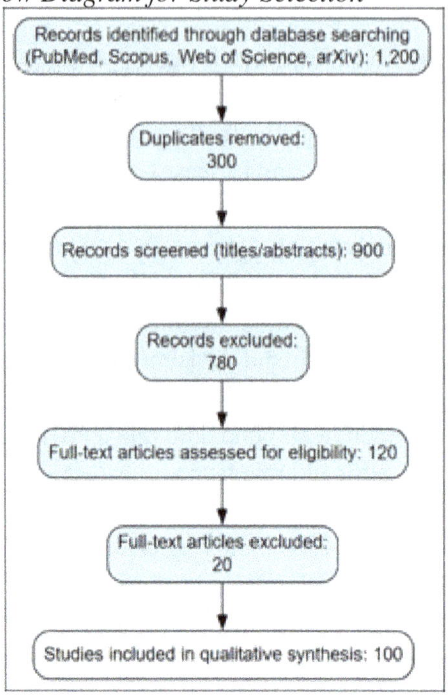

Figure 1 illustrate the systematic process of article identification, duplicate removal, screening, eligibility assessment, and final inclusion in the qualitative synthesis for this review.

DOMINANT DISCOURSE ON AI AND HEALTH INEQUALITY

Promise and Predominance of AI in Healthcare

Ubiquity and Applications of AI in Health

Over the past decade, artificial intelligence (AI) has evolved from a conceptual ambition to an everyday reality within global healthcare systems. This transformation is reflected not only in the exponential growth of academic publications, but also in the widespread integration of AI technologies into clinical workflows. According to the World Health Organization, more than 40 countries have launched national strategies for AI in health, while worldwide investment in healthcare AI is forecasted to exceed $45 billion by 2026, up from just $6.9 billion in 2021 (WHO, 2024).

The breadth of AI's application in healthcare is evident across numerous specialties and use-cases. In diagnostic medicine, deep learning algorithms now demonstrate accuracy rivalling—sometimes surpassing—human experts in radiology, dermatology, and ophthalmology (Whicher et al., 2023). Landmark studies have shown that convolutional neural networks can achieve dermatologist-level performance in skin cancer classification—a breakthrough rapidly emulated in detecting diabetic retinopathy and pneumonia from medical images (Gianfrancesco et al., 2018; Topol, 2019).

Beyond diagnostics, AI-powered predictive analytics are increasingly deployed to identify at-risk patients, anticipate disease outbreaks, and optimize health system resources (Esteva et al., 2017; Topol, 2019). Machine learning models derived from electronic health records are now used to predict hospital readmissions, treatment responses, or patient deterioration in intensive care, often with greater efficiency and scalability than conventional methods (Gianfrancesco et al., 2018). The COVID-19 pandemic, in particular, accelerated the adoption of AI, with hundreds of new algorithms developed for screening, triage, contact tracing, and vaccine distribution (Bullock et al., 2020).

AI has also found an essential role in healthcare administration, facilitating automated scheduling, claims processing, and patient communication through natural language processing and virtual assistants (Esteva et al., 2017). By the end of 2022, more than 165 FDA-approved AI or machine learning medical devices were actively used in the United States alone, encompassing imaging, cardiology, and digital pathology (Benjamens et al., 2020).

While regional differences in access and regulatory frameworks remain, the overarching trend is clear: AI is now ubiquitous throughout the healthcare value chain. This rapid and multidimensional expansion continues to inspire optimism about AI's transformative potential, but also sets the stage for urgent, nuanced debates on its impact, fairness, and contextual relevance.

Solutionism and the Technological Optimism Bias

Despite the rapid expansion and remarkable breadth of AI's applications in healthcare, a significant strand of both academic and policy discourse remains anchored in what scholars have termed "technological solutionism"—the inclination to frame complex health challenges as principally solvable through technological innovation (Morley & Floridi, 2020; Vayena & Blasimme, 2018). Within this paradigm, artificial intelligence is frequently cast as a panacea, capable of transcending human error, eradicating inefficiency, and advancing equity by virtue of its inherent capabilities (Whicher et al., 2023).

This form of solutionist optimism is evident in high-profile editorials, industry white papers, and policy briefs that portray AI as an engine of unprecedented progress, often with scant acknowledgment of the messy sociotechnical realities that shape health systems (Topol, 2019; WHO, 2024). The ongoing framing of AI as a neutral and universally effective tool relies on what could be called a "myth of efficiency", in which algorithms take precedence over clinicians in all contexts, independent of clinical context, quality of data, and characteristics of patients within that context. This assumption continues to persist, even with significant evidence that models that are trained on data from comparably well-resourced and more homogeneous populations often do worse—or outright fail—when placed in more diverse or resource-poor contexts (Obermeyer et al., 2019; Gianfrancesco et al., 2018).

Moreover, the prevailing tendency to spotlight AI "success stories" within the literature risks obscuring or downplaying the failures, unintended consequences, and contextual constraints that invariably arise in real-world practice (Abràmoff et al., 2023). The World Health Organization has cautioned that "an over-reliance on technological solutions may neglect the importance of local capacity, ethical safeguards, and the social determinants of health" (WHO, 2024). Empirical research further reveals that, in some cases, AI-powered interventions have unintentionally widened health disparities, with benefits disproportionately accruing to those populations already advantaged by robust digital infrastructure and healthcare access (Obermeyer et al., 2019).

Indeed, much of the optimism bias we see in literature with an optimistic focus on the myths of universal efficacy and algorithmic neutrality—has the potential to create unrealistic expectations and disillusions stakeholders from the realities of equity and implementation. A much more critical and context-sensitive approach to the complexities of power, diversity, and local realities is necessary if AI is going to deliver on its promises and not deepen inequalities. While there is still a prevailing literature suggesting that AI is a neutral and globally benevolent tool, there is emerging evidence documented in a series of recent, high-impact studies which analyzed cases of algorithmic intervention that failed to achieve the promise, added new risks, and exacerbated existing inequities. The following box outlines some representative cases to demonstrate the context and consequences of AI failures in real-life health care.

When AI Falls Short: Contexts and Consequences of Failure in Healthcare

While literature often foregrounds the transformative promise of artificial intelligence, an expanding body of empirical evidence exposes critical failures and unintended consequences that challenge this optimism. One landmark study by (Obermeyer et al., 2019) investigated a widely adopted risk scoring algorithm used to manage over 200 million patients in the United States. The authors found that the algorithm systematically underestimated health risks for Black patients compared to white patients with similar clinical profiles, a bias rooted in the algorithm's reliance on prior healthcare expenditures as a proxy for illness severity. Because Black patients, owing to systemic barriers, historically incur lower healthcare costs, this approach led to fewer referrals for advanced care—thereby amplifying pre-existing racial disparities in preventive service access (Obermeyer et al., 2019).

Similar disparities have been documented in AI-driven dermatology. Daneshjou et al. (2022) demonstrated that most training datasets for skin lesion classification are overwhelmingly composed of images from individuals with lighter skin tones, with more than 80% of samples drawn from such populations. Consequently, algorithms trained on these datasets exhibited reduced accuracy in detecting skin cancers and other conditions in people with darker skin, raising concerns about diagnostic equity and patient safety for ethnic minorities (Daneshjou et al., 2022; Groh et al., 2022; Morales-Forero et al., 2024; O'Malley et al., 2024).

The scale of these challenges is further highlighted by international adoption data. According to the World Health Organization, only 15% of low-income countries possess the infrastructure required to deploy clinically validated AI tools—a shortfall that both reflects and perpetuates global health inequities (WHO, 2024). Recent multi-center evaluations show that more than one-third of AI models developed for emergency triage lose at least 20% of their predictive performance when applied outside their original development population (El Arab & Al Moosa, 2025; Soltan et al., 2022; Yu et al., 2022). Despite frequent media celebration of "AI successes," (Rajkomar et al., 2019) note that most AI systems lauded in published studies are rarely scaled up or integrated into routine clinical practice, precisely because of their limited contextual adaptability. Collectively, these cases underscore that solutionist narratives, while compelling, often obscure the contextual realities and diversity that shape the real-world performance—and limitations—of AI in healthcare.

Myth of Algorithmic Neutrality

How Neutrality Is Framed in Scientific Literature

A defining feature of contemporary academic discourse on AI in healthcare is the persistent framing of algorithms as neutral and objective. Algorithms are often described as neutral tools that eliminate human bias and standardize clinical decision-making processes in an idealized way which suggests that outputs are inherently devoid of social, cultural, or institutional influences (McCradden et al., 2020; Lau, 2025). Such framings are supported by editorial norms that emphasize studies highlighting high algorithm evidence-based accuracy and technical "successes" while often downplaying more critical discussions of fairness, context, and equity (McCradden et al., 2020; Giovanola & Tiribelli, 2023).

In recent years, studies have been emphasized in many major scientific publications that document the instances where algorithms perform better than clinicians, thus advancing the misperception that machine learning is automatically more rational and less subjective than human judgement (Topol, 2019 ; McCradden et al., 2020). However, these depictions rarely reflect the social determinants of health, or the social realities of those creating these AI tools and how they might be used. Therefore, the literature usually supports the objective belief in data-driven, systems-based information and overlooks how algorithms often carry—and in some cases, compound—ingrained biases from the environment in which they have been trained (Gianfrancesco et al., 2018; Lau, 2025).

Editorial selection reinforces this normative bias of neutrality. In the rare instances where they do publish or report on algorithmic bias or algorithmic failure—especially when studies are focused on marginalized groups, vulnerable populations, or resource-limited settings—high impact journals are less likely to discuss systemic issues of justice or inclusion; unless of course, if it can be framed in the spectrum of isolated technical issues (Munk et al., 2024 ; Lau, 2025 ; Agarwal et al., 2023). The slight selection has a larger impact on the research program as it has bearing on the teleological priorities of the research questions, dispositions toward methodology, and how scientists and politicians understand both the promise of AI and the limitations of AI.

Limits of This Framing: What Is Left Out?

Table 1. provides a summary of the principal types of algorithmic bias identified in healthcare AI, along with concise definitions, illustrative real-world examples, and their potential impacts as documented in the recent literature.

Type of Bias	Definition	Examples / References	Potential Impact
Sample Bias	When training data do not represent the target population.	- AI dermatology models underperform on darker skin: (Adamson & Smith, 2018) (US)- Performance gaps on diverse images: (Daneshjou et al.,2022) (multi-country)	Misdiagnosis, health inequities
Measurement Bias	Systematic errors in how features/outcomes are measured or recorded.	- EHR errors bias AI predictions: (Gianfrancesco et al.,2018) Inconsistent imaging protocols: (Seyyed-Kalantari et al., 2020)	Inaccurate, unfair risk estimation
Label Bias	Ground truth labels reflect subjective or biased judgments.	- Biased outcomes in population health: (Obermeyer et al., 2019) Diagnosis labels in skin datasets: (Morales-Forero et al.,2024)	Discriminatory risk scores, misallocation
Algorithmic Bias	Biases introduced or amplified by model architecture or optimization.	- Model reproducing social biases: (Giovanola & Tiribelli, 2023) - Black box algorithms and ethical concerns: (McCradden et al., 2020)	Systemic inequities, trust loss
Deployment Bias	Biases that emerge when the AI is used in a new/ different environment.	- Sepsis model fails in new hospitals: (Wong et al.,2021)- COVID-19 model: performance varies across continents: (Mamandipoor et al., 2022)	Patient harm, unreliable predictions
Historical Bias	Bias inherited from past social or healthcare inequities in the data.	- Biased health resource allocation: (Obermeyer et al.,2019) - Structural racism in precision medicine: (Geneviève et al., 2020)	Perpetuates disparities, worsens injustice
Aggregation Bias	Errors from grouping or simplifying heterogeneous populations.	- Grouping masks subgroup risks: (Finlayson et al., 2021) - Aggregated COVID data hides differences: (Mamandipoor et al., 2022)	Missed risks, inequitable recommendations

While the narrative of algorithmic neutrality dominates scientific publishing, it often obscures the experiences and realities of vulnerable populations who are most at risk of being disadvantaged by AI-driven interventions. Literature's focus on technical performance frequently comes at the expense of investigating structural inequities or the lived consequences of deploying imperfect algorithms in complex, real-world settings (Adamson & Smith, 2018; Obermeyer et al., 2019).

One key limitation is the underrepresentation of empirical studies on algorithmic impact in diverse and low-resource populations. Most published research relies on datasets from affluent, homogenous groups, which not only limits the generalizability of findings but also risks perpetuating a form of "data colonialism" that privileges certain populations while marginalizing others (Gianfrancesco et al., 2018; WHO, 2024). Methodological reviews have highlighted that such practices can render the problems of minority groups invisible—either by excluding them from the dataset or by assuming that algorithms will function identically across contexts (Geneviève et al., 2020).

As (Munk et al., 2024) have demonstrated through extensive semantic analysis, macro-level literature rarely treats algorithms as contested or political artifacts, instead bias and discrimination are framed as technical bugs to fix and relegated to technical appendices from the methodological. This constrains both scientific inquiry as well as policy and regulatory approaches to addressing AI-driven inequities.

In other words, the myth of algorithmic neutrality does not persist because it is empirically validated, but because it is implicitly sustained, largely through institutional practices of research, publication, and policy making. To dismantle this myth, we need to consciously position the experiences of those who are most impacted by health disparities front and center, intentionally making the social, ethical, and political implications of algorithmic decision-making explicit.

Having unpacked the conceptual and methodological blind spots underlying the established narratives of algorithmic neutrality, we now turn to the burgeoning scholarship and practice that explicitly wrestles with these gaps and limitations. The following section explores how critical perspectives and new frameworks are challenging entrenched persistent constructions, making bias visible and striving for equity and laying platforms for more equitable approaches to AI in health care.

Critical and Emerging Voices

Rising Awareness of Bias and Health Inequality

Although popular literature still frames AI in healthcare as a neutral, universally beneficial innovation, an emergent cohort of researchers and practitioners is changing the conversation around algorithmic decision-making by emphasizing its real-world implications. Over the past couple of years, an increasing body of studies and systematic reviews have demonstrated how machine learning systems created from unrepresentative or biased datasets can reinforce, and even exacerbate, entrenched health inequity (Aquino et al., 2025 ; Haider et al., 2024).

For example, (Haider et al., 2024) offer a sweeping review of AI-driven clinical tools, uncovering robust evidence that racial, ethnic, and socioeconomic biases persist in widely adopted algorithms. These embedded biases often lead to unequal diagnostic accuracy and disparate health outcomes that are felt most acutely by historically marginalized communities. Similar patterns have been documented across gender, age, and language groups, illustrating how even the most well-intentioned and "neutral" algorithms can amplify inequity if issues of data representativeness and modeling practices are not rigorously addressed (Singhal et al., 2024).

Importantly, multi-country studies show that deploying AI in lower-income and resource-constrained settings often exposes a different set of challenges: digital infrastructure gaps, limited availability of local data, and contextual differences in disease burden or care pathways (WHO, 2024). These realities have fueled a mounting call—from both academic circles and patient advocacy organizations—for greater transparency, systematic equity audits, and, crucially, the meaningful participation of marginalized communities throughout the AI lifecycle (Ali & Nikberg, 2024).

From Technical Bias to Structural Inequality

This emerging body of research has sparked a fundamental and long-overdue debate: should algorithmic bias be understood simply as a technical flaw—an artifact that can be remedied by refining data and improving models—or as a manifestation of deeper, systemic inequities embedded in our health systems? Increasingly, scholars and practitioners argue for the latter perspective, cautioning that a purely technical focus risks obscuring the social, political, and ethical roots of health injustice (Panch et al., 2019; McCradden et al., 2020; Mergen et al., 2025).

Rather than seeing "debiasing" as a technical fix, these voices call for confronting the historical and institutional forces that have shaped, and continue to shape, patterns of inequitable health outcomes (Obermeyer et al., 2019; Giovanola & Tiribelli, 2023; Lau, 2025). This perspective is increasingly reflected in major policy frameworks, including those from the World Health Organization and prominent health equity scholars—which emphasize the need for participatory design, genuine community engagement, and strong regulatory mechanisms centered on justice, inclusion, and local context (WHO, 2024).

(Mergen et al., 2025), for instance, urge a fundamental reimagining of AI ethics—not merely "fixing the code," but rethinking how health technologies are conceived, developed, and governed from the outset. This critical stance reminds us that algorithms are never neutral or isolated from society; rather, they are deeply entangled with enduring questions of power, privilege, and justice. It is only by grappling with these broader forces that we can hope to realize the transformative potential of AI for health equity.

Synthesis and Transition

The previous review reiterates how contemporary narratives of technological promise, neutrality, and efficiency often dominate talk about AI in healthcare. These framings often erase or obscure the realities of vulnerable groups and the structural forces that sustain persistent health inequities. While an increasing amount of literature is producing algorithm-innovation stories, there remains a significant gap in that we still do not know nearly enough about how AI tools fare—and for whom—they are functioning, outside of the staged environments of clinical trials or demonstration projects. Recent critical and emerging perspectives also emphasize the dangers of striving for technical performance or the "debiasing" of algorithms. By treating bias only as a "technical problem" can inadvertently perpetuate entrenched social and institutional processes that create inequitable outcomes. In addition, the generally accepted "success stories" in research and policy discourse often distract from and to-and-from questions of justice and context and real-world dissonance. All of these limitations highlight the importance and need for more complex, contextually sensitive analyses instead of aggregate performance metrics. Future research should be anchored in empirical examinations of how the AI systems interact within the complex social, cultural, and economic determinants of healthcare delivery. This requires consideration of case-based, participatory, and interdisciplinary approaches, which will include the voices and experiences of the people most affected by digital innovation. The subsequent section addresses this call to action, turning attention to specific case studies and critical examples of bias and inequality in the use of healthcare AI.

BIAS AND INEQUALITY IN REAL-WORLD AI DEPLOYMENT

Algorithmic Bias in Practice

Clinical Case Studies

Despite the much-lauded theoretical promise of artificial intelligence to improve diagnostic accuracy and efficiency, real-world deployments have consistently revealed persistent—and sometimes severe—biases across multiple clinical domains. A widely cited example emerges from dermatology, where deep learning algorithms trained predominantly on images from individuals with lighter skin tones have been shown to underperform markedly when evaluating lesions on patients with darker skin. As Adamson & Smith demonstrated, such tools may overlook malignant melanomas in people of color, posing serious risks of delayed or missed diagnoses and further entrenching existing health disparities (Adamson & Smith, 2018).

Radiology presents similar cautionary lessons. For instance, Seyyed-Kalantari et al. (2020) found that leading chest X-ray interpretation algorithms not only learned to infer patient race from imaging data but also produced predictions with varying accuracy across demographic groups—even when images appeared visually identical to clinicians. This hidden encoding of demographic information raises the alarming possibility that AI systems may systematically disadvantage certain groups, thereby amplifying disparities in the detection of conditions such as pneumonia or cancer (Seyyed-Kalantari et al., 2020).

In cardiology, Obermeyer et al. (2019) identified a commercial risk-prediction algorithm used throughout U.S. health systems that consistently underestimated the health risks of Black patients, resulting in lower referral rates for advanced care. The root of this bias lay in the use of healthcare spending as a proxy for health needs—an approach that overlooks structural inequities shaping medical expenditures across racial groups (Obermeyer et al., 2019). Comparable challenges have emerged in mental health: natural language processing tools for suicide risk prediction or psychiatric triage often fail to accommodate dialect, culture, or linguistic variation, thereby limiting their effectiveness among diverse populations (Malgaroli et al., 2023).

Taken together, these cases illustrate that clinical AI systems—unless rigorously evaluated and deliberately tailored for demographic diversity—risk perpetuating or worsening disparities along lines of race, gender, age, and socioeconomic status.

These clinical findings are mirrored by similar patterns of bias at the administrative and system level, where algorithmic decisions can affect entire patient populations.

Administrative and System-Level Bias

Bias is not just at the clinical interface but is also evident in the administrative backbone of healthcare. AI-guided resource allocation, appointment organization, and triage will repeat biased outcomes if they are designed and implemented without taking the systemic inequities into account. For example, mult-center evaluations recently have shown that AI tools for triaging ER patients, when validated in new hospital contexts, dropped dramatically in predictive performance, especially for minority and low-income groups (Yu et al., 2022; El Arab & Al Moosa, 2025).

Insurance approval algorithms are another area of concern. Several reports highlight that predictive models used by insurers to authorize procedures or determine eligibility for programs may systematically deprioritize high-risk, marginalized groups if their historical data reflects biased practices (Lau, 2025). In the context of health system planning, machine learning models for forecasting resource needs can inadvertently channel more resources to well-served regions, reinforcing patterns of underinvestment in rural or disadvantaged communities. The broader implications are significant: when AI models automate or augment critical administrative decisions, any embedded biases can scale rapidly across large populations, cementing inequities in access, quality, and outcomes.

Structural Roots and Contextual Determinants of AI Bias

In order to appreciate these difficulties, it is necessary to examine where we might look upstream, beyond the algorithms themselves and therefore look at the bigger, structural challenges that shape the use, and reuse, of data. Exploring the roots of bias in healthcare AI clarifies that equitable innovation is built not only on technical design, but on the structural foundations of data infrastructures.

Data Infrastructures and Representation

Central to algorithmic bias in healthcare are the foundational concerns of data infrastructures—the sources, selection and curating of data that shapes how AI systems "see" the world. Most AI models are trained from larger datasets that reflect the data-richness of the population, clinical practices, and health system of where the model was developed; all of which can systematically encode the structural inequalities (Gianfrancesco et al., 2018; WHO, 2021).

A recurring concern is the chronic underrepresentation of minority groups, women, older adults, and those from low-resource settings in medical datasets. Daneshjou et al. (2022) demonstrated that dermatology image banks overrepresent light skin types, creating "data poverty" for populations with darker skin (Daneshjou et al., 2022). Similarly, Morales-Forero et al. (2024) found that widely used medical image datasets fail to capture the full diversity of real-world populations, perpetuating disparities in algorithmic performance (Morales-Forero et al., 2024). This problem extends to language, socioeconomic status, and geography. Natural language processing tools often fail to account for dialectal variation, further entrenching inequities (Malgaroli et al., 2023). Similarly, electronic health record (EHR) systems may omit social determinants of health, such as housing status or food insecurity, further institutionalizing disparities (Agarwal et al., 2023). Without deliberate strategies for inclusive data collection and critical scrutiny of sampling practices, AI in healthcare risks institutionalizing the very inequities it is purported to address.

Implementation Environments

The real-world performance of AI models, even when trained on comprehensive and heterogeneous datasets, is highly dependent on the contexts in which they are implemented. The transferability (or lack thereof) of AI tools across healthcare systems, regions, and patient populations has become a central concern, which is often labelled "algorithmic migration" failure (Yu et al., 2022). For instance, recent systematic reviews have demonstrated that AI triage systems validated in high-resource urban hospitals can lose substantial predictive power when deployed in lower-resource, rural settings (El Arab & Al Moosa, 2025). This drop in performance is often attributed to differences in patient demographics, disease prevalence, healthcare delivery models, and even local coding practices within EHR systems. Such discrepancies not only diminish the clinical utility of AI tools but also risk exacerbating health disparities—since the models may perform least well for those groups already underserved by existing infrastructures. International experience echoes this concern. COVID-19 predictive algorithms developed in Europe and North America, for example, often proved unreliable when applied in Sub-Saharan Africa or South Asia, where epidemiological patterns, healthcare-seeking behaviors, and data infrastructures differ markedly (Mamandipoor et al., 2022; WHO, 2024). The lack of transparency about the context of AI model development and testing further complicates efforts to identify and address these biases. Altogether, these challenges underscore the necessity of context-sensitive model development, continuous validation in diverse practice settings, and transparent documentation of data provenance and system limitations. To synthesize the critical points at which bias can emerge or be amplified, Figure 2 illustrates the main stages of the healthcare AI lifecycle, from data collection through clinical use, highlighting key vulnerabilities for bias introduction and propagation.

Figure 2. The AI Lifecycle in Healthcare and Key Points of Bias Emergence.

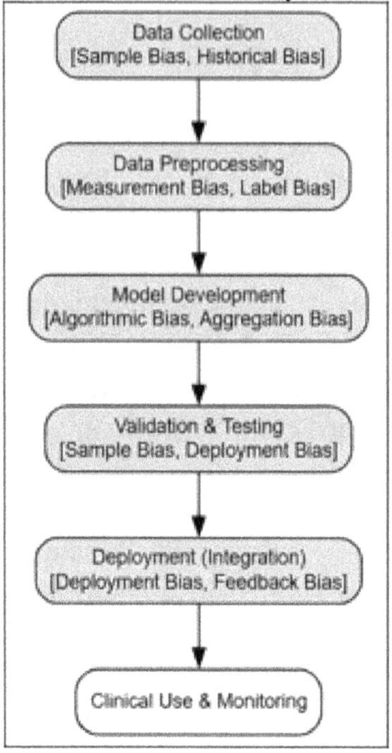

Each stage in the AI development and deployment process presents distinct risks for bias—from sample and historical bias during data collection, to measurement and label bias in preprocessing, algorithmic and aggregation bias during model development, and onward through deployment, integration, and ongoing clinical use. Recognizing these inflection points is essential for building more equitable and context-sensitive AI systems in health.

Lived Experience and Stakeholder Perspectives

Professional Experience

Although the existing literature on AI in healthcare is still primarily grounded in the measurement of technical performance, an emerging literature base has begun to document the lived experiences of clinicians and frontline workers who are tasked with introducing algorithmic-assisted patient care into their everyday practices. The qualitative narratives tell a complexity of stories—from hopeful optimism and deliberative repurposing to skepticism, frustration, and in some cases, outright resistance.

For example, in a recent international survey conducted by Amann et al. (2020), several clinicians expressed considerable concerns about "algorithmic opacity," or the issue of interpreting the decisions made by AI systems and their recommendations. Opacity prevented clinicians from defending or clarifying decisions made for patients or reconciling their own clinical judgement with the outputs of AI systems. This led to some clinicians demonstrating reticent behaviours (also known to researchers as algorithm aversion) in relation to AI tools and systems when the rationale for decision making was ambiguous, and where there were conflicts with medical expertise.

Similar challenges are echoed in other qualitative studies. For examples, a study by (Lombi & Rossero, 2024) with radiologists found that although some professionals saw AI as a valuable "second opinion," other professionals experienced concerns that if they become too reliant on AI or automated systems, they would lose their professional autonomy, or automated systems would deskill their profession. In some instances, healthcare clinicians described their exasperation with AI generated alerts or recommendations that only added to their administrative work and did not translate to meaningful improvement in patient care (Baillie et al.,2025).

Taken together, these perspectives make it clear that the successful adoption of AI in healthcare is not just a technical hurdle—it is also a deeply human, organizational, and cultural challenge. Building trust, ensuring transparency, and actively involving clinicians and frontline staff in the design, testing, and evaluation of digital tools are essential steps toward meaningful, sustainable integration.

These professional experiences find a parallel in the perspectives of patients and communities, whose trust in digital health innovation is equally shaped by issues of transparency, engagement, and real-world impact.

Patient and Community Perspectives

Patients and communities, too, experience the promises and pitfalls of AI-driven healthcare in ways that profoundly affect trust, engagement, and health outcomes. Studies show that awareness of algorithmic bias or a lack of transparency can undermine patient confidence in digital health interventions, particularly among historically marginalized groups (Agarwal et al., 2023). For instance, participatory research by (Carra et al., 2024) found that involving a diverse group of stakeholders—including patients, clinicians, and nurses—in the assessment of clinical AI applications helped surface concerns about fairness, transparency, and inclusion (Carra et al., 2024). Advocacy organizations and scholars have recommended participatory audits and feedback mechanisms that enable patients and stakeholders to identify and address algorithmic harms in real time (Panch et al., 2022).

Recent participatory frameworks and pilot studies—such as those described by Carra et al. (2024) and Panch et al. (2022) suggest that these models can increase trust, foster shared understanding, and help surface hidden biases that might otherwise go unaddressed. Ultimately, centering the lived experiences of clinicians, patients, and communities is not just an ethical imperative but a practical necessity for realizing the equitable potential of AI in healthcare. By shifting the focus from abstract performance metrics to real-world impact, we open the door to more responsive, just, and sustainable digital innovation. Building on these insights, the following section synthesizes key lessons and emerging best practices that can guide the development and implementation of fair, trustworthy, and context-sensitive AI in healthcare.

Lessons Learned and Emerging Best Practices

The case studies and stakeholder narratives reviewed above reveal several recurring patterns and actionable insights for addressing bias and inequality in healthcare AI. First, it is evident that algorithmic performance and fairness are deeply contingent on the quality, diversity, and contextual relevance of the data and settings in which systems are trained and deployed. Efforts to "debias" AI must therefore move beyond technical patching and embrace a holistic approach—one that recognizes the social, organizational, and ethical determinants of health technology outcomes (Gianfrancesco et al., 2018; De Manuel et al., 2023).

Synthesis of Key Case Study Findings

The evidence from diverse clinical and administrative settings underscores that algorithmic bias is inherently context-dependent and multi-layered. Models that achieve high performance in one environment frequently underperform—or may even harm—marginalized populations in others, owing to differences in local data, disease prevalence, and healthcare practices (Adamson & Smith, 2018; Iloanusi & Chun, 2024). Moreover, opaque or so-called "black box" systems erode the trust of both clinicians and patients. When the reasoning behind AI-generated recommendations is not transparent or explainable, users report significant difficulty in accepting, challenging, or contextualizing those outputs (Durán & Jongsma, 2021). Finally, the lack of meaningful stakeholder engagement consistently amplifies risk. AI systems developed in isolation from diverse communities and frontline professionals are much more likely to overlook critical sources of bias, as well as practical barriers to real-world implementation (Nadarzynski et al., 2024; Camacho et al., 2025). Collectively, these findings highlight that technical excellence alone is insufficient. Addressing the real-world complexities of healthcare AI requires openness, collaboration, and a deep commitment to equity at every stage of the technology lifecycle.

Practical Strategies for Bias Detection, Mitigation, and Co-Design

Building on the lessons from case studies and stakeholder experiences, contemporary research and international guidelines highlight a set of practical strategies essential for detecting, mitigating, and ultimately preventing bias in healthcare AI. Regular and diverse data audits are critical, ensuring that datasets are representative, inclusive, and free from systematic exclusions that disadvantage minority or underserved populations (Adamson & Smith, 2018; Finlayson et al., 2021). In parallel, contextual validation—systematic testing of models within the environments and populations where they will be deployed—remains vital for capturing local realities and adapting algorithms to real-world heterogeneity (Finlayson et al., 2021; Riley et al., 2021). Transparent and explainable AI approaches further support trust and accountability by making the reasoning behind algorithmic recommendations accessible to both clinicians and patients, while participatory co-design, involving stakeholders throughout the AI lifecycle, brings crucial lived experience and practical knowledge to bear on the development process (Panigutti et al., 2023; Schor et al., 2024; Camacho et al., 2025 ; Hermann et al., 2025). Beyond these technical and procedural advances, leading international organizations and regulatory bodies have developed comprehensive recommendations and standards for equity-oriented AI governance. Table 2 below synthesizes the principal frameworks from the World Health Organization, U.S. Food and Drug Administration, European Commission, National Academy of Medicine, and other key institutions, each emphasizing the need for human rights, transparency, data representativeness, multi-stakeholder oversight, and continuous monitoring as cornerstones of ethical and effective AI integration in healthcare.

Table 2. Key Recommendations from Major Institutions on AI, Bias, and Equity in Healthcare

Institution	Recommendation (Year)	Summary of Key Points	Reference
World Health Organization (WHO)	*Ethics & Governance of AI for Health* (2024)	Center human rights and equity in all AI health applications; ensure transparency, data representativeness, independent validation, and multi-stakeholder oversight.	(WHO, 2024)
US Food & Drug Administration (FDA)	*Proposed Regulatory Framework for Modifications to AI/ML-Based Software* (2019)	Require pre-market transparency, continuous monitoring, real-world performance auditing, and mechanisms to detect and address bias in AI-enabled medical devices.	(Benjamens et al., 2020; U.S. Food and Drug Administration, 2019)
European Commission	*Ethics Guidelines for Trustworthy AI* (2019)	Emphasize fairness, non-discrimination, explainability, and robust governance; advocate for regular bias audits and inclusive data practices in health AI.	(Busuioc, 2022 ; HLEG, 2019)
National Institutes of Health (NIH)	*Strategic Plan for Data Science* (2023)	Prioritize data diversity, FAIR principles (Findable, Accessible, Interoperable, Reusable), and explicit mitigation of bias at every stage of AI research.	(Arora et al., 2023; Chin et al., 2023)
US National Academy of Medicine (NAM)	*AI in Health Care: The Hope, the Hype, the Promise, the Peril* (2023)	Call for standards on data representativeness, inclusive design, regular external validation, and continuous post-deployment equity monitoring.	(Whicher et al., 2023)
UK National Health Service (NHS) AI Lab	*AI Ethics Initiative* (2022)	Mandate patient and public involvement, bias and fairness assessments, and publication of model documentation and evaluation results.	(Fletcher et al., 2021 ; Nazer et al., 2023)
World Economic Forum (WEF)	*AI Governance Framework for Health* (2022)	Encourage global standards, public-private collaboration, and explicit bias mitigation strategies in all stages of AI lifecycle.	(Bullard et al., 2022)

Collectively, these practical strategies and institutional guidelines underscore a crucial paradigm shift: moving from isolated technical "fixes" toward systemic, participatory, and justice-centered governance of AI. Only by embedding equity, transparency, and community engagement throughout the AI lifecycle can healthcare systems ensure that digital innovation serves to reduce, rather than reproduce, longstanding health disparities.

Implications for Research, Regulation, and Policy

Looking forward, advancing equity in healthcare AI requires moving beyond piecemeal technical fixes to embrace an interdisciplinary, participatory, and justice-centered research agenda. Future studies should be designed in collaboration with clinical practitioners, social scientists, ethicists, and most importantly, affected communities, ensuring that algorithmic harms are anticipated, measured, and meaningfully mitigated (Tariq, 2023). At the same time, robust regulatory oversight is essential—policymakers and governing bodies must mandate comprehensive algorithmic impact assessments, transparent public reporting of model performance across diverse groups, and enforceable standards for fairness and explainability (Selbst, 2021; Busuioc, 2022). To maintain accountability and adaptability over time, institutions should establish sustainable feedback and audit mechanisms, incorporating participatory audits and ongoing monitoring systems capable of detecting and correcting emerging biases as they arise (Krause, 2024). Ultimately, promoting equity in healthcare AI depends on a paradigm shift: from narrow technical optimization toward a context-aware, ethically grounded approach that centers inclusivity, justice, and the lived realities of patients and practitioners at every stage of digital innovation.

The empirical evidence examined here indicates a consistent pattern: the biases and inequities in healthcare AI are not purely technical nor accidental, but rather informed by larger social and structural, contextual dynamics. Clinical case studies, failures in administration, and the experiences of professionals and patients evince that often, AI algorithms reflect—and in some instances exacerbate—prior inequities rather than correcting them. This comes from a multitude of lens not only limited data/development, but also adversely affected by a lack of meaningful engagement with stakeholder and consideration for contextualization through the AI development lifecycle. Indeed, these findings illustrate a key limitation in current approaches to AI in health: narrowly technical or 'one-size-fits-all' approaches are not enough to achieve equitable outcomes. To address the issues of bias and inequality, we need to shift paradigms to an emphasis of interdisciplinary collaborations, participatory co-design, and justice-centered governing principles. This collaboration should draw on different disciplines, from clinical expertise, social science, ethics, and policy, while centering the voices of those communities impacted by digital health innovation. In the discussion, we will be looking at how these lessons can be converted into actual recommendations for research, practice and policy, paving the way for a more inclusive, transparent and accountable future for AI in global health equity.

DISCUSSION

This review reveals that while artificial intelligence (AI) continues to inspire optimism about its transformative potential in healthcare, its real-world deployment remains fundamentally constrained by the persistence of algorithmic bias and structural inequality. Despite impressive advances and widespread adoption, empirical evidence shows that algorithmic solutions alone are rarely sufficient to address the deeply rooted and context-dependent nature of health disparities.

A critical synthesis of recent studies highlights that the impacts of AI in healthcare are profoundly shaped by the data, contexts, and sociotechnical systems in which they operate. The myth of algorithmic neutrality has been steadily dismantled by cases of bias in clinical, administrative, and community settings. These cases emphasize the need for participatory design, rigorous validation, transparent reporting, and robust governance frameworks.

To distill the central findings of this review and to chart a path forward, Table 3 below synthesizes the key lessons learned, persistent gaps, and priority directions for future research and policy on bias and equity in healthcare AI.

Table 3. Key Lessons, Unresolved Challenges, and Future Research Directions in Healthcare AI Bias.

Key Lessons from Recent Literature	Persistent Challenges ("Gaps")	Directions for Future Research
Bias is multi-layered and context-dependent; "one-size-fits-all" debiasing rarely works.	Persistent underrepresentation of minority populations in training and validation data.	Systematic inclusion of diverse demographic, social, and clinical contexts in datasets.
Transparency and explainability are crucial for trust, adoption, and accountability.	Lack of standardized reporting and audit mechanisms for bias and fairness.	Development and implementation of open, reproducible auditing frameworks.
Participatory, stakeholder-driven co-design improves relevance and equity.	Limited engagement of patients, clinicians, and community groups in AI development.	Integration of participatory design methodologies throughout the AI lifecycle.
Real-world validation is essential: models must be tested in diverse settings.	Many AI systems remain "black boxes" with poorly documented deployment outcomes.	Longitudinal, post-deployment studies measuring real-world impacts on health equity.
Regulation and institutional guidance are evolving but fragmented across jurisdictions.	Fragmented or inconsistent regulatory approaches internationally.	Comparative analysis of global regulatory frameworks and harmonization of best practices.
Open data and open-source tools support reproducibility and equity.	Data privacy, governance, and ethical barriers to data sharing persist.	Innovations in privacy-preserving data sharing and federated learning models.

Contrary to narratives of neutrality that dominate much of the scientific and policy discourse, mounting evidence demonstrates that AI systems often reflect—and may amplify—the inequities embedded in the data, clinical practices, and health systems from which they arise (Gianfrancesco et al., 2018; Obermeyer et al., 2019; WHO, 2024). Multiple case studies highlight that diagnostic and prognostic algorithms trained on homogenous datasets or proxies, such as healthcare expenditures, systematically disadvantage racial minorities, women, the elderly, and those from low-resource settings, perpetuating health disparities rather than remedying them (Adamson & Smith, 2018; Rajkomar et al., 2019; Seyyed-Kalantari et al.,2020; Iloanusi & Chun, 2024). Such issues are further entrenched by methodological and editorial practices that prioritize technical novelty and reported "successes" over critical engagement with bias, context, and equity (De Manuel et al., 2023; Munk et al., 2024).

The illusion of algorithmic neutrality is sustained by the underrepresentation of marginalized groups in datasets, limited transparency about data provenance and modeling assumptions, and the frequent lack of context-sensitive validation across diverse healthcare environments (Gianfrancesco et al., 2018; Finlayson et al., 2021). Importantly, the transferability of AI models—often validated in well-resourced, homogenous settings—remains limited when these tools are deployed in different health systems or among patient populations with distinct epidemiological and social characteristics, leading to substantial drops in performance and unintended harms (Finlayson et al., 2021; Wong et al., 2021; Iloanusi & Chun, 2024). Qualitative research further reveals that both clinicians and patients express skepticism toward "black box" models whose recommendations lack transparency, interpretability, or alignment with professional expertise and lived experience (Durán & Jongsma, 2021; Rosenbacke et al., 2024). Absent genuine participation from healthcare workers, patients, and affected communities, efforts to "debias" algorithms remain insufficient, and trust in digital innovation is undermined (WHO, 2024; Camacho et al., 2025).

These findings highlight the urgent need for a paradigm shift in both research and governance. Technical fixes and fairness metrics, while important, cannot substitute for interdisciplinary, participatory, and justice-centered approaches that embed ethical reflection and contextual sensitivity throughout the AI development lifecycle (De Manuel et al., 2023; Tariq, 2023; WHO, 2024). Rigorous, continuous data audits and transparent reporting of model performance across demographic groups should become standard practice, complemented by the integration of social determinants and local knowledge into data infrastructures (Adamson & Smith, 2018; Finlayson et al., 2021). Furthermore, the creation of robust regulatory frameworks requiring impact assessments, participatory audits, and equity-focused oversight is essential to safeguard against the institutionalization of digital health inequities (Selbst, 2021; Busuioc, 2022; WHO, 2024). Finally, future research must prioritize cross-contextual and longitudinal studies, expand the inclusion of underrepresented populations and health systems, and develop participatory mechanisms for real-time monitoring, co-design, and accountability (Tariq, 2023; Camacho et al., 2025). Only through such comprehensive, context-aware, and justice-oriented strategies can the potential of AI in healthcare be harnessed to advance, rather than undermine, global health equity.

FUTURE RESEARCH

The rapid evolution of artificial intelligence in healthcare, although promising, reveals critical gaps that must be addressed by future work. First, academic research must move beyond controlled laboratory environments toward longitudinal impact studies conducted in real-world settings. It is essential to examine how diagnostic and triage algorithms influence clinical decision-making over the long term, with particular attention to their capacity either to reduce or to exacerbate health disparities among historically marginalized populations.

Moreover, overcoming the opacity of models—often described as "black boxes"—represents a major research priority. Future studies should explore interdisciplinary frameworks that combine computer science, ethics, and social sciences to develop "explainable AI" (XAI) that is contextually meaningful for practitioners. The objective is to transform purely mathematical performance metrics into transparent decision-support tools, enabling clinicians to understand the rationale behind algorithmic recommendations and to identify potential biases in real time.

Finally, a crucial dimension of forthcoming research lies in adopting participatory and intersectional approaches. Rather than analyzing biases in isolation (race, gender, or socioeconomic status), future researchers should investigate how these social identities intersect to generate unique forms of algorithmic discrimination. By involving patients and diverse stakeholders from the early stages of system design and data labeling, research can ensure that technological innovation is not only efficient but also fundamentally equitable and responsive to human diversity.

CONCLUSION

In conclusion, this review illustrates that while AI has transformational potential for health care, it risks not eliminating—existing health inequities if we indiscriminately scale it. AI system is not neutral or benevolent, and often disadvantages marginalized populations, when they do not incorporate context, variation and experience. In the face of these challenges, the persistent illusion of algorithmic neutrality—bolstered by methodological shortcomings and editorial convention—will continue to hide the inherently social nature of digital health innovation, and the nuanced realities of patients, practitioners and communities. Acknowledging the fair possibility of AI in healthcare thus requires a complete paradigm shift, from technical solutionism to participatory, interdisciplinary, and justice-oriented approaches. This entails thorough and continuous auditing of data and algorithms, public reporting, active regulatory auditing, and most critically, authentic engagement of communities directly impacted by AI and frontline practitioners throughout the whole AI lifecycle. By applying these practices throughout the lifecycle, we can make sure artificial intelligence becomes a vehicle for health equity, rather than a mechanism for introducing or catalyzing new or deepened disparities. The way forward is clear: as a global health community, we should be moving to a more just, inclusive, and accountable approach to AI – not just because it is warranted, but because it is critical.

DATA AVAILABILITY

This study is based on a literature review and does not involve the generation or analysis of original datasets. All data supporting the findings of this study are derived from previously published sources, which are properly cited in the reference list.

FUNDING

This work received no external funding.

CONFLICTS OF INTEREST

The authors declare no conflict of interest.

ACKNOWLEDGMENTS

The authors would like to sincerely thank all contributors for their invaluable support and insightful input throughout this study. We also extend our gratitude to ChatGPT for assistance with linguistic revision and improving the clarity and readability of the manuscript.

REFERENCES

Abràmoff, M. D., Tarver, M. E., Loyo-Berrios, N., Trujillo, S., Char, D., Obermeyer, Z., Eydelman, M. B., & Maisel, W. H. (2023). Considerations for addressing bias in artificial intelligence for health equity. *NPJ Digital Medicine*, *6*(1), 170. DOI: 10.1038/s41746-023-00913-9 PMID: 37700029

Adamson, A. S., & Smith, A. (2018). Machine learning and health care disparities in dermatology. *JAMA Dermatology*, *154*(11), 1247–1248. DOI: 10.1001/jamadermatol.2018.2348 PMID: 30073260

Agarwal, R., Bjarnadottir, M., Rhue, L., Dugas, M., Crowley, K., Clark, J., & Gao, G. (2023). Addressing algorithmic bias and the perpetuation of health inequities: An AI bias aware framework. *Health Policy and Technology*, *12*(1), 100702. DOI: 10.1016/j.hlpt.2022.100702

Ali, H., & Nikberg, N. (2024). *Bias in AI-driven healthcare: Navigating ethical challenges at an early stage.*

Aquino, Y. S. J., Carter, S. M., Houssami, N., Braunack-Mayer, A., Win, K. T., Degeling, C., Wang, L., & Rogers, W. A. (2025). Practical, epistemic and normative implications of algorithmic bias in healthcare artificial intelligence: A qualitative study of multidisciplinary expert perspectives. *Journal of Medical Ethics*, *51*(6), 420–428. DOI: 10.1136/jme-2022-108850 PMID: 36823101

Arora, A., Alderman, J. E., Palmer, J., Ganapathi, S., Laws, E., McCradden, M. D., Oakden-Rayner, L., Pfohl, S. R., Ghassemi, M., McKay, F., Treanor, D., Rostamzadeh, N., Mateen, B., Gath, J., Adebajo, A. O., Kuku, S., Matin, R., Heller, K., Sapey, E., & Liu, X. (2023). The value of standards for health datasets in artificial intelligence-based applications. *Nature Medicine*, *29*(11), 2929–2938. DOI: 10.1038/s41591-023-02608-w PMID: 37884627

Baillie, L., Stewart-Lord, A., Thomas, N., & Frings, D. (2025). Patients', clinicians' and developers' perspectives and experiences of artificial intelligence in cardiac healthcare: A qualitative study. *Digital Health*, *11*, 20552076251328578. DOI: 10.1177/20552076251328578 PMID: 40534891

Benjamens, S., Dhunnoo, P., & Meskó, B. (2020). The state of artificial intelligence-based FDA-approved medical devices and algorithms: An online database. *NPJ Digital Medicine*, *3*(1), 118. DOI: 10.1038/s41746-020-00324-0 PMID: 32984550

Benjamens, S., Dhunnoo, P., & Meskó, B. (2020). The state of artificial intelligence-based FDA-approved medical devices and algorithms: An online database. *NPJ Digital Medicine*, *3*(1), 118. DOI: 10.1038/s41746-020-00324-0 PMID: 32984550

Braveman, P., Arkin, E., Orleans, T., Proctor, D., & Plough, A. (2017). *What is health equity? And what difference does a definition make?* Robert Wood Johnson Foundation.

Bullard, N., et al. (2022). Ethics by design: An organizational approach to responsible use of technology.

Bullock, J., Luccioni, A., Pham, K. H., Lam, C. S. N., & Luengo-Oroz, M. (2020). Mapping the landscape of artificial intelligence applications against COVID-19. *Journal of Artificial Intelligence Research*, *69*, 807–845. DOI: 10.1613/jair.1.12162

Busuioc, M. (2022). AI algorithmic oversight: New frontiers in regulation. In *Handbook of regulatory authorities* (pp. 470–486). Edward Elgar Publishing.

Camacho, M., Perramon, J., Puig-Bosch, X., Dang, V. N., Díaz, O., & Lekadir, K. (2025). Stakeholder engagement: The path to trustworthy AI in healthcare. In *Trustworthy AI in medical imaging* (pp. 471–493). Elsevier. DOI: 10.1016/B978-0-44-323761-4.00038-9

Carra, G., Kulynych, B., Bastardot, F., Kaufmann, D. E., Boillat-Blanco, N., & Raisaro, J. L. (2024). Participatory assessment of large language model applications in an academic medical center. *arXiv*. https://doi.org//arXiv.2501.10366DOI: 10.48550

Chin, M. H., Afsar-Manesh, N., Bierman, A. S., Chang, C., Colón-Rodríguez, C. J., Dullabh, P., Duran, D. G., Fair, M., Hernandez-Boussard, T., Hightower, M., Jain, A., Jordan, W. B., Konya, S., Moore, R. H., Moore, T. T., Rodriguez, R., Shaheen, G., Snyder, L. P., Srinivasan, M., & Ohno-Machado, L. (2023). Guiding principles to address the impact of algorithm bias on racial and ethnic disparities in health and health care. *JAMA Network Open*, *6*(12), e2345050. DOI: 10.1001/jamanetworkopen.2023.45050 PMID: 38100101

Daneshjou, R., Vodrahalli, K., Novoa, R. A., Jenkins, M., Liang, W., Rotemberg, V., Ko, J., Swetter, S. M., Bailey, E. E., Gevaert, O., Mukherjee, P., Phung, M., Yekrang, K., Fong, B., Sahasrabudhe, R., Allerup, J. A. C., Okata-Karigane, U., Zou, J., & Chiou, A. S. (2022). Disparities in dermatology AI performance on a diverse, curated clinical image set. *Science Advances*, *8*(32), eabq6147. Advance online publication. DOI: 10.1126/sciadv.abq6147 PMID: 35960806

De Manuel, A., Delgado, J., Parra Jounou, I., Ausín, T., Casacuberta, D., Cruz, M., Guersenzvaig, A., Moyano, C., Rodríguez-Arias, D., Rueda, J., & Puyol, A. (2023). Ethical assessments and mitigation strategies for biases in AI-systems used during the COVID-19 pandemic. *Big Data & Society*, *10*(1), 20539517231179199. Advance online publication. DOI: 10.1177/20539517231179199

Durán, J. M., & Jongsma, K. R. (2021). Who is afraid of black box algorithms? On the epistemological and ethical basis of trust in medical AI. *Journal of Medical Ethics*, *47*(5), 329–335. DOI: 10.1136/medethics-2020-106820 PMID: 33737318

El Arab, R. A., & Al Moosa, O. A. (2025). The role of AI in emergency department triage: An integrative systematic review. *Intensive & Critical Care Nursing*, *89*, 104058. DOI: 10.1016/j.iccn.2025.104058 PMID: 40306071

Esteva, A., Kuprel, B., Novoa, R. A., Ko, J., Swetter, S. M., Blau, H. M., & Thrun, S. (2017). Dermatologist-level classification of skin cancer with deep neural networks. *Nature*, *542*(7639), 115–118. DOI: 10.1038/nature21056 PMID: 28117445

Finlayson, S. G., Subbaswamy, A., Singh, K., Bowers, J., Kupke, A., Zittrain, J., Kohane, I. S., & Saria, S. (2021). The clinician and dataset shift in artificial intelligence. *The New England Journal of Medicine*, *385*(3), 283–286. DOI: 10.1056/NEJMc2104626 PMID: 34260843

Fletcher, R. R., Nakeshimana, A., & Olubeko, O. (2021). Addressing fairness, bias, and appropriate use of artificial intelligence and machine learning in global health. *Frontiers in Artificial Intelligence*, *3*, 561802. DOI: 10.3389/frai.2020.561802 PMID: 33981989

Geneviève, L. D., Martani, A., Shaw, D., Elger, B. S., & Wangmo, T. (2020). Structural racism in precision medicine: Leaving no one behind. *BMC Medical Ethics*, *21*(1), 17. DOI: 10.1186/s12910-020-0457-8 PMID: 32075640

Gianfrancesco, M. A., Tamang, S., Yazdany, J., & Schmajuk, G. (2018). Potential biases in machine learning algorithms using electronic health record data. *JAMA Internal Medicine*, *178*(11), 1544–1547. DOI: 10.1001/jamainternmed.2018.3763 PMID: 30128552

Giovanola, B., & Tiribelli, S. (2023). Beyond bias and discrimination: Redefining the AI ethics principle of fairness in healthcare machine-learning algorithms. *AI & Society*, *38*(2), 549–563. DOI: 10.1007/s00146-022-01455-6 PMID: 35615443

Groh, M., Harris, C., Daneshjou, R., Badri, O., & Koochek, A. (2022). Towards transparency in dermatology image datasets with skin tone annotations by experts, crowds, and an algorithm. *Proceedings of the ACM on Human-Computer Interaction*, *6*(CSCW2), 1–26. DOI: 10.1145/3555634

Haider, S. A., Borna, S., Gomez-Cabello, C. A., Pressman, S. M., Haider, C. R., & Forte, A. J. (2024). The algorithmic divide: A systematic review on AI-driven racial disparities in healthcare. *Journal of Racial and Ethnic Health Disparities*. Advance online publication. DOI: 10.1007/s40615-024-02237-0 PMID: 39695057

Hermann, J., Jansen, N., & Dogangün, A. (2025). We need to understand where the data comes from: Co-designing transparent AI systems for caregiving. In *Companion Proceedings of the 30th International Conference on Intelligent User Interfaces* (pp. 105–109). ACM. DOI: 10.1145/3708557.3716354

Iloanusi, N.-J., & Chun, S. A. (2024). AI impact on health equity for marginalized, racial, and ethnic minorities. In *Proceedings of the 25th Annual International Conference on Digital Government Research* (pp. 841–848). ACM. https://doi.org/DOI: 10.1145/3657054.3657152

Krause, D. (2024). Addressing the challenges of auditing and testing for AI bias: A comparative analysis of regulatory frameworks. SSRN *Electronic Journal.* https://doi.org/DOI: 10.2139/ssrn.5050631

Lau, P. L. (2025). *Rewriting the narrative of AI bias: A data feminist critique of algorithmic inequalities in healthcare.* Law, Technology and Humans., DOI: 10.5204/lthj.3845

Lombi, L., & Rossero, E. (2024). How artificial intelligence is reshaping the autonomy and boundary work of radiologists: A qualitative study. *Sociology of Health & Illness, 46*(2), 200–218. DOI: 10.1111/1467-9566.13702 PMID: 37573551

Malgaroli, M., Hull, T. D., Zech, J. M., & Althoff, T. (2023). Natural language processing for mental health interventions: A systematic review and research framework. *Translational Psychiatry, 13*(1), 309. DOI: 10.1038/s41398-023-02592-2 PMID: 37798296

Mamandipoor, B., Bruno, R. R., Wernly, B., Wolff, G., Fjølner, J., Artigas, A., Pinto, B. B., Schefold, J. C., Kelm, M., Beil, M., Sigal, S., Leaver, S., De Lange, D. W., Guidet, B., Flaatten, H., Szczeklik, W., Jung, C., & Osmani, V. (2022). COVID-19 machine learning model predicts outcomes in older patients from various European countries, between pandemic waves, and in a cohort of Asian, African, and American patients. *PLOS Digital Health, 1*(11), e0000136. DOI: 10.1371/journal.pdig.0000136 PMID: 36812571

McCradden, M. D., Joshi, S., Mazwi, M., & Anderson, J. A. (2020). Ethical limitations of algorithmic fairness solutions in health care machine learning. *The Lancet. Digital Health, 2*(5), e221–e223. DOI: 10.1016/S2589-7500(20)30065-0 PMID: 33328054

Mergen, A., Çetin-Kılıç, N., & Özbilgin, M. F. (2025). Artificial intelligence and bias towards marginalised groups: Theoretical roots and challenges. In Vassilopoulou, J., & Kyriakidou, O. (Eds.), *International perspectives on equality, diversity and inclusion* (pp. 17–38). Emerald Publishing Limited., DOI: 10.1108/S2051-233320250000012004

Morales-Forero, A., Rueda Jaime, L., Gil-Quiñones, S. R., Barrera Montañez, M. Y., Bassetto, S., & Coatanea, E. (2024). An insight into racial bias in dermoscopy repositories: A HAM10000 data set analysis. *JEADV Clinical Practice, 3*(3), 836–843. DOI: 10.1002/jvc2.477

Morley, J., & Floridi, L. (2020). An ethically mindful approach to AI for health care. *Lancet, 395*(10220), 254–255. DOI: 10.1016/S0140-6736(19)32975-7 PMID: 31982053

Munk, A. K., Jacomy, M., Ficozzi, M., & Jensen, T. E. (2024). Beyond artificial intelligence controversies: What are algorithms doing in the scientific literature? *Big Data & Society*, *11*(3), 20539517241255107. DOI: 10.1177/20539517241255107

Nadarzynski, T., Knights, N., Husbands, D., Graham, C. A., Llewellyn, C. D., Buchanan, T., Montgomery, I., & Ridge, D. (2024). Achieving health equity through conversational AI: A roadmap for design and implementation of inclusive chatbots in healthcare. *PLOS Digital Health*, *3*(5), e0000492. DOI: 10.1371/journal.pdig.0000492 PMID: 38696359

Nazer, L. H., Zatarah, R., Waldrip, S., Ke, J. X. C., Moukheiber, M., Khanna, A. K., Hicklen, R. S., Moukheiber, L., Moukheiber, D., Ma, H., & Mathur, P. (2023). Bias in artificial intelligence algorithms and recommendations for mitigation. *PLOS Digital Health*, *2*(6), e0000278. DOI: 10.1371/journal.pdig.0000278 PMID: 37347721

O'Malley, A., Veenhuizen, M., & Ahmed, A. (2024). Ensuring appropriate representation in artificial intelligence–generated medical imagery: Protocol for a methodological approach to address skin tone bias. *JMIR AI*, *3*, e58275. DOI: 10.2196/58275 PMID: 39602221

Obermeyer, Z., Powers, B., Vogeli, C., & Mullainathan, S. (2019). Dissecting racial bias in an algorithm used to manage the health of populations. *Science*, *366*(6464), 447–453. DOI: 10.1126/science.aax2342 PMID: 31649194

Panch, T., Duralde, E., Mattie, H., Kotecha, G., Celi, L. A., Wright, M., & Greaves, F. (2022). A distributed approach to the regulation of clinical AI. *PLOS Digital Health*, *1*(5), e0000040. DOI: 10.1371/journal.pdig.0000040 PMID: 36812520

Panch, T., Mattie, H., & Atun, R. (2019). Artificial intelligence and algorithmic bias: Implications for health systems. *Journal of Global Health*, *9*(2), 020318. DOI: 10.7189/jogh.09.020318 PMID: 31788229

Panigutti, C., Beretta, A., Fadda, D., Giannotti, F., Pedreschi, D., Perotti, A., & Rinzivillo, S. (2023). Co-design of human-centered, explainable AI for clinical decision support. *ACM Transactions on Interactive Intelligent Systems*, *13*(4), 1–35. DOI: 10.1145/3587271

Rajkomar, A., Dean, J., & Kohane, I. (2019). Machine learning in medicine. *The New England Journal of Medicine*, *380*(14), 1347–1358. DOI: 10.1056/NEJMra1814259 PMID: 30943338

Riley, R. D., Debray, T. P. A., Collins, G. S., Archer, L., Ensor, J., van Smeden, M., & Snell, K. I. E. (2021). Minimum sample size for external validation of a clinical prediction model with a binary outcome. *Statistics in Medicine*, *40*(19), 4230–4251. DOI: 10.1002/sim.9025 PMID: 34031906

Rosenbacke, R., Melhus, Å., McKee, M., & Stuckler, D. (2024). How explainable artificial intelligence can increase or decrease clinicians' trust in AI applications in health care: Systematic review. *JMIR AI*, *3*, e53207. DOI: 10.2196/53207 PMID: 39476365

Schor, B. G. S., Kallina, E., Singh, J., & Blackwell, A. (2024). Meaningful transparency for clinicians: Operationalising HCXAI research with gynaecologists. In *Proceedings of the 2024 ACM Conference on Fairness, Accountability, and Transparency* (pp. 1268–1281). ACM. DOI: 10.1145/3630106.3658971

Selbst, A. D. (2021). An institutional view of algorithmic impact assessments. *Harvard Journal of Law & Technology*, *35*, 117.

Seyyed-Kalantari, L., Liu, G., McDermott, M., Chen, I. Y., & Ghassemi, M. (2020). CheXclusion: Fairness gaps in deep chest X-ray classifiers. In *Biocomputing 2021: Proceedings of the Pacific Symposium* (pp. 232–243). World Scientific. https://doi.org/DOI: 10.1142/9789811232701_0022

Singhal, A., Neveditsin, N., Tanveer, H., & Mago, V. (2024). Toward fairness, accountability, transparency, and ethics in AI for social media and health care: Scoping review. *JMIR Medical Informatics*, *12*(1), e50048. DOI: 10.2196/50048 PMID: 38568737

Soltan, A. A., Yang, J., Pattanshetty, R., Novak, A., Yang, Y., Rohanian, O., Beer, S., Soltan, M. A., Thickett, D. R., Fairhead, R., Zhu, T., Eyre, D. W., Clifton, D. A., Watson, A., Bhargav, A., Tough, A., Rogers, A., Shaikh, A., Valensise, C., & Muthusami, V. (2022). Real-world evaluation of rapid and laboratory-free COVID-19 triage for emergency care: External validation and pilot deployment of artificial intelligence-driven screening. *The Lancet. Digital Health*, *4*(4), e266–e278. DOI: 10.1016/S2589-7500(21)00272-7 PMID: 35279399

Tariq, S. (2023). AI and ethics: Interdisciplinary perspectives on algorithmic transparency and bias. *Multidisciplinary Research in Computer and Information Systems*, *3*(4), 256–266.

Topol, E. J. (2019). High-performance medicine: The convergence of human and artificial intelligence. *Nature Medicine*, *25*(1), 44–56. DOI: 10.1038/s41591-018-0300-7 PMID: 30617339

U.S. Food and Drug Administration. (2019). *Proposed regulatory framework for modifications to artificial intelligence/machine learning (AI/ML)-based software as a medical device (SaMD): Discussion paper and request for feedback.*

Vayena, E., & Blasimme, A. (2018). Health research with big data: Time for systemic oversight. *The Journal of Law, Medicine & Ethics*, *46*(1), 119–129. DOI: 10.1177/1073110518766026 PMID: 30034208

Whicher, D., Ahmed, M., Israni, S. T., & Matheny, M. (2023). Artificial intelligence in health care: The hope, the hype, the promise, the peril.

WHO. (2024). World Health Organization. Ethics and governance of artificial intelligence for health: WHO guidance. Geneva: World Health Organization; 2021. ISBN 9789240029200. Disponible sur https://iris.who.int/handle/10665/341996

Wong, A., Otles, E., Donnelly, J. P., Krumm, A., McCullough, J., DeTroyer-Cooley, O., Pestrue, J., Phillips, M., Konye, J., Penoza, C., Ghous, M., & Singh, K. (2021). External validation of a widely implemented proprietary sepsis prediction model in hospitalized patients. *JAMA Internal Medicine*, *181*(8), 1065–1070. DOI: 10.1001/jamainternmed.2021.2626 PMID: 34152373

Yu, J. Y., Xie, F., Nan, L., Yoon, S., Ong, M. E. H., Ng, Y. Y., & Cha, W. C. (2022). An external validation study of the Score for Emergency Risk Prediction (SERP), an interpretable machine learning-based triage score for the emergency department. *Scientific Reports*, *12*(1), 17466. DOI: 10.1038/s41598-022-22233-w PMID: 36261457

KEY TERMS AND DEFINITIONS

Algorithmic Bias: Systematic and repeatable errors in a computer system that create unfair outcomes, often by privileging one group over another, typically resulting from biased data, flawed model design, or inappropriate deployment.

Artificial Intelligence (AI): Computational systems that perform tasks typically requiring human intelligence, such as learning, reasoning, and problem-solving, including applications in diagnosis, prediction, and decision support in healthcare.

Contextual Validation: The process of testing and confirming the reliability, accuracy, and fairness of AI models in the actual settings and populations where they will be used, accounting for local contexts and variations.

Fairness in AI: The principle that algorithms and AI systems should operate in a way that is impartial and just, minimizing discriminatory outcomes and promoting equal opportunity across diverse populations.

Health Equity: The absence of avoidable, unfair, or remediable differences among populations or groups defined socially, economically, demographically, or geographically.

Machine Learning (ML): A branch of AI in which algorithms improve their performance on a given task through experience, learning patterns from large datasets rather than relying on explicit programming.

Stakeholder Engagement: The meaningful involvement of diverse individuals and groups—including patients, clinicians, developers, and affected communities—at all stages of AI design, validation, and deployment, to ensure relevance and trustworthiness.

Chapter 9
Streaming Motherhood: A Digital Ethnography of Postpartum Voices on Social Media

M Siva Vidhya
http://orcid.org/0000-0003-3242-7298
SASTRA University, India

K Sunanda
http://orcid.org/0009-0001-3803-9977
SASTRA University, India

ABSTRACT

The article explores how short-form video platforms like Instagram reels and YouTube shorts reflect and support the emotional journey of postpartum mothers in India. The research uses qualitative thematic analysis of over 300 comments across 15-20 popular postpartum themed videos along with the validation from interviews with 10 mothers. The research uncovers recurring themes such as sleep deprivation, emotional exhaustion, lack of empathetic support, culture and family pressure, and self-doubt. These stories are often narrated in sentimental, amusing or caustic way that provides a sense of belonging and validation. In a setting, where candid conversations about postpartum difficulties are frequently stigmatized, the study concludes that these digital platforms serve as an unofficial, cultural based support network. By combining digital discourse analysis with real voices, this paper highlights how language, culture and community intersect in shaping maternal mental health in India.

DOI: 10.4018/979-8-2600-0939-0.ch009

INTRODUCTION

Postpartum, a crucial phase in woman's life involves complex, physical, emotional and psychological adjustments. This period significantly impacts maternal and infant health, family dynamics and overall well-being. Despite advances in medical care, many women continue to face challenges such as postpartum depression, anxiety and social isolation (Eo et al., 2020). Clinical aspects of postpartum deals with physical and mental screening of mothers and its treatment options; whereas sociological research examines family support and community roles (Dennis et al., 2007). However these studies often overlook the way the mothers express their experiences especially through language and cultural practices. Culture shapes maternal experiences and expectations. In many societies, traditional rituals, beliefs and community support play a fundamental role in recovery.

India is rich in diverse cultural contexts where postpartum practices vary widely across regions, religions and communities. Despite this diversity, there is a limited qualitative research that explores how Indian mothers communicate and construct their postpartum experience. Social media usage among young mothers is growing rapidly which offers a new avenue for expression and support in India. Existing literature lacks in-depth analysis of the linguistic and cultural dimension of postpartum in Indian context. There is also a scarcity of studies examining how digital media influences maternal experiences and emotional expression. This study aims to fill the identified gap by exploring postpartum experiences shared by Indian mothers on digital forums such as Instagram reels and YouTube shorts. The study analyse the language, cultural references and emotional context embedded in these narratives.

BACKGROUND TO THE STUDY

Postpartum Depression (PPD) is the most challenging phase that consists of severe physical, emotional and psychological needs and changes in the mother's body. The pattern of postpartum experience is not uniform among all the women and it is greatly influenced by traditional practices, cultural beliefs, expectation of the society on the mother to be self-sacrificing agent, insufficient family care, pressure due to expectation of typical maternal role, etc. Also, women are criticised for genuinely expressing their mental state or it is often labelled as 'normal' or 'temporary'.

Many researches have been made on PPD, anxiety and stress among young mothers after childbirth. 22-28% of Indian mother experience PPD according to the recent research. Adding to that, the awareness, diagnosis and treatment remains unknown or ignored due to the social stigma about mental health especially after childbirth. Therefore, this unsupportive environment for the mothers makes them feel unrecognised and disconnected. Currently the social media which is popular among young mothers depicts the mental state and sleeplessness of the mothers. New mothers express their state through reels and short videos. The video includes the sleeplessness, lack of family support, cultural stigma, gender stereotyping, etc. through both emotional and humorous videos. In the comment section, one can view the comments of many new moms sharing their feeling of togetherness.

In the past few years, the growing social media apps like Instagram and YouTube which contain short form videos that are visually engaging and have become a source of entertainment and education. For the mothers who feel completely left out, emotionally disconnected or have fully engaged time schedule, these platforms help them feel connected and recognised through the contents related to maternity and postpartum recovery. Relatable contents such as breastfeeding struggles, sleepless nights, emotional breakdowns, depiction of daily chaotic schedule, etc., help them deeply understand the pattern. Also, these platforms act as a mediator to expose their journey and struggles more freely than in offline. Though, if not posting contents of their journey, many women find relief when commenting in the relatable reels or just by reading or seeing the struggles of other mothers of same condition. This helps the others to internalise their emotions and opinions without judgements.

The global perspective of Postpartum Depression focuses on many aspects of the individuals experiencing stress, anxiety and feeling of isolation. The intervention of short-form video content in reducing stress, PPD and anxiety has not been explored much in many research. Existing research primarily focuses on methods of clinical intervention like Cognitive Behavourial Therapy (CBT), Psychodrama Therapy and Internet-based Support Programs (ISP). Although, these interventions benefit the young mothers greatly, they are of typical therapy style of treatment which makes the mothers feeling diagnosed. These interventions also do not consider the everyday emotional reflections of the mothers. But, the social media and the short-form videos greatly aid the mothers by embracing their internal feelings and emotions through the relatable content.

PPD has multiple aspects that influence its effect profoundly. The earlier studies focus on improving mother's psychological conditions. But, there is rarely any study that explores how Indian mothers use digital discourse to fulfil emotional needs. Especially, how the short-form videos influence the collective aspects of postpartum experience. Adding to that, there is also lack of qualitative analysis or exploration. The previous studies mostly focus on surveys or clinical reports and limited researches made on real-life case studies.

This chapter focuses on analysing the introduction of short-form video contents in the academic scenario of PPD recovery. Through a qualitative thematic analysis, the study also deepens the insights on short-form videos and their growing recognition. If these visual aids help in reducing the stress and providing emotional relief, they can be strategically used to diagnose the mental issue of postpartum period along with the therapeutic sessions. This methodology can offer new insights to health practitioners, NGOs, and support groups in creating awareness and motivating new mothers for early help-seeking.

Social media can best support human health when it is used intentionally as a heath communication space rather than a site of excessive or passive consumption. In specific contexts, such as work-related stress, social isolation during COVID period, social media demonstrates a meaningful engagement through shared experiences, emotional expression and mutual reassurance. Studies by Damra et al., 2024 and Jin et al., 2025 indicate that social media use helps in coping the stress and loneliness arising from social isolation during COVID pandemic. Wegmann, E et al., 2023 deals with the way the social media helps in handling the stress. Moreover, Gómez-Casillas & Gómez Márquez claim that social media especially youtubes can function as an effective channel for climate change awareness. Thus when used positively and purposefully social media can help reduce loneliness, stress and emotional burden and strengthens social connectedness. Guaranteed health benefits can be achieved if individuals encounter shared lived narratives that normalize distress, reduce self-blame and facilitate cognitive reframing of personal struggles as common and manageable. Thus, the progressive role of social media in supporting human health does not lie in the intrinsic nature of the medium itself but rather hinges on its purposeful and moderated use that complements formal health care systems. The effective implementation of social media in public health platform is demonstrated through various studies discussed in the following literature survey.

LITERATURE REVIEW

Clinical and Digital Intervention in PPD:

The study by Eo et al. (2020b) conducted study about 250 mothers in Nigeria through an interview-based questionnaire, including Edinburgh Postnatal Depression Scale (EPDS). The mothers were analysed on their PPD (Prevalence and Postpartum depression) while attending healthcare centres after six weeks following childbirth. The study examined the data using a cross-sectional design and the score identified is ≥ 13. This indicates a rapid downfall of mental health conditions among the mothers in early stages of postpartum. PPD is 35.6% contributed by many factors such as caesarean delivery, maternal ill-health after birth, breastfeeding, etc. Multivariable Logistics regression used in this research categorised four major themes, such as intimate partner violence, experiencing postpartum blues, lack of support in infant care, and unsupportive partners. This clearly showcases the psychosocial conditions of PPD which are quite common among new mothers irrespective of demographic factors. Challenges such as having an unsupportive partner or lack of assistance in infant care strongly contribute to the mental distress of mothers. Therefore, the study suggests considering Nigerian Postnatal women mental health with an emphasis on these factors. It also recommends regular screening for postpartum depression, addressing domestic violence, strengthening support systems for new mothers, etc. to ensure early identification and better management of postpartum mental health issues.

Pettman et al. (2023) conducted a study on examining the maternal stage after postpartum by using Cognitive Behavioural Therapy (CBT). Various factors are analysed, such as anxiety, stress, social support and many others that contribute to the increasing or decreasing maternal depression. This study has reviewed 31 studies, which include a total of 5291 women participants, through randomised and controlled trial sessions of 26 trials that significantly contribute to the meta-analysis. The trials also included other CBT components such as Problem Solving Therapy, Behavioural Activation, Traditional CBT methods, etc. The data collected by CBT are analysed through systematic review and meta-analysis to measure its effectiveness. The correlation of bias was assessed by using the ROB 2.0 tool. Through this methodology, the authors found that there is a significant reduction in anxiety, stress, and lack of social support. The impact of CBT is considerably relevant and works well in reducing depression during the perinatal period (a period extending from pregnancy to postpartum). There are a few factors that influenced the working of CBT, such as the type of control group, the kind of CBT used and the agent of delivering the therapy (psychologist or counselling member). However, the result derived is only at a moderate level due to many other complexities in utilising CBT. It can be concluded that the difference in working of CBT is due to various contexts of measuring in different formats (online, grouped, ungrouped, individual). But the researcher again emphasises the fact that CBT is effective during and after childbirth. If the issues are addressed, better and more consistent research can be conducted.

Another case study by Appleton et al. (2025) showed how the eight-week Tresillian group psychotherapy program helped the mothers in PPD. This course is also added with a complementary program 'Circle of Security Perentng, COS-P' to check for any extra improvement in reducing anxiety and depression. The study is conducted in two metropolitan sites between the years 2017 and 2019. It has taken 141 consented women participants. Approximately 101 women travelled till end of the evaluation which opens a new research gap of missing data. The research shows a significant reduction in anxiety and depression level even after four weeks of the programme. The results were assessed using EPDS and EPDS-3A and the scores have dropped from 14.11 to 9.99. Also, women with history of family depression also showed similar improvement as those of the other women. Also the COS-P did not contribute any additional improvement but on the whole the therapy session yielded considerable improvement despite the drawbacks of incomplete data.

Branquinho et al. (2022) reported that using Blended Cognitive Behavioural Therapy (CBT) can significantly reduce the postpartum depression (PPD). In a CBT program called 'Be a Mom Coping with Depression' online sessions and sessions with psychologists were conducted to ease the mothers who struggle to attend typical therapy sessions. The case study reveals the identity of the person involved in the experiment. The investigation deals with a 31-year old woman named Sofia who experienced PPD, anxiety and exhaustion due to many factors such as low confidence as a mother, relationship struggles and isolated feeling. This intervention continued for 13 weeks of 7 psychologist sessions and 6 online modules. This program helped the young mother to cope up with her thoughts, emotions, values, social support and coping strategies. Through this controlled session, Sofia learnt to control negative thoughts, self-compassion, clear communication with partner and to carry out meaningful activities. With these significant improvements, the EPDS scores dropped from 19 to 8 evidently showing the psychological flexibility and improved self-compassion.

Maternal Mental Health

Yaqoob et al. (2024) in their study, analyses many risk factors related to postpartum depression (PPD) among women of Asian Countries. The factors are psychological, biological, cultural and socio-demographic related issues. The researchers have taken academic publications on PPD published between the years 2007 and 2023 which includes 90 studies from 14 Asian Countries such as India, Japan, Turkey, South Korea, Nepal and Iran. The study shows that 0.82% to 93% of PPD is seen among the maternal population after cut-off scores or eliminating the measurement gap. The risk factors are categorised into five categories. They are socio demographic factors, cultural factors, psychological factors, obstetric factors and biological or physical factors. The research concludes that Asian maternal population is highly influenced by its culturally sensitive intervention and inconsistent diagnosis measures.

Wang et al. (2021) conducted a large-scale meta-analysis and a systematic review on postpartum depression prevailing at global level. The researchers have taken 565 studies across 80 countries. The data has covered almost 12,36,365 postpartum women to understand the factors contributing to PPD across regions. Using authentic screening tools, mostly Edinburg Postnatal Depression Scale, the study has found that 17.22% of global prevalence is found. In other words, about 1 in 5 women worldwide experiences PPD every day. Adding to that, the prevalence of PPD varies due to different factors such as geographical region, cultural beliefs, traditional practices, etc. For example, a country like South Africa shows high rate of PPD, which is about 40%. Contrasting to that, developed countries of high income showed significantly lower PPD rate, which is around 14-15%. On the other hand, low and middle class income countries had much higher rates. Therefore, health system differences according to cultural, socio-economic, and traditional values followed by the region. The study also highlighted some of the key factors that highly contribute to PPD globally. They are low education, financial difficulties, smoking or alcohol use, intimate partner violence, unplanned pregnancy, low social support, very low involvement of the partner, unsatisfactory living conditions, death of the infant, poor breastfeeding experiences, etc. Some other biological factors like the mode of delivery, pre-term birth, adolescent motherhood, sleep difficulties have also increased the risk of PPD among women.

Zhu et al. (2025) conducted a study to analyze the help-seeking behaviour of women after positive intervention about mental health awareness. The study has identified many factors that influence the help-seeking behaviour of women. And the study is conducted in two Maternal and Child Health MCH hospitals in Shanghai, China. This quantitative survey consisted of 516 women, and there was also a qualitative interview with 22 stakeholders like women, husbands, service providers, and administrators. The factors identified aligned with Anderson's behavioural model that examines the predisposing factors, enabling factors, and the need factors. The findings of the study show that 45.5% of women did not seek any mental health service after positive intervention on mental health awareness whereas 54.5% of women sought help such as counselling, stress management sessions, referred services, etc. The factors that contributed to the decline in percentage of mothers seeking mental health awareness are: multiparous women, i.e. women who have already given birth, so they are less likely to seek any help, next the higher education level that surprisingly reduced the level of service seeking due to self-reliance or time constraints. The poor awareness of community mental health service location also acts as a factor for low likelihood accessing of any mental health services. Low partner support is one of the strongest barriers from attending programs to reduce PPD. From the qualitative survey, it is concluded that there are low awareness of maternal mental health, stigma around seeking help for mental health, lack of proper service provider or more systematic protocol to be followed in the healthcare systems. This always led to mistrust in healthcare services. The study concludes that maternal mental health services are still underutilized due to many of the determinants like personal structural barriers, social or increasing social stigma.

Impact of Social Media in Overcoming Depression

Y. Xu et al. (2023) used transactional stress and coping model to analyse coping mechanism of people in China during COVID-19. The lockdown restrictions boosted the stress among people and suitable coping strategies were found in social media platforms such as Tik Tok, Bilibili, Douyin, etc., by the people. Through online survey, 1569 responses were collected across 31 provinces after a few months of lockdown regulations. To measure the anxiety level, GAD-7 is used; EFC (Emotion-focused coping) and PFC (Problem-focused coping) were used to measure coping mechanism and fluctuations in interaction and behavioural traits of the people. The results show that people are stressed at the initial stages of lockdown for about 1-2 months. Therefore, the users increased their screen timing for short videos of entertainment aspect. The structural equation modelling used in the study states that these stress levels during COVID-19 indirectly increased the video watching time as a form of coping mechanism.

Paleri et al. (2023) investigated whether breathing techniques can reduce stress and negative emotion among young adults especially during COVID-19. The study used quasi-experimental pre-post design. A total of 30 dental college students were included in the demographic case study. Among them, 26 students filled the entire questionnaire. 13 students in the total gave hair samples for cortisol analysis. All the participants are made to watch 8-minute video that contains three major parts. They are:

1. Introduction to stress.
2. Hazards of excessive screen time.
3. Practice session in diaphragmatic breathing.

The data on stress level measured using DASS-21 stress scale. All the negative emotions were measured using Chronic stress biomarkers and Likert-Scale questionnaire via Hair Cortisol Concentration. The findings of the study show a significant reduction in stress level after intervention. Hair Cortisol levels decreased from 36.37 to 30.64 pg/mg which still statistically requires at least 6 weeks to show measurable shift. However, the researchers conclude that even one session video intervention along with daily practice effectively reduced perceived stress and negative emotions despite the sample size and biomarker collection.

Y. Zhang et al. (2023) conducted a randomised controlled trial on 242 primiparous women admitted in two hospitals in Shenzhen. There were two groups in which intervention group experiences ISP plus routine postpartum care and the controlled group experience timely care to check whether the internet-based support program (ISP) can reduce PPD, increase social support for the first-time mothers especially during COVID-19 period. ISP added group had only five extra components. They are communication forum for peer support, a baby story sharing space, reminder systems, learning forum for parenting knowledge and an ask-the-expert-forum. This experiment has taken place for three months for twice per week. The data collected were analysed through three stages: baseline (T0), after three months of intervention (T1) and three more months after T1 period (T2). The results support that mothers who used ISP comparatively has high maternal self-efficacy (MSE) and reduced PPD at T1 and T2 than the other controlled group. Also, higher time spent on platforms resulted in higher self-efficacy, higher social support and reduced depression scores.

K et al., (2024) have done a project called SAMBHAV on mothers attending immunisation clinic in Bengaluru, India. This project involves video-based intervention to create awareness among the young mothers about PPD. The study shows that 22% of mothers in India experience PPD, but only 50% of them have awareness about it. The factors such as poor health literacy, stigma, limited mental health services, cultural beliefs, etc., delayed acknowledgement of the issue, and thereby delayed the treatment. The researchers have taken 130 postpartum mothers (within 6 months of childbirth) and analysed the challenges faced by them through quasi-single-group design. The 130 mothers will watch educational video that particularly relates with their region, language and cultural context. All the videos are obtained based on the literature review and group discussions involving mothers and healthcare experts on various areas of postpartum experience (stigma, help-seeking barriers, realistic view of symptoms, etc.) The impact of this method is measured using Postpartum Depression Literacy Scale (PoDLiS) before the intervention and t-test and ANOVA test after 4-8 weeks of intervention. Feedbacks about the videos were collected through PHQ-9 questionnaire form. The results of the study show significant improvement in eliminating the stigma, early identification of PPD in young mothers, improved awareness among the mothers and the related caretakers, etc. The study lacks control group and only the knowledge-based outcomes are discussed. Further, the study can analyse how video can be adopted for community use and long-scale awareness of maternal mental health across India.

Social media has become an important digital tool that helps in improving digital wellness, relief and emotional well-being. Chung et al. (2025) in their study examine how short-form video clip apps like Tik Tok and Douyin have an effect on life satisfaction among Chinese healthcare workers of young age. This study examines whether these short-form video clips helps in reducing anxiety level, occupational burnout, and stress and whether it creates sense of belongingness, overall life satisfaction and other rewards such as leaning, relaxation and enjoyment. The demographic structure of the study consists of 362 healthcare workers of age between 18-34 that includes nurses, physicians and other med interns. The data were analysed using regression and mediation models such as PROCESS Model 4 and 6. The findings of the study show that the healthcare workers reduce their occupational burnout by watching short-form video apps as a form of coping mechanism. The short-form video clips also promote two psychological factors. They are sense of community (sense of belongingness with peer group in online community) and intrinsic rewards

Figure 1. Conceptual Model

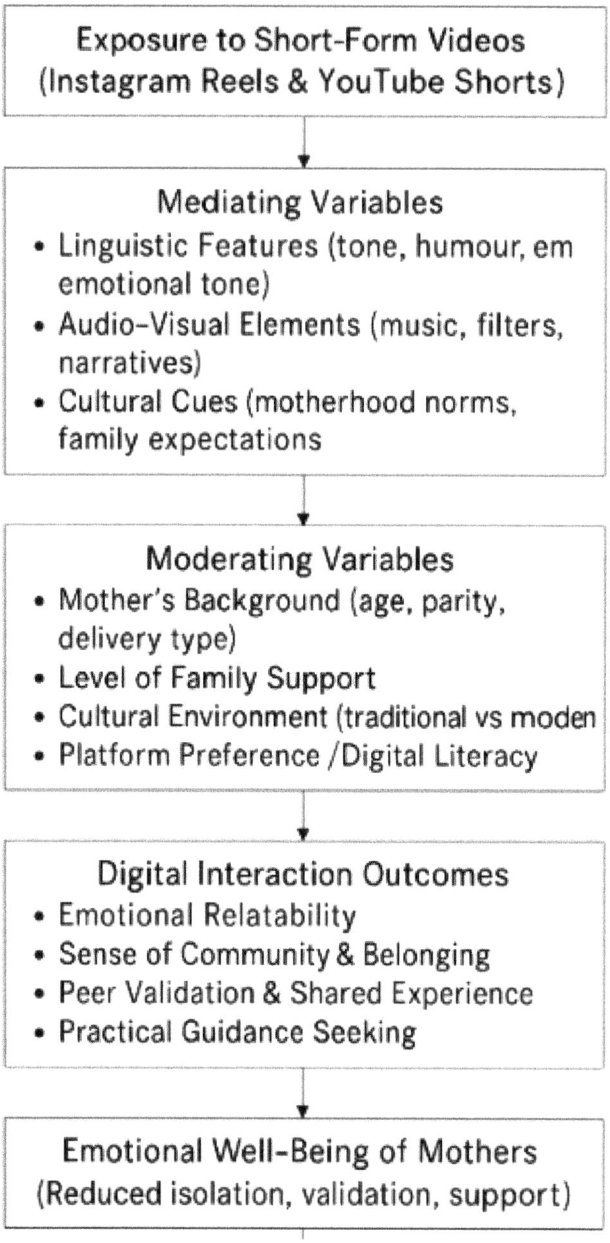

This figure shows the conceptual framework followed in this chapter

RESEARCH METHODOLOGY

The paper adopts qualitative study by examining the language, cultural elements and community sentiments present in postpartum-themed reels in India. Adding to that, a systematic literature review is followed to understand the findings of the previous studies on PPD and the contributing factors.

Data Collection

Platform selection

Instagram reels and YouTube shorts are chosen for their popularity among young mothers.

Sampling Criteria

- Reels focus on postpartum experiences with key words such as 'postpartum', 'new mom', 'mom life', etc. Around 15-20 Reels and shorts uploaded by Indian mothers (individual mothers or mom influencers) are considered for sampling. The study limits with 15 to 20 reels because the comments received from each reaches up to 300.
- A qualitative thematic analysis of 300+ user comments was collected from Instagram and YouTube shorts that focus on postpartum experiences.
- Manual coding was conducted to identify recurring emotional, psychological and cultural themes. The thematic categories were derived from the data through iterative reading.

Analysis Framework

Linguistic Features

- Analysis the frustrated, humorous, hopeful, emotional and sarcastic tone used in reels and shorts.
- Identifying the use of repeated phrases and rhetorical questions like "Who has not slept?"

Cultural References

- The analysis explores traditional gender roles and family expectations such as role of father and in-laws

- It also discusses social taboos that prevents crying, expressing anger and seeking help

Sentiment and Thematic analysis

- Sentiment expressed in reels are categorized as solidarity, exhaustion, humor, self -doubt and empowerment
- Major themes observed in reels include sleep deprivation, body image, comparison with ideal mother, unsolicited advice

Validation

15 new mothers are invited for an informal interview or focus group discussion to validate the interpretation of reels' emotional and cultural impact. Moreover, the comment section in the shorts and reels are also considered to check their impact.

Ethical consideration

Though the data collected for language reviewing are available in the open forum like YouTube and Instagram comments, their identities are hidden.

The mothers who are interviewed are also informed about the purpose of the interview and their identity is also concealed.

Findings

Nine distinct themes emerged from the analysis. The most prevalent themes were sleep deprivation, lack of support, and mental health and depression. Many commenters expressed a strong emotional connection to the video, often stating phrases like *"I too feel the same"* or *"It happened to me."* Several mothers also mentioned that they were unsure where to voice their struggles, highlighting a deep sense of isolation. Comments frequently overlapped, reflecting a common interplay between physical exhaustion, emotional strain, and social neglect.

The theme "Mother as Saviour" appeared consistently, showcasing the irreplaceable role of maternal support in the postpartum period. Meanwhile, "Cultural and Social Expectations" revealed the burden placed on new mothers by traditional beliefs and unsolicited advice.

The following section presents the nine themes in detail, along with representative comments that illustrate the lived experiences of postpartum mothers.

Theme 1: Lack of Support

- "No one had ever said that to me, ever. Even my mom."
- "Same problem, I took care of my baby by myself from the time it was born."
- "My mom never did that and I went into depression recovering still."
- "No one is there to take care of my baby... I gave bath to my 5-day-old baby..."
- "Nobody say this to me I had physical and mental problems because of sleeplessness."

Total Comments: 50+

Theme 2: Sleep Deprivation

- "I sleep just for 2 to 3 hours a day."
- "I hardly sleep 2 to 3 hrs a day."
- "Still I am not allowed to sleep."
- "When works get done baby wake up I got no rest."
- "I can't sleep until my baby sleeps."

Total Comments: 75+

Theme 3: Mother as Savior

- "Mom is real God. Who just lives for us."
- "My Amma.. Without her I am nothing."
- "My mom is a really God in disguise."
- "Only amma will say this."
- "It's my mother who says like that."

Total Comments: 40–50

Theme 4: Mental Health & Depression

- "Feeling so depressed."
- "I fall in deep postpartum depression."
- "Sometimes I feel like I've got a curse from God."
- "I am going through the same stress..."
- "Started getting severe migraine..."

Total Comments: 50+

Theme 5: Cultural & Social Expectations

- "Expert advice by some relatives."
- "They tell me to wake up at 4 a.m. and do housework."
- "In joint families, when the baby sleeps, you have to do housework."
- "My in-laws are scolding me for buying baby items early."

Total Comments: 30–45

Theme 6: Self-Reliance / Learning Alone

- "I learned everything by myself."
- "I handled my baby alone with stitches."
- "I gave bath to my new born without knowing how."
- "No one helped me but told me what to do."
- "I'm not going to be like them—now I help others."

Total Comments: 25–30

Theme 7: Requests for Help / Advice

- "Please give tips on how to make baby sleep."
- "Do we have a forum to discuss depression?"
- "Can you please tell how to stop breastfeeding?"
- "Can we eat pineapple after delivery?"
- "Which belt is best post-delivery?"

Total Comments: 20–25

Theme 8: Love for Baby / Motivation

- "Every struggle goes off when we see baby smile."
- "Love my baby."
- "This baby is my life."
- "Even with heavy blood loss, I managed out of love."
- "Baby alone motivates me."

Total Comments: 20–32

Theme 9: Anger / Sarcasm / Frustration

- “What a way to get rid of responsibility.”
- “Why the hell you make bad faces… irritating.”
- “That’s why it’s good to have two wives.”

Total Comments: 5–7

Figure 2.

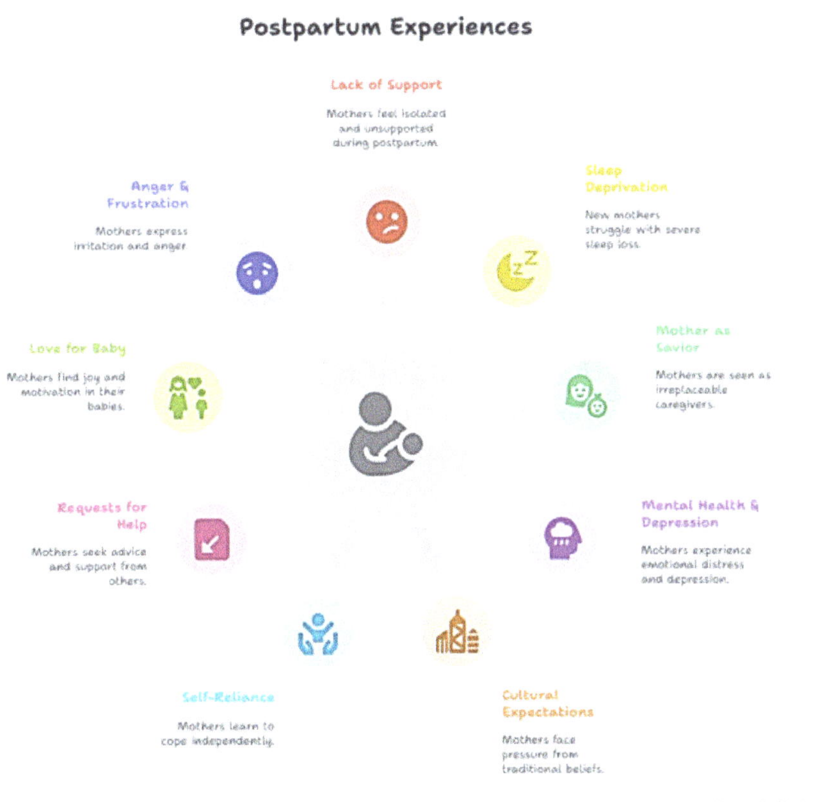

This figure shows various kinds of emotions the new and young mothers undergo and the different factors influencing it.

Table 1. Final Summary Table

Theme	Approx. Comment Count
Lack of Support	50+
Sleep Deprivation	75+
Mother as Saviour	40–50
Mental Health & Depression	50+
Cultural & Social Expectations	30–45
Self-Reliance / Learning Alone	25–30
Requests for Help / Advice	20–25
Love for Baby / Motivation	20–32
Anger / Sarcasm / Frustration	5–7

RESULTS AND DISCUSSION

The results of this study provide a detailed insight of how Indian postpartum moms express their emotional pain, look for support, and question cultural norms through short-form internet platforms. The most common themes—insufficient sleep, a lack of support, and mental health issues—reflect a profound and frequently overlooked layer of emotional toil that new moms bear. These reels and the comment sections that go with them serve as informal, peer-led emotional places in contrast to conventional treatment. Through humour, sarcasm, and emotionally charged language, mothers reveal their weaknesses, and they frequently find solace in the experiences of others who have gone through similar things. Digital connections provide not only relevancy but also emotional relief and identity validation, as demonstrated by statements such as "I too feel the same" and "It happened to me."

One cultural phenomenon that was exclusive to Indian family settings was the notion of "Mother as Saviour." Many moms cited their own mothers as their sole source of strength, despite feeling unsupported by their partners or in-laws. This reveals gendered disparities in household duties and reflects intergenerational caregiving patterns. The on-going weight of cultural expectations was another important realization. Advice such as "Do housework when the baby sleeps" or "Wake up at 4 a.m." demonstrates how conventional norms still take precedence over emotional health. These results are consistent with sociological ideas that contend that the ideal of the "self-sacrificing mother" frequently restricts women's ability to express their emotions.

The birth of hope and perseverance is very potent. Among the pleas for assistance and mental weariness, there were a few remarks that sounded like "this too shall pass." Reassuring new moms with phrases like "It gets better," "Now my child is grown, and I sleep," or "Hang in there," women who formerly battled now come back to discuss how they overcame that stage. The digital environment becomes a spontaneous, non-clinical, but profoundly therapeutic kind of group therapy as a result of this communal remembering and forward-looking energy. In this sense, language becomes a means of healing rather than just a means of expression. Externalizing guilt, exhaustion, and loneliness, rhetorical inquiries, exaggeration, self-deprecating humour, and slang turn reels into micro-narratives of struggle, release, and healing.

While literature supports CBT and clinical interventions, this study contributes to a growing body of research recognizing the role of peer-led, culturally grounded digital communities in maternal mental health. These digital micro-communities provide emotional first-aid, proving that healing may also be crowd sourced, particularly in India, where mental health is still stigmatized and clinical access is restricted.

Reflection Beyond the Screen Validating Digital Narratives Through Personal Testimonies

In addition to the examination of reels, shorts and comments sections, short-form interviews with 15 postpartum mothers were also incorporated into this study to further examine the emotional journeys. The personal testimonials gave the findings a more intimate human voice. The elements found in digital content such as emotional isolation, tiredness and the strength of peer narratives were reaffirmed. The mothers opened up the feeling of emotionally exhausted, unsupported and overwhelmed by physical changes; yet they express deep love and strength drawn from their child. Several mothers mentioned that their emotions were unrecognized or dismissed leading to the feeling of being unheard. The theme of resilience emerged from these narratives- one mother mentioned that she meditated to stay sane and another uttered that she survived on self-talk and hope. Many mothers articulated that they were not even aware that they were experiencing depression. The interviews brought depth, narrative continuity and emotional clarity, making visible what is often buried under the surface of smiling pictures and expected joy.

Interview Validation of Digital Findings

The experiences of mothers that included insomnia, emotional exhaustion, lack of sympathetic support and a sense of invisibility closely reflected the stories seen in reels and shorts comments. Mothers described the mental battle using words like "not feeling like myself even after a year" and "the burden of handling everything alone" confirms their emotional exhaustion. One mother highlighted, "nobody understood what I was going through emotionally" emphasizes emotional isolation mentioned earlier. Their statements confirmed that the emotional realities portrayed online are firmly anchored in actual experiences. Thus these reflections serve as a reminder that the digital traces and real voices together form a more complete picture of postpartum life especially within the cultural context of Indian motherhood, where silence is often mistaken as strength.

Digital Engagement Among Interviewed Mothers

Almost all mothers interviewed had engaged with short-form video content during their postpartum phase either through Instagram reels or YouTube shorts. Digital platforms not only gave comfort to these mothers but also a space for the mothers where they can represent themselves emotionally. Several respondents mentioned that in digital space they "felt seen" or "found someone exactly saying what I couldn't express". The tone and language can be emotional, humorous or sarcastic that helped them cope during their difficult days. One mother mentioned, "Those videos made me to cry and laugh on the same day- it was a relief". These reflections highlight how digital space plays an important role in supporting the emotional well-being of new mothers.

Themes That Overlap With one Another

The themes identified from the studies are not of individual cause, but they overlap with one another, and they interconnect in many ways. For example, the prominent interconnection can be seen in two themes, such as sleep deprivation and mental health struggles. Mothers who have reported 2 to 3 hours of sleep also expressed high levels of anxiety, irritation, hopelessness, and a feeling of being isolated or on the edge. Due to the exhaustion of physical strength, there was also a weakness prevailing in the emotional resilience of the mothers. Having a daily routine challenges their emotions. Here, sleep deprivation is not just a physical strain, but also a psychological impact on depression symptoms. The other significant themes that intersect are cultural expectations and the lack of support. Due to cultural and societal stigma, many new mothers are simultaneously compelled to carry on household duties while also taking care of the child. This drains their resting period. Some mothers report that they are expected to wake up by 4 am to do daily household work as well as to take care of the baby. This leads to a high emotional breakdown, and it is always hidden behind their normal routine. So the cultural norm and the ideas such as the 'self-sacrificing mother' also led to suppress their emotional needs, a lack of a support system, and a low help-seeking behaviour.

Therefore, mothers feel lonely even in a joint family, and the physical presence of the people doesn't really correlate with their emotional and practical care. A third intersection can be seen in the themes of self-reliance and emotional isolation. Mothers who say that they can handle everything alone or that they learned everything by themselves often have a sense of independence. This independence is not a form of empowerment in most of the cases, but a form of survival. Due to the absence of empathetic partners, their self-reliance is shaped by internalized pain and pressure to manage everything alone. This feeling is combined with emotional negligence and unspoken expectations.

Thematic Saturation

The analysis of this study has a clear view of thematic saturation. Across the 10-15 reels and more than 300 comments, the core themes identified are sleep deprivation, emotional exhaustion, lack of societal support or familial care, cultural expectations and mental health struggles. These themes came in variations in first few rounds of the coding. Adding to that, the comments reviewed do not have any new major theme, but a multiple variation and emotional intensities of existing themes. The saturation was higher in themes such as sleep deprivation and lack of emotional or domestic support. Although the comments are from different cultural and linguistic backgrounds within India, there was a similarity that existed in content of their experiences. Some other themes like anger, sarcasm, and frustration were less frequently viewed, but it contained some important significance to the overall analysis. These themes do not have numerical dominance, but very useful in analyzing deeper suppressed emotions, such as a resentment towards unrealistic societal expectation, dismissive family members or partners. There were also low frequency themes which are not much taken in the studies, but it analytically given more significant insights to understand the hidden emotional tension of many mothers who are hesitant to express their emotions explicitly. The combination of most important themes and minor themes reflects a holistic understanding. It also helps to understand the emotional impact found in short form video platforms that are not coincidental, but a consistent representation of lived postpartum experience of many Indian mothers.

Short-form Video Platforms as Shared Emotional Ecosystems

The study derives its data from YouTube Shorts and Instagram Reels. The emotional patterns, linguistic expressions, and forms of interaction in these platforms were similar and there were no significant distinction in how postpartum mothers engage with and respond to the content. So, instead of considering these two platforms as separate or contrasting digital environments, both platforms can be collectively regarded as a shared emotional ecosystem. In both the platforms mothers expressed vulnerability, and seek validation. The narratives conveyed in these spaces exhibits similar tones of exhaustion, emotional exposure, resilience, humour, and solidarity which indicates that the platforms express lived emotional experiences. Thus, this study treats YouTube and Instagram as interconnected spaces that facilitate the same psychosocial function enabling mothers to transform private suffering into shared emotional discourse. This unified approach helps in collective meaning-making processes by focusing on the emotional content, and language patterns, rather than considering technological distinctions. Thus two different platforms do not significantly alter maternal engagement or emotional outcomes.

The Convergence of Online and Offline Data Collected

The emotional aspects found in the Reels, Shorts, and the comment sections directly has a significant convergence with the digital expressions of postpartum mothers and their offline life. It is identified through the interviews conducted. Although the platforms provide narrative freedom, humor, and creativity to the content-creating mothers, it also strongly projects how the mothers emotionally feel. Therefore, the emotional content showcases the recognized predictors of postpartum depression in the earlier literature. Also, the digital data never dilutes or dramatizes the maternal struggle projected. It always captures the unfiltered aspects of postpartum life that are often rejected or ignored in real-world environments due to many aspects of social expectations, cultural silence, etc.

Many themes such as sleep deprivation, lack of support from partners or family, lack of support from in-laws, self-doubt, anxiety, etc., are consistently showed in the digital data collected. This emotional statement directly aligns with Wang et al., (2021), who emphasized on sleep disturbances, lower partner involvement with socio-economic pressure as a major problem that creates postpartum depression. The mothers commenting online often recorded that "I sleep barely 2-3 hours a day" and also states "handling everything alone". These statements strongly emphasize on the same patterns of exhaustion and emotional depression among the mothers, which is clearly stated in clinical studies, therefore the alignment of these findings with the recognized symptoms deepens the methodological validity of digital comments as a meaningful data source.

The theme of Emotional Invisibility is shown as an important element in both literature and the findings of the study, Zhu et al., 2025, shown in their study that many mothers hesitate to ask for mental health support. They are often misunderstood or ignored within their family circle due to typical mindset of the society and the normalization of post-partum depression. The study also includes the insight of the mothers such as "nobody understands what I am going through" or "I cry silently while doing my work", showcases how culturally women are suppressed, especially the mothers, into a feeling of isolation. Their dependence on online videos compensates their space of unfilled emotional support. This indicates that digital platforms also work as therapeutic spaces within the context of social stigma and ignored mental health care.

Many reels depict sleep battles, chaotic baby routines, or domestic conflicts in a humorous or exaggerated manner. And also the commenters responded with emotional validation, sarcasm, or laughter. This usage of humor, sarcasm, or exaggeration showcases that online humor becomes a psychological space of healing that helps the mothers to process their stress without directly confronting it. This made the postpartum mothers to transform their frustration into content or narratives to allow them to feel relieved, connected, or understood. Here the digital environment becomes a coping mechanism as stated by Xu et al., (2023).

A Psychological Paradox in Maternal Digital Expression

The evolution during motherhood is often characterized by a profound psychological apprehension. While traditional systems recommend emotional recovery through close-knit and private support systems such as family and local peers, many mothers find these intimate spaces psychologically threatening. This behavioural shift among mothers gives way to a psychological paradox in which mothers retreat from their immediate social circles to disclose their vulnerabilities in a public forum of strangers. This transition can be called the Intimacy-Anonymity Paradox. Usually, intimacy occurs with a close person or evolves from long-term trust. But in the postpartum period, mothers are anxious about expressing their problems to their husbands or mothers because they are scared of judgement. These mothers share their deepest psychological problems with strangers because they believe that the anonymity of the forum provides safety. Thus, the belief that trusts in strangers will relieve the emotional vulnerability and can be termed the Intimacy-Anonymity Paradox. This behaviour is driven by Superwoman Syndrome, where the society expects mother to be perfect which creates an environment where honest disclosure to family feels like an admission of failure. To resolve this inner conflict, the mother uses digital spaces to bypass the fear of local judgement. By posting about their stress and externalizing the dissonance and by seeing other mothers validating their experiences, the "Superwoman" mask is dropped. This reduces the psychological tension because she no longer needs to perform emotional perfection. This paradoxical movement from silence within intimacy to disclosure in anonymity prepares the ground for understanding how digital platforms mediate postpartum psychological distress.

The clinical hallmark of postpartum depression is often social withdrawal that is the mothers become silent because they feel their pain is a burden. But digital media provides a unique low-stakes environment that circumvents their psychological barrier. This happens through a mechanism called asynchronous Communication. Face-to-face communication often requires immediate emotional energy but a digital space allows a mother to compose her thoughts at her own pace which removes this pressure. This also leads to a transition in the psychological state of the depressed mother. Depressed mothers begin in silence as lurkers but when they see other mothers describing their feelings, it provides linguistic forms for their unspeakable sufferings. The forum acts as an external voice for their internal pain and they feel seen even without speaking yet. Thus, the final post a mother shares in social media is not simply a chat but externalization of her psychological self, making a shift from silence to emotional sharing.

When a mother struggles with postpartum depression, she often needs to handle fear, panic and stress. This makes her feel trapped because she is worried about being judged by someone who is closer to her which creates high-stress state in her mind which in turn constantly bumps out cortisol, the stress hormone. So, joining in a digital community acts like a circuit breaker for this stress. Once, the mother receives a message from a stranger replying with kindness automatically her brain releases oxytocin which soothes the panic. Since she cannot find peace within herself, she tries to outsource it by connecting with other mothers. When she sees and reads the conditions of other mothers in social media, her brain says, "I recognize that pain, I am just like her and I am not a broken machine". This thought makes the brain realizes that the situation is not a personal emergency but a shared experience. The brain finds a way to process its problems which was previously too heavy to carry alone.

Influence of Setting in the Online Data

Neuro-networking and Public Health Marketing in Digital Maternal Communities

Neural responses moulded and structured within networked environments, through repeated social and emotional interactions are referred to as neuronetworking. In the context of postpartum mothers, digital platforms act as neuro-emotional ecosystems because through repeated exposure to shared narratives, emotional pathways are processed. Depressed mothers frequently encounter posts that talk about fear, exhaustion, guilt, and recovery. These repeated narratives allow mothers to map their own emotions onto shared experiences which help them understand that their grief is neither unique nor abnormal and is not permanent. When mothers read posts by peers describing their struggles, it results in emotional mirroring. This mirroring is capable of normalizing distress without direct interaction and reduces emotional isolation. By seeing others narrating their emotions by giving language and structure, depressed mothers can cognitively organize their distress that was previously vague and overwhelming. Thus, the repeated exposures to these digital interactions gradually shift emotional responses from vulnerability to safety. Neuronetworking clearly shows how digital maternal communities serve as primary emotional support system.

Neuronetworking clearly addresses the psychological regulation that occurs within digital maternal communities and it also reveals how these spaces function as informal sites of public health marketing. From a public health marketing perspective, digital maternal communities function as peer-driven healthcare communication systems that uphold emotional well-being of postpartum mothers. Usually health campaigns are designed by experts following the authorities or institutional guidelines. But this unconventional digital platform propagates shared coping strategies and recovery trajectories generated by the mothers through their lived experiences. Through recurrent exposure to these narratives on digital platforms, mothers adopt positive messages such as the normalization of postpartum stress, acceptability of emotional vulnerability, and seeking support. These messages align with the central goals of public health marketing. These transformations occur in the absence of overt persuasion or clinical framing, allowing the changes to occur naturally. Thus by combining neuronetworking and public health marketing, digital maternal communities serve as low-cost, accessible, and culturally sensitive public health environments that support postpartum mental health.

Aesthetic and Visual elements in Reels

The setting of the postpartum-themed shorts and reels also influences the emotional impact on mothers facing PPD. The combination of music and filters that soften the harsh realities, editing styles that carries humor and sarcasm, camera angles, and narrative voiceover also contributes to mothers' feelings, emotional response, etc. These aesthetic elements are indirect tools that make the private feeling of postpartum depression into a public, relatable, approachable, and less isolating one.

POV Video formats

POV Style Storytelling or Point of View Storytelling is another important mode of Reel or Shorts creation. These type of preens puts the viewer in the shoes of mothers, and the camera angles such as looking down at a crying baby or sitting awake at 3am, or also listening to advices from the relatives, showcases the emotional relativity between the creator and the viewer. Also, these type of reels make the viewers to feel the experiences of the content creator. This methodology reflects Zhang et al. (2023) who emphasizes on peer support dynamics to reduce PPD, increase self-efficacy, and emotional relief.

Identity Construction in Digital Motherhood

These reels and shots help the mothers to negotiate and reflect their identities as a mother. Motherhood in Indian cultural context is associated with self-sacrifice, emotional endurance, and silent resilience. This social stigma leads to frustration, vulnerability, exhaustion, and humor. However, the short-form videos help the mothers to openly articulate their struggles that eventually led to the criticism of culturally set idea of 'ideal mother' identity.

Through the comments posted by the mothers, "I don't feel like myself anymore", "I'm just surviving", "I'm still learning every day", etc., shows how mothers redefine their socially prescribed roles into what they really feel. Also, the blend of humorous, sentimental, and sarcastic tones and the linguistic tool of the video helps the mothers to openly criticize the unrealistic standards of perfection demanded by the society and the family surrounding. The traditional expectations of mothers to silently work as a caretaker but the digital environment helps them openly state their contradiction of loving the baby and simultaneously fighting with the mental battle. This helps in eliminating the normalization of postpartum complexities.

Adding to that, there is also a form of acknowledgement observed in the comment section. The comments like, same here, me too, you spoke my heart, validates the experiences of mothers and their struggles. This validation is a form of psychological mechanism that helps the mothers to regain their identities. Therefore, instead of considering themselves as a failing or overwhelmed person, they start to recognize the struggles faced by them and accept their emotions as a normal one. This identity construction also forms a digital sisterhood that differentiates judgments and acceptance in their offline environments.

Table 2. A Comparative insight of Literature Review and Comments analysis:

Concept / Theme	Literature Review Insight	Comment Section Insight
Partner Support	Lack of partner involvement is a major predictor of PPD (Eo et al., 2020; Yaqoob et al., 2024).	Mothers repeatedly mention absent, unsympathetic, or unhelpful husbands.
Family / Social Support	Low social support increases depression; support improves outcomes (Pettman et al., 2023).	Mothers express being left alone, handling baby without help from in-laws or family.
Sleep Deprivation	Sleep difficulties are strongly linked to PPD and emotional instability (Wang et al., 2021).	Most frequent comment theme: mothers report sleeping only 2–3 hours.
Cultural Pressure	Cultural expectations and stigma affect help-seeking and mental health (Yaqoob et al., 2024).	Mothers share pressure to wake at 4 a.m., do chores, hide emotions, follow rituals.
Emotional Isolation	Many women do not seek help due to stigma and not being understood (Zhu et al., 2025).	Comments describe feeling "unheard," "crying alone," and "emotionally invisible."
Mental Health Struggles	High prevalence of PPD; symptoms include anxiety, hopelessness, irritability (Global meta-analyses).	Mothers openly say "I'm depressed," "I feel cursed," "I'm losing myself."
Self-reliance caused by lack of support	Women often cope alone due to limited resources or absence of help (Appleton et al., 2025).	Mothers say they "learned everything alone," "handled baby with stitches," etc.
Need for Accessible Support	Digital or video-based interventions help reduce stress and increase awareness (Zhang et al., 2023; SAMBHAV, 2024).	Mothers use reels/shorts for emotional relief, validation, and parenting tips.
Peer Community Benefit	Peer support programs improve maternal well-being (group therapy, ISP forums).	Comments show mothers feel comfort when others say "same here," "me too."
Impact of Emotional Expression	Expressing emotions reduces stress but is culturally restricted (Dennis et al., 2007).	Mothers use comments to vent feelings they cannot express at home.
Role of Mother's Mother (Intergenerational Support)	Maternal family often provides primary emotional support in postpartum (cultural studies).	Many comments praise their mother as "the only support," "God in disguise."
Need for Awareness	Low awareness of PPD and symptoms delays treatment (Zhu et al., 2025).	Many mothers didn't know they had depression until seeing relatable reels.
Practical Knowledge Seeking	ISP programs show mothers seek guidance on infant care and routine.	YouTube comment sections filled with questions about breastfeeding, sleep, diet.
Stress from Household Workload	Studies show domestic burden contributes to PPD, especially in traditional cultures.	Mothers report being forced to do housework even when exhausted, sleep-deprived.
Emotional Coping Through Media	Short videos and relaxation techniques improve stress outcomes (Paleri et al., 2023).	Mothers say reels make them "laugh and cry," help them feel understood.

The table shows a strong overlap between research findings and mothers' lived experiences shared in digital platform which proves that clinical themes are repeatedly mentioned in shorts and reels. The theoretical medical diagnoses have been transformed into personal stories in comment sections which makes PPD visible beyond medical language. The digital platforms serve as a site for collective storytelling and shared emotional processing. Also, it acts as a mediator for expressing pain, and exhaustion in simple terms. The emotional vocabulary of mothers reflects an urgent need for empathy. New mothers feel recognized and heard due to the shared experience. Thus, these alignments highlight how digital discourse validates and reinforces real-life emotional struggles. Finally, the study proves that emotional experiences discussed in informal digital forum, transforms the private suffering to shared understanding. The interaction among mothers reflects an organic support mechanism operating alongside formal healthcare systems.

Validity and Reliability of the Study

Methodological Validity

This study has used thematic analysis, which directly aligns with emotional, cultural expressions and linguistic aspect of the postpartum theme reveals and the user comments. The themes are derived manually through iterative reading and manual coding to ensure the authenticity of the findings represented through the data rather than preconceived assumptions.

Systematic coding used in the study

The study has followed a transparent coding structure described in the methodology. Repeated readings and the comparative checks are used to detect the similar patterns. The similar patterns were consistently recorded to indicate that the data was sufficient. The repeated emotional expressions in the comments of the reels also shows stable postpartum experience among the mothers.

Theoretical alignment with previous studies

The themes identified in the study also align with the findings of the previous study such as Eo et al. (2020), Wang et al. (2021), Yaqoob et al. (2024), and Appleton et al. (2025). This consistent alignment ensures validity of the study on cultural, emotional, and psychological aspect of the digital data that reflects the empirical analysis of PPD predictors.

Ethical Reliability

All the online data are publicly available. The user identities are concealed to maintain ethical standards of the study. Also, the interview participants are informed about the purpose and confidentiality of the study before the study or the interview starts. This again ensures the reliable and responsible data collection followed in the study.

Platform Reliability

Both the selected platforms such as Instagram Reels and YouTube Shorts showcases similar emotional patterns. This thematic overlap and a consistent emotional pattern showcases that the findings are not platform specific but a shared postpartum experience.

FURTHER RESEARCH

This chapter has concluded with many themes related to postpartum depression. But there are many independent factors that can be changed with proper intervention. The independent causes of PPD, such as unsupportive fathers or partners, and low support from family groups, can be modified through proper intervention. The current study focuses on the mothers, but analyzing the views and reactions of other stakeholders related to the young mothers, such as fathers, partners, family members, societal members, can help in deeper understanding of socio-cultural expectations and to fulfil the gap in shared responsibility and accountability of parenting. Understanding the partner involvement can help in designing more inclusive digital micro-interventions and modifications in mental health care systems. Further research can also be done on promoting digital micro-interventions sponsored and supported by mental health care centres. The mode of giving such content knowledge to mothers improves the rate of help-seeking, reduces anxiety, and increases emotional literacy among the postpartum women. This will also become a meaningful contribution by the healthcare centres.

Future studies can focus on comparing the cultural context. For example, studies conducted in South Asian countries like Pakistan, Bangladesh, Sri Lanka, and East Asian countries like China, Japan, Korea, or Western societies can be compared which helps in understanding the differences in postpartum narratives based on the cultural differences. This comparative work will help to understand PPD at a global level and other themes identified in this chapter like cultural expectations, digital motherhood, or emotional expression. A quantitative approach can be made in analyzing the rate of PPD. The qualitative measure can also be done which includes Natural Language Processing, Sentiment Analysis, Machine Learning-based Emotion Detection, and Digital Ethnography. These tools can help to identify the themes along with some numerical measures on areas like distress, sarcasm, self-doubt, hope, etc. across thousands of comments. This mode of quantitative analysis can help in promoting a general analysis with numerical terms to identify pattern and further experiments in computational methods.

MANAGERIAL IMPLICATIONS

The findings of the study contribute to many managerial implications for healthcare providers, NGOs, policy makers, and digital platform managers. For policy makers, the findings help to formally recognize digital media as a form of supplementary mental health resource. Many government interventions like RMNCH+A, LaQshya and PMMVY can incorporate these short-form videos into the routine. This will help to maintain a routine check up on PPD reduction. Also, the state-level health departments can encourage the local language influencers to give validated content on family support postpartum emotional changes, signs of PPD, signs of anxiety and depression, ways to maintain sleep hygiene, etc.

Similarly, the influencers, creators, and digital platform managers on Instagram and YouTube can promote supportive postpartum content to reduce harmful myths and to provide empathetic mental health resource prompts. We can also encourage collaboration between platforms and public health bodies to strengthen the responsibility and accountability of content creation and reduce misinformation. On the other hand, the health care managers can promote traditional health education with audio-visual content. From the study, it is seen that mothers strongly relate themselves to other emotional narratives in the form of audio-visual content. So it is suggested that many hospitals can create verified information channels on Instagram and YouTube to educate the mothers as well as the other stakeholders on postpartum depression, encourage screening through EPDS, share breastfeeding guidance, and de-promote the cultural pressure or misinformation and myths. This initiative can help many mothers in gaining information about postpartum depression or awareness on how to protect them from it and also to build trust among the maternal community.

Community Health Organization and other NGOs can use the insights of this study to build a community engagement strategy to reduce the cultural barriers. The identified themes like isolation, emotional invisibility, lack of support, etc. showcases that there is a need for safer space to express distress of the young mothers. Therefore, creating digital peer networks, WhatsApp communities, or online support groups which are handled by trained counsellors or ASHA workers can significantly reduce the emotional gap between mothers and the healthcare systems. This also provides a non-judgmental space which is similar to the analysis found in the comment section of Instagram Reels and YouTube Shorts.

This chapter suggests that short-form videos are a mode of indirect or informal emotional counselling spaces utilized by young mothers during the phase of post-partum depression. This is a great opportunity for the mental health care centres to integrate this digital micro-intervention with existing mental health programs. This can also be collaborated with content creators, psychologists, and digital educators to provide early help-seeking to the mothers despite the cultural drawbacks, social stigma or cultural practices. These low-cost contents yet reaching public widely enhance the rate of intervention in reducing PPD.

CONCLUSION

This chapter examined how short-form videos from Instagram Reels and YouTube Shorts helps mothers facing postpartum depression in expressing their emotional struggles, validation seeking and negotiating cultural expectations. The study has analysed more than 300 comments and interviews with 15 new mothers to identify major themes related to PPD, such as sleep deprivation, depression, emotional exhaustion, lack of familial support, identity loss, cultural pressure, etc., which are often ignored or silenced in the offline environments. Apart from providing entertainment, the short-form videos work as a form of informal way of therapy spaces, where the mothers find collective empathy, emotional relief, and relatability. The study also included literature survey that helps in understanding how social media works as a supplementary mental health resource, especially in societies where there are limited support or social stigma exist. Also the chapter reinforces the healthcare systems and policy makers to promote valuable tools for early intervention to reduce the causes of PPD. The insights provided in the chapter also helps in designing maternal healthcare efforts, policy decisions, collaborative efforts of digital media platforms and healthcare resources, etc. Further, it can be concluded that short-form videos help in understanding the unheard voices, hidden struggles, and reality of the postpartum journey and promote a solution that transforms the isolation into community power.

The current chapter clearly exposes why mothers experiencing postpartum depression gravitate towards lived –experience- based peer support. However, it is essential to clarify that digital experience sharing is not a replacement of professional clinical therapy; rather it functions as a preliminary and transitional intervention. It takes a long run for many mothers to leap from suffering in silence to sitting in a therapists' office. Digital community spaces act as a psychological bridge, provides early emotional stabilization and subsequent help-seeking behaviour. Since, the peer-based content sharing relatable, mothers begin to realize that their emotional experiences are normal and shared rather than isolated or pathology. Early normalization and emotional regulation may lessen the symptoms of some mothers, thereby reducing the need for clinical intervention, while still allowing way for clinical intervention if the symptoms persist. Instead of intimidating or pathologizing mothers' struggle, peer interaction softens the stigma surrounding mental health. It acts as an apparatus for normalization of the struggle in the world of mental health care. Acknowledging that not every mother is able to access clinical care immediately due to emotional and social factors, digital peer communities emerge as timely and accessible early stage support system offering immediate emotional containment while complementing, rather than competing with, formal clinical intervention.

RECOMMENDATION

Paediatricians and maternal health practitioners should be attentive to the early signs of maternal emotional distress because paediatricians are the first point of contact for the mothers regarding the sleeplessness and prolonged crying of babies, and breastfeeding difficulties. However, this maternal mental health concern is often dismissed culturally. When a mother repeatedly laments her sleeplessness, exhaustion and emotional struggle during the consultations, clinicians should facilitate access to trusted maternal networks that can normalize the emotional disruption. At this early stage, intensive clinical intervention is not necessary because it is more a situational adjustment rather than a diagnosable condition. These peer interactions among mothers offer emotional stabilization, reduce stigma and encourage acknowledgement of shared experiences thereby helping mothers regulate emotions before it escalates. Thus by integrating informal peer support into routine maternal care, healthcare systems can provide early, culturally sensitive and responsive interventions. The study recommends structured peer interactions such as maternal well-being camps or guided group sessions within the community that can provide space for shared narratives, emotional support, and early psychological stabilization. Therefore, the peer-based initiatives help mothers realize the commonality of the experiences while maintaining clear pathways for clinical intervention when the symptoms persist. In the contemporary world, such peer-interactions can increasingly occur through digital mediated community spaces which extend the support network beyond physical settings. Since attending physical meeting is often difficult for mothers caring new born babies, due to time consumption, fatigue and mobility limitations, mobile phone provides immediate and flexible access to peer support. Although health care system may not have access to these digital spaces, their functions allow the clinicians to understand how independently mothers seek help for their emotional regulation at the early stage.

REFERENCES

Appleton, J., Fowler, C., Latouche, L., Smit, J., Booker, M., & Fairbrother, G. (2025). Evaluation of group therapy intervention for anxiety and depression in the postnatal period. *Maternal and Child Health Journal*, *29*(4), 537–548. DOI: 10.1007/s10995-025-04076-9 PMID: 40138124

Branquinho, M., Canavarro, M. C., & Fonseca, A. (2022). A Blended Cognitive–Behavioral Intervention for the Treatment of Postpartum Depression: A case study. *Clinical Case Studies*, *21*(5), 438–456. DOI: 10.1177/15346501221082616

Chung, D., Meng, Y., & Wang, J. (2025). The role of Short-Form Video apps in Mitigating occupational burnout and enhancing life satisfaction among healthcare Workers: A Serial Multiple Mediation model. *Health Care*, *13*(4), 355. DOI: 10.3390/healthcare13040355 PMID: 39997230

Damra, J. K., Akour, M. M., & Al Omari, O. (2024). Stress and loneliness: Exploring adolescents' use of social media as a coping strategy during COVID-19. *Nursing Children and Young People*, *36*(1), 26–32. DOI: 10.7748/ncyp.2023.e1456 PMID: 37211812

Dennis, C., Fung, K., Grigoriadis, S., Robinson, G. E., Romans, S., & Ross, L. (2007). Traditional Postpartum Practices and Rituals: A Qualitative Systematic review. *Women's Health (London, England)*, *3*(4), 487–502. DOI: 10.2217/17455057.3.4.487 PMID: 19804024

Eo, A., Eo, O., Oj, K., Om, I., & Ka, O. (2020). Prevalence and predictors of postpartum depression among postnatal women in Lagos, Nigeria. *African Health Sciences*, *20*(4), 1943–1954. DOI: 10.4314/ahs.v20i4.53 PMID: 34394261

Instagram (n.d.) Cultural expectations faced by new mothers [Reel]. Available at: https://www.instagram.com/reel/DIgX70NSHkH/?igsh=MWNmYWI0MHN3Y3hzcQ== (accessed 10 June 2025).

Instagram (n.d.) Emotional reel about postpartum exhaustion and healing [Reel]. Available at: https://www.instagram.com/reel/DEucL-UTlah/?igsh=MW85emtucDZ3ZGViZQ== (accessed 10 June 2025).

Instagram (n.d.) Relatable postpartum struggles shared by Indian mom [Reel]. Available at: https://www.instagram.com/reel/CurGHCBIbxS/?igsh=MXE5eGJlZTZleHFtNg== (accessed 10 June 2025).

Jin, J., Zhang, Z., & Luo, C. (2025). From perceived threat to coping strategies: Exploring the role of social media and its impact on loneliness and anxiety during the COVID-19 quarantine. *Frontiers in Psychology*, *16*, 1514669. DOI: 10.3389/fpsyg.2025.1514669 PMID: 40918271

K, L., Ganjekar, S., S, M. K., S, V. H., Philip, M., G, S., Rajaram, D., Acharya, S., Vaiphei, K., & R, S. A. (2024). Study on awareness and management based health action using video intervention (SAMBHAV) for postpartum depression among mothers attending immunisation clinic in a tertiary medical college hospital: Study protocol. *PLoS ONE, 19*(4), e0301357. https://doi.org/DOI: 10.1371/journal.pone.0301357

Paleri, R. J., Meena, K. S. M., Sharma, M. K., Ravish, H., Krishnamurthy, L., Joshi, R. K., & Lepcha, R. (2023). Efficacy of video-based relaxation technique to minimize stress in young adults during the COVID-19 pandemic. *Journal of Neurosciences in Rural Practice*, *14*(3), 544–546. DOI: 10.25259/JNRP_68_2023 PMID: 37692799

Pettman, D., O'Mahen, H., Blomberg, O., Svanberg, A. S., Von Essen, L., & Woodford, J. (2023). Effectiveness of cognitive behavioural therapy-based interventions for maternal perinatal depression: A systematic review and meta-analysis. *BMC Psychiatry*, *23*(1), 208. DOI: 10.1186/s12888-023-04547-9 PMID: 36991389

Wang, Z., Liu, J., Shuai, H., Cai, Z., Fu, X., Liu, Y., Xiao, X., Zhang, W., Krabbendam, E., Liu, S., Liu, Z., Li, Z., & Yang, B. X. (2021). Mapping global prevalence of depression among postpartum women. *Translational Psychiatry*, *11*(1), 543. DOI: 10.1038/s41398-021-01663-6 PMID: 34671011

Wegmann, E., Schiebener, J., & Brand, M. (2023). Social-networks use as adaptive or maladaptive strategy for coping with stress. *Scientific Reports*, *13*(1), 11895. DOI: 10.1038/s41598-023-39042-4 PMID: 37482602

Xu, Y., Wang, J., & Ma, M. (2023). Adapting to Lockdown: Exploring stress coping strategies on short video social media during the COVID-19 pandemic. *Psychology Research and Behavior Management*, *16*, 5273–5287. DOI: 10.2147/PRBM.S441744 PMID: 38170068

Yaqoob, H., Ju, X., Bibi, M., Anwar, S., & Naz, S. (2024). A systematic review of risk factors of postpartum depression. Evidence from Asian culture. *Acta Psychologica*, *249*, 104436. DOI: 10.1016/j.actpsy.2024.104436 PMID: 39142256

YouTube. (n.d.) Crying at 3AM and nobody knows why [Short video]. Available at: https://youtube.com/shorts/9Jfd7qq-2nI?si=GM64SqLEky1Kph4k (accessed 11 June 2025).

YouTube. (n.d.) Husband's response to postpartum meltdown [Short video]. Available at: https://youtube.com/shorts/n-wbQF67lEU?si=_WtWchCPUnQYB8SG (accessed 11 June 2025).

YouTube. (n.d.) Postpartum reality no one talks about [Short video]. Available at: https://youtube.com/shorts/QeCpZ_mQUcU?si=ybDTvSsnu5OcmN06 (accessed 11 June 2025).

YouTube. (n.d.) POV: New Mom's Daily Routine [Short video]. Available at: https://youtube.com/shorts/VwXAPNTdWiM?si=-kYP-PYZqrn-tn0o (accessed 11 June 2025).

YouTube. (n.d.) The things in-laws expect after childbirth! [Short video]. Available at: https://youtube.com/shorts/JnxaEpQ3JBk?si=EL-esARvdxhNVm8C (accessed 11 June 2025).

YouTube. (n.d.) When visitors say "You look tired!" after delivery [Short video]. Available at: https://youtube.com/shorts/v873qYRtkIk?si=U454jXB0mAi5P50 - (accessed 11 June 2025).

YouTube. (n.d.) You will sleep when baby sleeps they said [Short video]. Available at: https://youtube.com/shorts/MMZqHfWbog0?si=0__pnXZ1W8dvGJUA (accessed 11 June 2025).

Zhang, Y., Zhu, J., Li, S., Huang, L., Fang, Q., & Zheng, X. (2023). The effectiveness of an internet-based support program on maternal self-efficacy, postpartum depression and social support for primiparous women during the COVID-19 pandemic: Randomized controlled trial. *Frontiers in Public Health, 11*, 1035872. DOI: 10.3389/fpubh.2023.1035872 PMID: 36844811

Zhu, Z., Wang, H., Zhu, T., Wang, Z., Shen, Y., Xiong, C., & Jiang, H. (2025). Mental health service utilization among pregnant and postpartum women: Status, determinants, and insights from a mixed-methods study. *BMC Public Health, 25*(1), 1942. DOI: 10.1186/s12889-025-23132-1 PMID: 40420041

Chapter 10
Bidirectional LSTM Modeling for Predicting Breast Cancer Cell Motility and Wound Healing Dynamics

Sheik Mohideen Shah
http://orcid.org/0000-0002-6998-2247
SASTRA University, India

S. Meganathan
http://orcid.org/0000-0003-4570-8259
SASTRA University, India

P. Umamaheswari
http://orcid.org/0000-0003-2007-697X
SASTRA University, India

K. Venkatesh
SASTRA University, India

ABSTRACT

One of the most prevalent causes of death due to cancer worldwide, breast cancer is often linked to the ability of cells with cancer to proliferate and invade nearby organs. This study looks at the dynamics of how cells move in breast cancer, focusing on wound reconstruction processes since they offer a helpful model for understanding cancer cell migration. The primary objective of this research is to use

DOI: 10.4018/979-8-2600-0939-0.ch010

a Bidirectional Long Short-Term Memory (Bi-LSTM) model to predict the wound healing patterns in breast cancer cells. The Bi-LSTM algorithm has been trained using both artificial and actual wound pictures to provide reliable performance in a range of scenarios. The results from the two approaches are combined using a fusion technique to produce more precise and trustworthy estimates of wound reconstruction dynamics. In order to determine the predictive efficacy of the suggested framework, its performance is thoroughly examined using common metrics such as precision, recall, precision, and F1-score.

1. INTRODUCTION

Breast cancer is among the greatest diseases that affect women all over the world. Successful treatment of the cancer requires early diagnosis and understanding of its development and progression. Although laboratory tests are useful in detecting malignant cells early and scans also assists this process, it is not usually able to detect the dynamic nature of the malignant cells as time goes by. In a bid to address this, this study utilizes two sophisticated neural network models namely Conv-LSTM and Bi-LSTM. Bi-LSTM provides the deep understanding of the cell functioning considering the input processing in a directional way to consider both present and future data. Conv-LSTM uses the sequence of photos to detect the position and development of cancer cells. The prediction of how cancer will develop is more accurate when such models are used and could guide physicians to tailor therapies and enhance patient outcomes. Breast cancer is a type of disease that is most prevalent and has the capacity to kill women and in rare situations, men can develop breast cancer. It starts when the abnormal cells of the breast tissue start multiplying out of control to create a lump or tumor, which can further extend into the surrounding tissues or even spread to other body parts. The breast consists of lobules (glands that produce milk), ducts (milk passageways), and connective tissues; in either case, the cancer may begin in any of those locations, however, ductal carcinoma occurs primarily in the ducts, or lobular carcinoma occurs primarily in the lobules.

The precise cause of breast cancer is still unknown with a number of risk factors being relevant in the development of breast cancer. These are genetic mutations (BRCA1 and BRCA2), hormonal factors, family history, age, obesity, the effects of many years of exposure to estrogenic, and lifestyle-associated factors (alcohol intake or lack of exercises). Early identification based on routine screening procedures such as mammography, ultrasound and biopsy is very essential as it influences a better survival rates and treatment outcomes. Medical research has come to the forefront with introducing several types of treatments such as surgery, radiation therapy, chemotherapy, hormone therapy, targeted therapy as well as immunotherapy. The choice of the treatment is based on the stage of the cancer, molecular subtype, and conditions of the patient.

Artificial intelligence and deep learning models have also been used over the years to enhance the accuracy of the diagnosis process through the examination of medical images and prediction of the tumor behavior. The mortality has also been minimized through the public awareness and early screening programs through timely intervention. Breast cancer is still an issue of high concern in the world, but the current efforts of research, technology, and personalized medicine are increasing survival chances and life quality in cancer patients with early detection and treatment, which is a positive step in the right direction.

Breast carcinoma is the most common disease identified in women across the world with an approximate of 2.3 million new cases each year and still ranks as one of the leading causes of cancer related deaths. The rising cases across all countries, small and large are globally due to the ageing populations, improved ways of identification and alterations in risk factors. As an illustration, in the year 2025, 316,950 women alone in the United States will be diagnosed with invasive breast cancer. The factors are age, hormones, parental and reproduction history, genetic predispositions including BRCA changes, and lifestyles such as alcohol consumption and obesity which are considered to be of great risk. Some of the molecular classifications that can be used to customize their therapy regimens and predict prognoses include HER2-enriched, basis-like, luminal B, and luminal A. The major screening method is mammography, MRI and ultrasound screening and contrasting agents are added as risky screening methods. Artificial intelligence is advancing technologies that improve early diagnosis and reduce unnecessary diagnoses by modulating screening rate based on the risk of the individual. The multimodal therapies involve hormone therapy, radiation therapy, chemotherapy, surgery and specific biologic therapy. The current clinical trials and in particular the ones announced during ASCO 2025 point to a movement of more personalized, biomarker-based therapies that do not need as much generic chemotherapy as possible. Combination therapy, involving focused and immune-modulating drugs, have demonstrated better outcomes, especially for aggressive cancer types such as HER2-positive and triple-negative tumours.

The worldwide burden of breast cancer is expected to rise sharply by 2050 as a result of differences in early diagnosis and access to healthcare, with lower-income countries bearing a disproportionate share of this burden. To fully utilize scientific advancements, it will be essential to address issues such as the availability of biomarker testing, financial limitations, validation in real-world settings, and equitable care. In the meantime, studies are still being conducted to enhance patients' quality of life, deal with treatment resistance, and improve individualized methods of managing breast cancer. Models that can capture temporal dependencies in both past and future states are necessary for the prediction of breast cancer, especially when using sequential or time-dependent data like wound healing images or measurements of cellular features. Bi-LSTM networks are bidirectional networks that can handle sequential data, and thus can be particularly effective with breast cancer prediction. This two-way processing enables the model to discern the temporal patterns in a better way. Bi-LSTMs are especially useful in the following tasks, where the sequential or time-dependent data is needed. They will be able to enhance accuracy in predicting the stages of wound healing and aggressive behavioural changes of cancer by comparing historical and later time points to determine changes in wound size, colour, and morphology that are subtle. Bi-LSTMs can be effectively used to monitor the dynamics of cell migration and proliferation of datasets consisting of sequences of cellular or tissue images. It is a powerful model that is resistant to irregular or non-linear trends which are common in the behavior of the cancer cell since it predicts the future state whilst considering previous trends. Bi-LSTMs are especially effective in modeling quantitative features extracted out of pictures, such as the variation in texture, density of cells, and the area covered by a wound. The network is also able to accurately differentiate benign tissue development, malignant tissue development, and normal tissue development since sequential dependencies are detected.

Benefits of Bi-LSTM used in Breast Cancer Prediction is a better insight into complicated biological sequences by learning both forward and backward temporal dependencies. It uses the information in the whole sequence to reduce the error in classification as opposed to unidirectional models and Supports components of spatiotemporal images as well as quantitative features sequences efficiently, particularly along with ConvLSTM layers. Also it is capable of modeling the non-linear and hysterical patterns of cell motions or wound healing that we often find in cancerous tissues. DL is a disruptive field in machine learning that has been utilized to investigate the behavior and maturation of cancerous cells. The conventional methods, such as manual microscopy and classical machine learning are typically designed to operate merely on manually designed features and fail to meet the high dimensionality and complexity of biological data. In fact, deep learning algorithms are more precise and predictive because they automatically derive abstractions and hierarchical structure in raw data including multi-omics data, histopathology images, and time-lapse microscopy images.

Recent deep learning designs include convolutional neural networks (CNNs), recurrent neural networks (RNNs), and long short-term memory (LSTM) networks and have greatly contributed to the accuracy of cancer cell prediction. Through these models, it is possible to classify precisely the benign, carcinoma-prone and malignant cells and predict the cell movement, its invasion and its possible metastatic ability over the period of time. Furthermore, deep learning allows combining genomic and imaging data, which helps in the personalized prediction of cancer and targeted treatment methods. Deep learning has become an important strategy in modern cancer studies, improving the process of diagnosis, prognosis, and therapy planning by improving prediction accuracy and speeding up high-throughput analysis.

2. RELATED WORK

An attempt to predict breast cancer, scholars have critically examined numerous techniques in machine learning such as K-Nearest Neighbors (KNN), Support Vector Machines (SVM), Artificial Neural Networks (ANN), Random Forests (RF), XGBoost and Auto ML models. The results show that KNN models as well as Auto ML models such as H2O-XGBoost are predominantly truly precise, often above 95 percent on fashionable datasets. Stacked ensemble models, which integrate feature extraction with convolutional neural network (CNNs) and feature classifiers such as SVM, RF, Naive Bayes, and Logistic Regression also have over 90% accuracy and AUC of about 0.93. Certain hybrid classifiers have enhanced predictions by combining features and fusion models in the prediction space leading to an accuracy of above 96 in tests. Furthermore, ensemble deep learning methods that utilise multiple model architectures usually have a higher accuracy rate than a single machine learning model.

2.1 Traditional Approaches

The primary form of X-ray visualization- mammography has been a common screening tool in the detection of breast cancer, as it is effective in locating early tumor stages and micro-calcium, which are small deposits of calcium. Ultrasound involves the use of high-frequency sound waves and is used in the biopsy of tissues as well as distinguishing solid tumors and fluid-filled cysts. During use of ultrasound, it is common to use it alongside mammography. Due to the high-resolution images of the breast of magnetic resonance imaging (MRI), the method is applicable in individuals who are at high risk or have dense breast tissue. Bayesian networks are used to detect and predict cancer and survival based on such datasets as Wisconsin Provincial Breast Cancer Diagnostic Dataset because K-Nearest Neighbors (KNN), Support Vector Machines (SVM), Random Forests (RF), Decision Trees (DT), Logistic Regression (LR), and Naive Bayes (NB) are examples of machine learning classifiers that have been extensively used in computational analysis to classify tumors as benign or malignant. Whereas Deep Learning algorithms such as Artificial Neural Networks (ANN) and Convolutional Neural Networks (CNN) achieve higher accuracy and generate complex hierarchical patterns using raw data, ensemble-based algorithms such as the Random Forests and AdaBoost algorithms are more effective at improving the accuracy of classification using multiple decision-trees.

2.2 Hybrid Approaches

The hybrid model relies on convolutional neural networks (CNNs) to perform classification and on the Random Forests (RFs) to select relevant features. By applying the two-stage approach, prediction accuracy is enhanced with the initial step of the approach being the selection of the most relevant features followed by grouping the features with the aid of deep learning. This model was better than the traditional methods and was able to detect malignant tumours with an AUC-ROC of 0.95 and a success rate of approximately 93.5%. The other technique combines meta-learning and artificial neural networks (ANN). In this approach, meta-models are fed with various machine learning algorithms such as logistic regression, SVM and KNN.

This architecture achieved accuracy scores of up to 98.74% and an F1-score of 98.02%, outperforming individual models through improved feature selection and stacking integration.

Some research employ hybrid models, which combine conventional machine learning algorithms with naturalistic optimization techniques, to improve feature selection and classifier training. This improves resilience as well as accuracy. Additionally, ensemble hybrid frameworks like Meta-Health Stack leverage the benefits of many algorithms by combining different models and learning strategies, resulting in a more precise prediction of breast cancer. To improve interpretability, hybrid models that combine ML and DL approaches can be used for breast cancer diagnosis and prognosis.

By analyzing both geographical and temporal information, current research uses computational models and machine learning techniques to categorize the course of wounds. To follow wound closure, high-resolution time-lapse microscopy pictures are used for image-based feature extraction, which quantifies characteristics such wound area, perimeter, color intensity, and edge roughness. Conv-LSTM and other temporal modeling techniques successfully portray the progression of wounds across several time points by capturing spatiotemporal variations in wound pictures. By analyzing sequential quantitative features—such as wound size, shape, and color—in both forward and backward directions, sequence analysis utilizing Bidirectional LSTM (Bi-LSTM) networks improves predictive accuracy.

Data augmentation techniques, including as rotation, scaling, segmentation, and synthetic image synthesis, are used to improve model generalization under various experimental situations. Additionally, spatial and temporal information are integrated via fusion models that blend Conv-LSTM and Bi-LSTM outputs, resulting in more thorough and reliable prediction performance. Numerous research have used bidirectional LSTM to forecast breast cancer cell movement through deep learning methods. By building deep learning models using current knowledge, (Anderson et al., 2021) reduced the variability for predictors of breast cancer subtypes. This paper's primary focus is on knowledge curation: incorporating knowledge into machine learning. Inference reduces predictor variability, which reliably improves generalization and reliability. (Slimi et al., 2024) developed sophisticated deep learning methods for examining breast cancer photos. The study employs cutting-edge deep learning algorithms to evaluate breast cancer photos utilizing MobileNetV2, InceptionV3, and DenseNet121. With a 99.1% accuracy rate on the MIAS dataset, it might enhance the diagnosis of breast cancer. (Kirelli et al., 2023) proposed the cascading deep learning network as a successful technique for breast cancer detection. The study demonstrated how ResNet50 could assist radiologists in effectively and efficiently detecting cancers while also potentially facilitating early detection by using it for classification tasks and evaluating metrics such as F1 score and specificity. (Elaraby et al., 2024) tested deep learning algorithms with traditional machine learning techniques to identify breast cancer early. (Asadi & Memon, 2023) investigated breast cancer ultrasonography using deep learning, taking into account a variety of diagnoses, including molecular subtype prediction, lymph node assessment, and chemotherapy efficacy evaluation. This study shows that using these models with successful treatment increases patients' quality of life and survival rate. (Martinez & van Dongen, 2023) used a fusion deep learning framework to predict the rank of breast cancer from pathological images using architectures such as ResNet-50, DenseNet-121, and Inception Net.

Benign tumors are abnormal cell growths that remain confined to their original site. They do not penetrate adjacent tissues or disseminate to other parts of the human body. Benign tumors often have distinct borders, develop slowly, and are not life-threatening. However, they could pose problems if they grow sufficiently big to crush nearby organs or structures. Uterine fibroids and cutaneous lipomas that occur are two examples. The results revealed the high accuracy, reliability, and the efficiency of the framework in the prediction of the grade of breast cancer, which highlights its therapeutic significance.

(Tao, 2023) improved radiation research and used sciences through the application of deep learning to determine the change in breast cancer volume after neoadjuvant chemotherapy (NAC). The study sought to describe the spatial distribution of TP53 in breast cancer using deep learning tools with pre-trained models on H&E-stained whole-slide images (WSIs) followed by the use of deep learning tools, including ResNet18 and ResNet34. The results proved that the ability to predict abnormal TP53 expression using next-generation sequencing (NGS) and immunohistochemistry (IHC) was effective and enhanced the efficiency of the biomarker analysis. To enhance the success of surgery, they conducted their research based on the analysis of DCE-MRI images of breast cancer patients with the help of DenseNet-201 architecture. NAC reduces the size of tumors before surgery. The deep learning model was also effective in tracking the alterations in the volume of tumors, which is important information on the effectiveness of treatment.

Based on the CNN-based deep learning methodology, Jianchun Kong, Xiongbin You, and their colleagues designed a system to forecast the tumour response to NAC in breast cancer (Frascarelli et al., 2024). The model had the correct tumour responsiveness to chemotherapy by training convolutional neural networks (CNNs) on medical images taken before and after treatment, including MRI or ultrasound images.

This simple and data-driven method promotes the early clinical decision, tailored planning of treatment, and enhances patient outcomes as a result of the effective analysis of complex datasets and the ability to predict therapeutic outcomes. (Gu et al., 2024) developed a small deep convolutional neural network (CNN) to classify breast cancer and it was successful because it was able to differentiate between benign and malignant tumours using mammographic or histological images. Due to its high accuracy and low processing needs the portable CNN model can be applied in real-time diagnostics and in the environment with limited resources in healthcare fields. This method enhances the care delivery of patients through better early diagnosis and clinical decision-making.

3. PROPOSED FRAMEWORK

Traditional techniques tend to miss the complicated behavior of cancer cells and primarily, their locomotion and alterations as observed in medical images in various time periods. A predictive and accurate method is in high demand, in order to analyse this time-based images information and predict the future dynamics of a cancer cell. The proposed project will focus on creating a deep learning model that combines both Conv-LSTM and Bi-LSTM networks so that the future behavior of breast cancer could be analysed and evaluated more effectively. Among the leading causes of death among women world over is breast cancer. The traditional methods do not always completely describe the multifaceted activity of cancer cells, especially with respect to their mobility and the changes that can be seen in medical images obtained at various times. Such time based image data needs a reliable and predictive methodology so that the future dynamics of cancer cells can be predicted.

The paper is intended to create a deep learning algorithm that uses the Conv-LSTM and Bi-LSTM networks to more effectively evaluate and predict future behavior of breast cancer cells by using sequential picture data. This will be useful in assisting clinicians to make improved treatment recommendations by establishing both the spatial patterns in the images and the temporal variation with time. The Bi-LSTM networks are used in this work to predict the future behavior of the breast cancer cells. To illustrate the movement and alteration of cancerous cells at a given time, first, there will be collection of time-lapse images. Conv- LSTM element is able to identify the patterns in these images analyzing not only the time feature (the way the cells have been changed over time) but also the space feature (how the cells were seen). Subsequently, when the data are considered both forward and backward, the Bi-LSTM compares these sequences, and this method helps the model to understand the activity of cancer cells in a better way.

This is a holistic approach that intends on coming up with a model that can effectively predict where cancerous cells in the breast can grow or progress so as to guide physicians in making improved treatment choices. It aims at developing a deep learning model predicting the motion and progression of breast cancer cells with time based on a combination of two neural networks; each Bi-LSTM to analyze alterations in the previous and future context and Conv-LSTM to detect spatial patterns in cell movement images. Such synergy assists the physician in formulation of improved treatment strategy by enhancing the precision of prediction and the awareness of the model towards cancer cell dynamics. The cells or tumors of the body can be divided as normal, benign and malignant cells on their condition or activity. Normal cells, cells that are in excellent health and undergo a regulated division, expansion and death without aberrant growth are those that make the tissue structure of the body and facilitate its normal functioning.

Malignant tumors are composed of cells that can spread to other regions of the body through the circulation of blood or lymphatic system, proliferate uncontrollably, and invade surrounding tissues. They can have uneven shapes, grow quickly, and endanger human life. Malignant tumors often require radiation, chemotherapy, or surgery because they disrupt normal physiological functions. Examples include carcinomas and sarcomas. Malignant tumor cells are often either not well differentiated or unstructured in comparison to normal cells. The method begins with collecting data, which entails obtaining both real biological data and synthetic information, mostly images of the multiple phases of cancer-related wound healing.

A diverse dataset is essential since it reduces bias and allows the model to learn in the way of various patterns. The second step is data pre-processing that involves segmentation (with the help of special tools, such as SAM or Med SAM to isolate the wound area), augmentation (adding the flips, rotations, and brightness alterations to the dataset), and normalization (standardizing the inputs in 0-1 range). Such processes guarantee the model receives good quality and structured data. When implementing the algorithm steps three critical deep learning techniques are employed namely Conv-LSTM which uses the sequences of wound images which capture the temporal dynamics of the healing process and also spatial aspects of an image like size and shape. Bi-LSTM also takes numeric features such as area, perimeter, and texture which are used to capture the pattern of healing.

The Fusion Layer is a combination of the Conv-LSTM and Bi-LSTM outputs, whereby the two features are blended (numerical and visual). Conv-LSTM, Bi-LSTM, and Fusion are the three components that undergo testing on unseen samples after being trained on the data. Using the combined traits from the prediction stage, the breast cancer wounds are then classified as benign, normal, or malignant. Finally, the assessment step computes performance using metrics including accuracy, precision, recall, and F1-score to assess model performance. The obtained results were drawn in graphic form in charts and graphs so that to provide a proper analysis in light of the performance of the model and to focus on the areas of improvement. This is done to convert raw data to the right breast cancer wound category.

3.1 Conv-LSTM Algorithm

Figure 1. Conv-LSTM Methodology

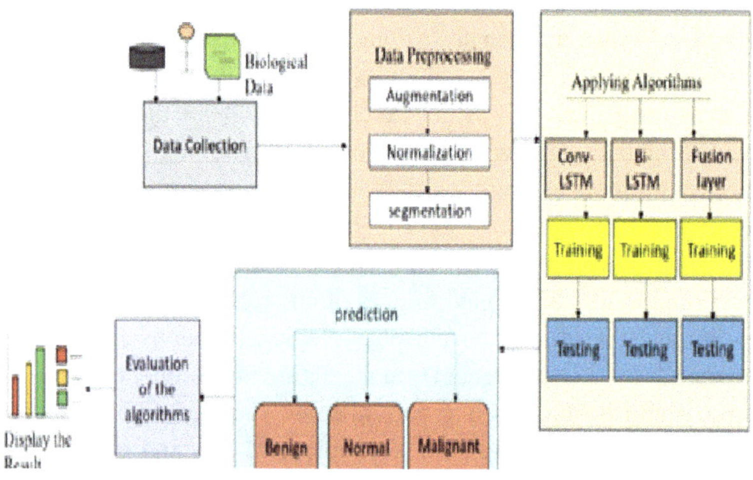

A modified deep learning architecture called Convolutional Long Short-Term Memory (Conv-LSTM) unites the advantages of Long Short-Term Memory (LSTM) networks and Convolutional Neural Networks (CNNs) as shown in Figure1. By assimilating convolutional operations into the LSTM gates, Conv-LSTMs process inputs as two-dimensional spatial data, such as images, in contrast to standard LSTMs, which consider inputs merely as flat vector representations. In sequential image data, this allows Conv-LSTM to simultaneously learn temporal dynamics—how spatial features such as patterns and textures evolve over time—along with the spatial information itself. In Conv-LSTM, convolutional operations replace the traditional matrix multiplications used in LSTM, preserving the spatial relationships between pixels while modelling their progression across time steps.

Conv-LSTM is thus very applicable in sequential imaging activities, such as medical imaging, wound-healing assessment, and video prediction. Conv-LSTM has been successfully applied in the wound-healing analysis of breast cancer that is able to meet key spatial structures to track the temporal evolution of wounds while making more accurate predictions of healing and providing the ability to distinguish benign, malignant, and normal healing processes. Along with that, a counterpart neural network model, the Bidirectional Long Short-Term Memory (Bi-LSTM) is defined to take sequences of data both forward and backwards and provide a more detailed view of the temporal dependencies. A Bi-LSTM has the benefit over a traditional LSTM that it can learn more complex temporal patterns due to its bidirectional processing as opposed to past information alone. The Bi-LSTM assists in giving a detailed picture of the wound-healing process by analyzing the wound properties including wound size, shape, and colour change with time. In order to obtain a more accurate representation, results of Conv-LSTM and Bi-LSTM are usually aggregated, usually by concatenation. The Bi-LSTM is critical in the breast cancer wound analysis by the ability to model the time change in extracted features, including wound area, perimeter, and texture, which enables it to track subtle and complex trends in healing. This deeper understanding enables more accurate classification of wounds into normal, benign, or malignant categories based on the observed healing patterns.

The working principle of Bi-Directional LSTM is as follows

$$f_t = \sigma\left(W_f \cdot [h_{t-1}, x_t] + b_f\right) \tag{1}$$

$$i_t = \sigma\left(W_i \cdot [h_{t-1}, x_t] + b_i\right) \tag{2}$$

$$\widetilde{C}_t = \tanh\left(W_C \cdot [h_{t-1}, x_t] + b_C\right) \tag{3}$$

$$C_t = f_t \cdot C_{t-1} + i_t \cdot \widetilde{C}_t \tag{4}$$

$$o_t = \sigma\left(W_o \cdot [h_{t-1}, x_t] + b_o\right) \tag{5}$$

$$h_t = o_t \cdot \tanh\left(C_t\right) \tag{6}$$

Where:

- f_t, i_t, o_t are the forget, input, and output gates, respectively.

- C_t is the cell state, and h_t is the hidden state.
- W_f, W_i, W_C, W_o are the weight matrices, and b_f, b_i, b_C, b_o are the bias terms.
- σ and tanh are activation functions (sigmoid and hyperbolic tangent).

$$h_t^{\text{bi}} = \left[h_t^{\text{forward}}, h_t^{\text{backward}}\right] \tag{7}$$

Where:

- h_t^{forward} is the hidden state from the forward LSTM layer.
- $h_t^{\text{backward}}$is the hidden state from the backward LSTM layer.
- h_t^{bi} is the concatenated bidirectional hidden state.

$$h_t' = h_t \cdot \text{Bernoulli}(p) \ (8)$$

Where:

- h_t is the output after applying dropout to the hidden state ht.
- Bernoulli(p) is a Bernoulli random variable with probability p, the dropout rate (e.g., p=0.2).

$$y_{\text{pred}} = W_{\text{out}} \cdot h_T + b_{\text{out}} \tag{9}$$

Where:

- y_{pred} is the prediction at the next time step.
- W_{out} is the weight matrix for the output layer.
- h_T is the final hidden state from the bidirectional LSTM.
- b_{out} is the bias term for the output layer.

3.2 Fusion Layers (Concatenation)

The main objective of the fusion layer is to unite outputs from various model components. Conv-LSTM is used in this work to process image data, whereas Bi-LSTM analyzes wound-related characteristics, such as size, to generate distinct outputs. Using concatenation, the fusion layer unites these two outputs, enabling the model to incorporate both numerical wound-measurement data and visual information extracted from images. This method maintains the integrity of key information. The final prediction is moulded by running the combined data through dense layers after it has been fused. By allowing the model to consider both image-based and numerical features and it also progresses the model's intelligence and calculation accuracy. Fusion layer role is more crucial while uniting several data types into a solitary model.

3.3 Evaluation of Algorithms

Three deep learning networks, LSTM, Bi-Directional LSTM (Bi-LSTM), and a Fusion Layer Model, were applied and put in comparison with each other in terms of competence to predict and cluster the behaviour of breast cancer cells based on sequential imaging information to determine the effectiveness of the proposed framework. In order to ensure uniformity and comparative inequalities, identical pre-processed dataset was used to train both models. Model evaluation encompasses the standard performance measures that are Accuracy, precision, recall, F1-score, and ROC-AUC. The combination of these measures gives the unified assessment of the models performed on the measure of reliability, generalization potential and classification power. In order to have a greater insight into the discriminative performance of each model, was also employed to examine the distribution of the samples that were correctly and incorrectly classified as benign, normal and malignant. The capability to understand long-range temporal dependencies within sequential cellular image frames was also viewed as a strength of the Long Short-Term Memory (LSTM) network.

The model may not capture contextual information of the subsequent time steps, however, since it processes information in only one direction. Its capacity to resolve dynamic morphological changes that require bidirectional temporal context was a bit low though its accuracy was admirable. In parallel processing of input sequences in both directions, the Bi-Directional LSTM (Bi-LSTM) model was found to be superior to the traditional LSTM. Due to the bidirectional processing of sequences, deeper contextual connections and accuracy in classification were achieved. To enhance the knowledge of time, the model was effective in utilizing both past and future data frames. This increased the accuracy and the value of recollection, especially in differentiating the manner of the cancerous cells. The Fusion Layer Model also pooled together, Conv-LSTM and Bi-LSTM network feature representations to have access to both time and location-based learning features. This combination approach allowed a more detailed description of the data through a combination of geographic pattern recognition capabilities of Conv-LSTM, with the sequential modeling capabilities of Bi-LSTM. The fusion architecture was superior in general, and both ROC-AUC and F1-Score were found to have high improvement and also a higher classification durability, generalization and robustness. Even though the LSTM has been successful in capturing temporal relationships, a comparison study has shown that its unidirectional aspect limited its prediction capabilities. Bi-LSTM enhanced the accuracy and consistency because it utilized the information of both directions, i.e., forward or backward. Fusion Layer model considerably improved the performance and provided the most stable and precise predictions in order to classify the behavior of the breast carcinoma cells through fusing the complimentary spatial and temporal variables.

4 PERFORMANCE ANALYSIS

4.1 Accuracy

Accuracy in deep learning of a model is its ability to categorize examples. It is evaluated by dividing the number of the cases predicted correctly by the total number of cases. A higher accuracy indicates better performance, however, the imbalanced datasets may not be suitable in its application. It is a simple evaluation measurement that is applied to identify the overall effectiveness of a deep learning model.

Accuracy = Number of Correct Predictions / Total Number of Predictions

4.2 Precision

Precision in deep learning is the percentage of true positive predictions of all the positive predictions of the model. It depicts the way the model can avoid false positives in which it becomes nearly correct when the model makes a prediction. Precision is a vital measure in an activity such as detecting fraud or a medical condition where false positives are costly or harmful. When the precision is larger, better performance in the recognition of positive cases is observed.Precision = True Positives / True Positives + False Positives

4.3 Recall

In deep learning, recall estimates the proportion of actual positive examples of the data, which the model correctly fits. It assesses the effectiveness of the model in reducing the false negatives by including all the relevant positive cases. Greater recall even at the cost of more false positives demonstrates that the model identify do well detect most of the positive cases. It is also important in activities such as anomaly detection and medical diagnosis in which missing positive cases are essential.

Recall = True Positives / True Positives + False Negatives

4.4 F1- Score

F1-score of deep learning is a harmonic mean of precision and recall. It can be useful when evaluating the performance of the model in a binary classification problem since it provides a single score and balances the precision and the recall. The greater F1-score reflects the greater overall performance, both in terms of false positives and false negatives.

F1-Score = 2 × (Precision × Recall) / (Precision + Recall)

Table 1. Predicting Breast Cancer Cell Migration Using Bidirectional LSTM Results

	Precision	**Recall**	**F1-score**	**Support**
Benign	0.92	0.99	0.95	90
Malignant	1.00	0.86	0.92	42
Normal	0.88	0.85	0.86	26
Accuracy			0.93	158
Macro avg	0.93	0.90	0.91	158
Weighted avg	0.93	0.93	0.93	158

Figure 2. Sample Breast cancer images

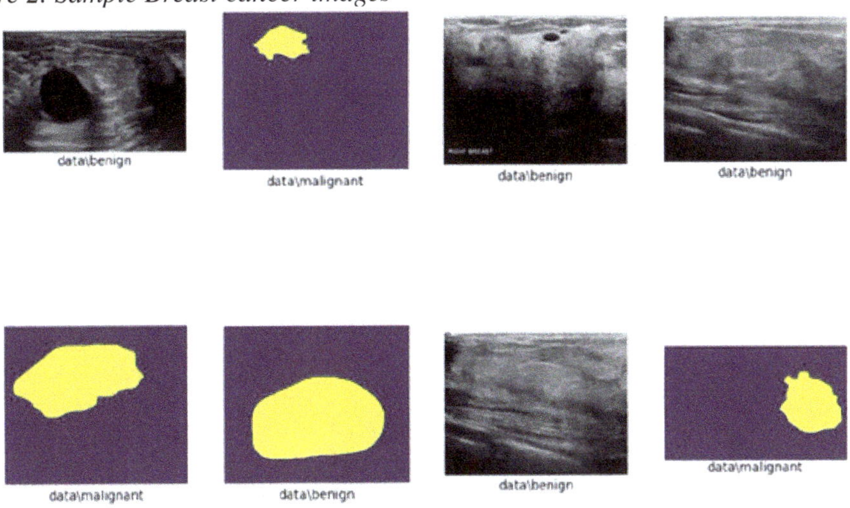

Figure 2 illustrates that structural characteristics of breast tissue are reflected in the grayscale ultrasound images. Overall, the benign samples (labeled as data-benign) are characterized by homogenous textures within and sharp and clear edges. Conversely, malignant samples (designated as data-malignant) are heterogeneous echotextural, spiculated, and irregular in shape, which are all features of cancerous lesions. These morphological and textural differences are crucial when isolating benign and malignant body tissue. Each ultrasound image comes with a corresponding segmentation mask, the yellow regions denote sections of a tumour manually annotated. The separating of the lesion or region of interest (ROI) against other irrelevant tissue is done with the segmentation masks. The purple background illustrates the areas without lesion. With proper background noise elimination and better classification, accurate segmentation also provides better performance. To guarantee high precision and dependability, domain experts prepared the segmentation ground truths. In order to extract lesion patches and help the learning algorithms precisely identify tumour boundaries, these expert annotations are used during the pre-processing stage.

Additionally, as indicated by the labels (data\benign, data\malignant), the dataset is methodically arranged into separate directories for each class. Effective data loading, labeling, and management are made possible by this hierarchical structure during the training and testing procedures. During experimental evaluation, it also facilitates robust cross-validation and balanced sampling. An efficient and non-invasive method for early breast cancer detection is ultrasound-based lesion segmentation and classification. The suggested deep learning framework can concurrently learn boundary information and spatial characteristics by utilizing both raw ultrasound imagery and segmentation masks, improving diagnostic precision and model generalization.

Figure 3. Breast Cancer Dataset: Image Count Summary

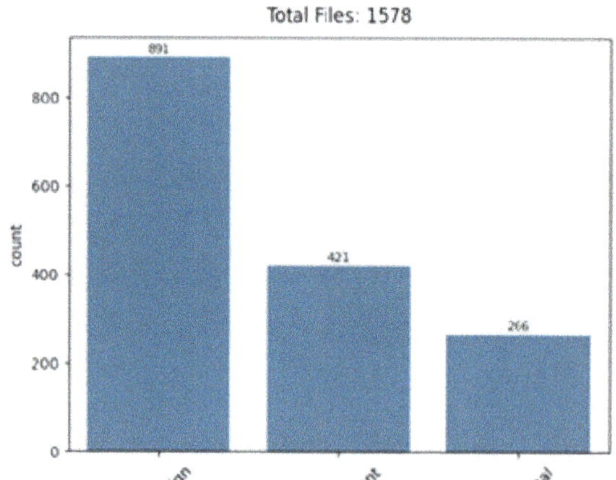

4.5 The Dataset Composition for Image Categories

The benign category has the largest number of 891 images. The malignant group consists of the 421 images, and the normal group has the 266 images. This distribution has a class imbalance. Compared to both the malignant and the normal classes, the benign class is overrepresented. Such imbalances ought to be considered when training the models to be able to obtain such fair and unbiased results in classification. The dataset in this study contains 1,578 images divided into three categories.

Figure 4. Model Training and Validation Performance

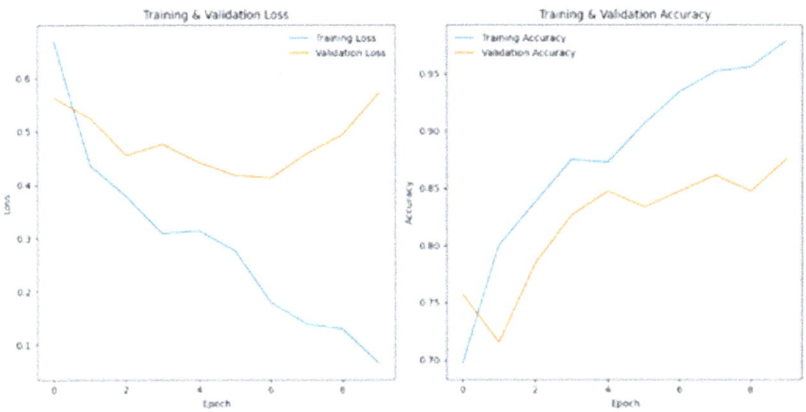

4.6 The Epoch-wise Training and Validation Analysis

The graph shows the general training developments. The model is highly effective, on training data, with a decreasing loss of training slowly on the left. Nonetheless, the validation loss starts increasing after a preliminary drop, which could indicate that the model can overfit, and cannot generalize well to new, unseen data. Validation set shows uneven performance on the right because the accuracy of the validation is not consistent, and which points to non-uniform performance, and to further reduce the probability of overfitting on the validation set, the model might still need specific strategies, including early stopping, dropout regularization, or other data augmentation techniques.

Performance of the classification model is given by the confusion matrix, which compares predicted against actual class labels. It shows the model's error and its accurate predictions. This is the confusion matrix structure. (False Negative): The model predicts a negative value when it is actually positive. False Positives, or FPs, occur when a model predicts a positive outcome when it is actually negative.

Figure 5. Evaluation of Classification Accuracy using Confusion Matrix

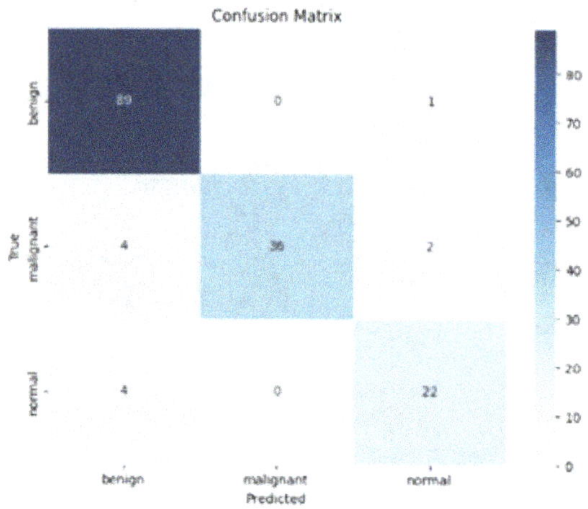

4.7 Model Performance Visualization

The figure represents a confusion matrix of a model to classify medical images of three different types which are benign, malignant and normal. The classes that are predicted appear in the columns of this matrix and the rows are associated with the actual class names. The actual performance of the model is carefully evaluated due to the fact that every cell in the matrix will represent how many times a certain true class was classified as a certain predicted one. The model is exceptionally accurate in benign cases where it correctly identified 89 cases. Each of the samples had not been erroneously identified as malignant and only one benign sample had been misidentified as normal. This can be interpreted to mean that the model is highly precise in picking up the non-cancerous growths thus critical in reducing unnecessary medical interventions. Four of the malignant samples were wrongly identified as a benign case and two as a normal case, whereas the model correctly identified 36 cases in the malignant group. Twenty two samples were correctly identified and four were identified as benign, and none were identified as malignant. This indicates that though the model is effective in identifying most of the cancerous ones, there is some cross contamination between the malignant and other ones which may have clinical implications in case the undetected cancer is classified under the normal category. It means that some slight misclassification, even in normal tissues, may still occur despite the fact that it is usually identified properly, which may be minimized by further training or a better model structure. On the whole, the confusion table demonstrates a good performance of the model, particularly in identifying benign cases, as well as a reasonable accuracy of both normal and malignant classes. The misclassifications noted especially in the cases of normal and malignant samples indicate the areas where the model can be improved further to enhance its application in clinical decision-making in medical imaging analysis, reduce diagnostic errors and enhance accuracy.

4.8 DenseNet121-BiLSTM Hybrid Architecture

Figure 6. Flowchart of Deep Learning Model Architecture.

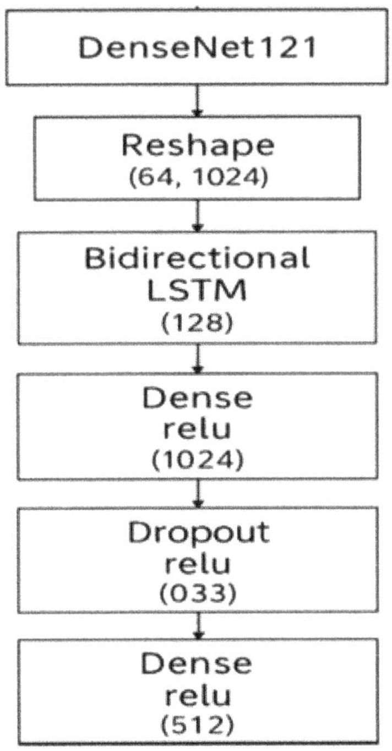

Being an example of machine learning, deep learning has grown to be a trusted method of computation regarding the recognition of complex patterns in large volumes of information. Deep learning provides a direct recovery of relevant features in raw input data by hierarchically training neural networks, unlike other more traditional machine learning methods that heavily use manually defined features. The ability has triggered vast improvements in various areas, including biomedical research, computer vision, natural language processing and speech recognition. The key building block of deep learning is known as Artificial Neural Networks (ANNs), which are inspired by the structure and the processes of the human brain. These networks are made up of an input layer, multiple hidden layers and an output layer which are made up of interconnected neurons. The more hidden layers there are, the deeper the network will be and it will be able to deal more effectively with complex and high-dimensional data (images, audio, and time-series inputs) with sequential time-series inputs. The deeper architecture of this model allows the model to simplify or simplify more complex patterns in the data.

To provide the training of the deep learning models, data should be propagated through the network, and the errors in the predictions should be measured with the help of the loss function, and the network parameters should be optimized with the help of the gradient-based optimization method and the backpropagation technique. Advancements in architectures such as transformers, Long short-term memory networks (LSTMs), recurrent neural networks (RNNs), and convolutional neural networks (CNNs) have greatly extended the use of deep learning to a number of new sophisticated areas of research. These architectures are now important in fields like drug discovery, genomic prediction and analysis, and detection of diseases using medical image not to mention that they are increasingly providing more accurate, efficient, and data-driven insights to each contributing field. Two key advantages of deep learning as a research perspective are its generalization ability when it has been trained on large and diverse datasets and how it can fit complex nonlinear relationships that are challenging with traditional methods. It has since become the central tool in the contemporary computational studies and the stimulus to the development of the theoretical as well as practical spheres.

A Dense Net, also known as a Densely Connected Convolutional Network is a type of convolutional neural network, which, as opposed to classical CNNs, does not use connections between layers in a cascade manner. DenseNet or Densely Connected Convolutional Network is a type of CNN architecture where, unlike canonical CNNs, all layers are inter-connected in a feed-forward fashion.DenseNet is a CNN architecture in which each layer is connected directly to all layers in front of it, rather than through indirect connection to the layer it connects to. This sparse pattern of interconnections provides the network with the ability to recycle existing features learned in the past, aiding in the elimination of the vanishing-gradient problem and the amount of parameters required overall in deep learning networks.

In neural network architectures like Dense Net, multi-dimensional feature maps are normally reorganized or flattened to a single-dimensional vector and afterwards, forwarded to the fully connected (dense) layers, which are used to perform classification. Once an experienced linear transformation has been applied, dense layers (usually combined with the ReLU activation function) introduce non-linearity by converting negative values to zero, leaving positive ones alone. This step of flattening is done after the last convolutional or dense block and is done to make sure that the features extracted can be processed effectively by the dense layers. The dense layer finds the weighted averages of these inputs but ReLU enables the model to capture the versatile and complicated decision boundaries with the final result being more accurate and predictive predictions. One of the most important aspects of such architectures as Dense Net is this approach, which makes it possible to transition the process of extracting the spatial features in a convolutional layer into the more complex inference and decision-making steps enabled by the dense layers and nonlinear activation.

Randomly "dropping out" (turning off) a share of neurons during training, prevents overfitting by applying a regularisation technique named as dropout. This forces the network to not rely too heavily on any one neuron. ReLUs (Rectified Linear Units), which create non-linearity by zeroing out negative inputs while keeping positive ones intact, and are generally applied immediately following the activation stage. ReLU and Dropout combine to create a more robust network that more effectively generalizes to new data by first activating neurons with ReLU and then randomly disabling some of these activated outputs during training with Dropout. Although the model weights are frequently adjusted to account for the dropout effect during training, dropout is disabled and all neurons are active during evaluation or inference. In conclusion, Dropout adds noise during training by randomly deleting neurons, whereas ReLU supplies the non-linear activation, minimize overfitting and enhances model's volume for generalization.

The design of a deep learning model is depicted in the pictures below. DenseNet121, a potent neural network, starts the process by extracting significant features from the input images. After that, the extracted data is transformed into a sequential format so that it can be handled similarly to a time series. To capture more thorough patterns, a Bidirectional LSTM (Bi-LSTM) then reads this sequence both forward and backward. The Bi-LSTM's output travels through dense layers, which are fully connected layers that enable the learning of increasingly intricate features. A dropout layer is inserted in between these dense layers to keep the model from overfitting. Ultimately, the model generates a conclusion, like assigning the picture to a particular category.

Figure 7. The Classification Result: Normal Tissue

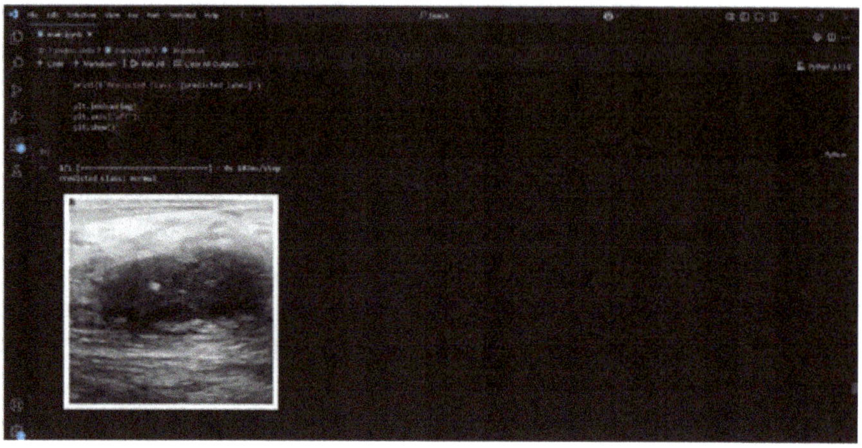

The result of applying a deep learning model to a medical image—likely an ultrasound scan—is depicted in the figure. The Python notebook code that represents the series of steps the model takes to process the input image is displayed at the top of the screen. The image is loaded first, pre-processed, and then fed into the deep learning network that has been trained. The model predicts the medical condition shown in the scan by analyzing the image using its learned features and hierarchical representations. Following the analysis, the model predicts that the input image falls into the "normal" category. According to the model's learned criteria, this classification indicates that the tissue or organ being examined appears to be healthy because no anomalies or pathological signs were found in the ultrasound scan. The prediction is clearly visible, giving the user or clinician instant feedback. The matching black-and-white ultrasound image is displayed beneath the prediction, enabling visual verification and comparison with the model's evaluation.

The model finished the prediction in about 183 milliseconds, according to the output's performance metric, which also highlights the deep learning framework's effectiveness and quick inference speed. This illustrates how these models can offer diagnostic assistance in almost real-time, which is especially helpful in clinical workflows where precision and speed are crucial.

The figure demonstrates the process of analyzing a medical image, presumably, an ultrasound scan, with the help of a deep learning model. The medical image in this case is p1.png and the trained neural network, that has been trained to classify medical images based on the presence of pathological conditions, is used to process the input image. The algorithm involves processing the input image, and feeding the information into the deep learning model, which incorporates the minor details in the scan and spatial characteristics to come up with the correct prediction. Upon processing, the model gives a prediction that the input image falls in the category of the malignant. This categorization reveals that the model revealed the features present in the scan that are associated with cancer or malignant tissue development, which to indicate a potential pathological phenomenon that may require further clinical evaluation. The prediction results, displayed above the image, gives clear and immediate feedback of the evaluation of the model. The prediction is seen alongside the real black-and-white ultrasound scan under the image, thus allowing the visual confirmation and comparison with the interpretation of the model. Also, the output shows that the prediction took approximately 229 milliseconds, which proves the ability of the model to be fast in making an inference. This fast and accurate examination explains how deep learning models can assist physicians to diagnose and make decisions rapidly, particularly in the environment in which it is vital to analyze imaging data promptly.

Figure 8. The Classification Result: Malignant Tissue

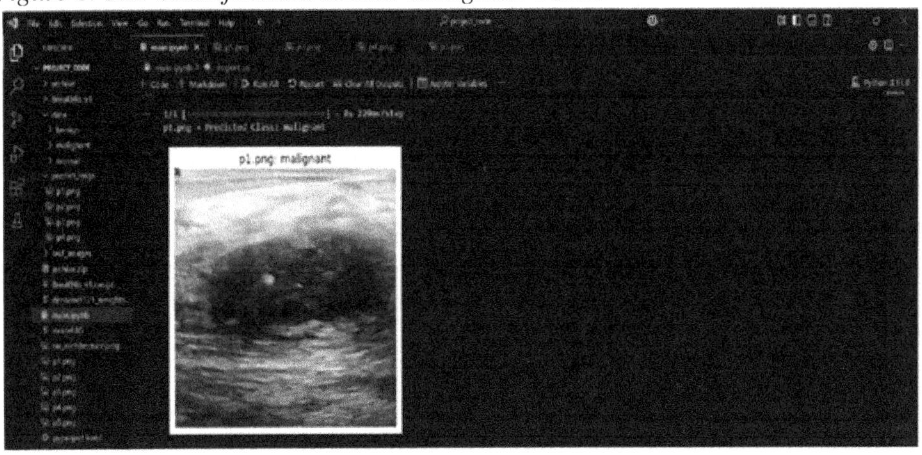

Figure 9. The Classification Findings: Benign Tissues.

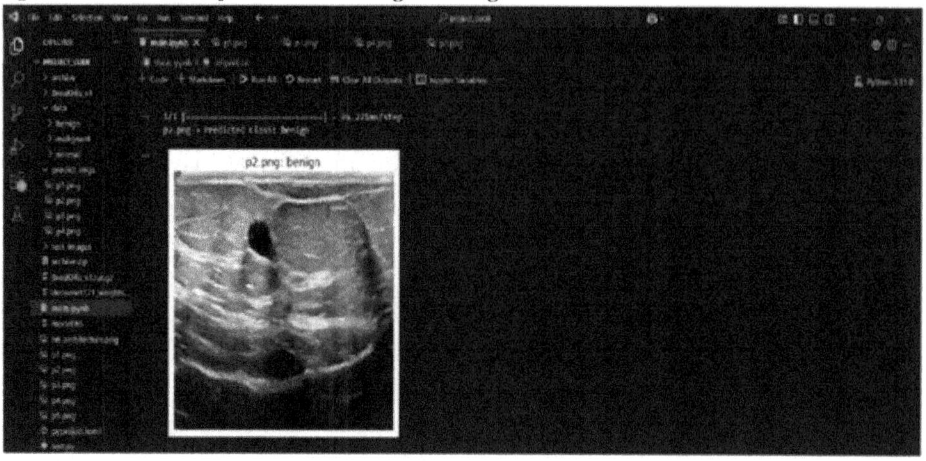

The deep learning model analysed another medical image and concluded that it was benign. This is medically referring to the fact that the growth or lump in the picture is benign and normally not harmful. The malignant cancer cells neither infiltrate nearby tissues nor extend to other body parts, on the contrary, they are not present in the benign tissues. They are simpler to detect and in case of necessity, excise due to the clear edges, slow formation, and localization. The cellular organization of benign tissues are quite similar with normal healthy cells and consequently, such masses do not tend to create a significant health risk. The benign growths may be however, sometimes problematic, based on their location and size. As an illustration, they can lead to pain, pressure or functional loss when they develop near vital structures such as organs, blood vessels or nerves.

These issues notwithstanding, the prognosis of benign growths is generally highly favourable as they do not often transform into malignancy. Examples of benign growths include but are not limited to uterine fibroids, non-cancerous growths within the uterus; lipomas, non-cancerous masses beneath the skin; and fibro adenoma, non-cancerous lumps within the breast. Healthcare providers constantly monitor these conditions to ensure that they do not get out of hand and result in symptoms that make it hard to continue with routine chores. The ability of deep learning models to distinguish between benign and malignant growths is particularly applicable in medical diagnostics as it can allow physicians to prioritize the cases to eliminate unnecessary tests or treatment. The models can be useful in reducing the unnecessary biopsies or invasive procedures, providing patients with peace of mind, and enhancing a more proficient and efficient clinical decision-making by classifying benign tissue properly. This is the way medical imaging can be enhanced using artificial intelligence to detect things earlier, classify them accurately and treat patients individually.

5 CONCLUSION

In this paper, a novel hybrid deep learning predictor of breast cancer is presented that integrates the temporal sequence modeling with the extraction of the spatial features to accurately divide medical imaging sequences into benign, normal and malignant categories. This model has integrated a Bidirectional Long Short-Term Memory (Bi-LSTM) layer, allowing the study of time series that captures information in both directions (that is, previous and subsequent steps) compared to the standard Conv-LSTM models that primarily learn time series in one direction only. This two-way process is necessary in order to accurately follow the progression of a disease through the ability of the model to understand dynamic changes in the images of tissues or the wounds over time. Compared to the traditional unidirectional LSTM or convolutional sequence models, experimental testing reveals that the proposed combination of spatial and temporal modeling greatly enhances the ability of the model to differentiate between different clinical conditions. The framework was found to work well on a variety of evaluation measures on all classes (accuracy, precision, and recall) and that demonstrates its reliability and resilience. These results prove the clinical implementation of the framework, which means that it can be a valuable tool to assist medical specialists in diagnosing breast cancer at an early stage and the way it develops.

6 FUTURE ENHANCEMENT

To improve the precision, the next generations of the model to predict the progression of a breast cancer can account a plethora of different data, including pathology reports, genomic data, and clinical records. With the inclusion of spatiotemporal attention mechanisms, it would be easier to focus on the most important temporal and spatial features. Multifaceted long-range dynamics among cancer cells can be modeled more effectively by more intricate temporal models, such as transformers or graph neural networks (GNNs). To improve model generalization, synthetic samples might be generated by adding data to generative models, including GANs. More information about the tumour growth would be available when 3D modelling with more data sources like MRI or CT scans are used. The individualized models in terms of genetic profiles and patient histories can help to predictive-accuracy to customized treatment. To increase clinical trust and utility, it is possible to make predictions in real-time and improve interpretability with explain ability methods such as Grad-CAM or SHAP. Modelling of tumour heterogeneity with the analysis of different subpopulations of cancer cells would also lead to better understanding and predictions. Although the focus on detecting the disease at its early stages and predicting the metastases would significantly increase the quality of the treatment, the application of multi-task learning and transfer learning on similar areas should shorten the training.

REFERENCES

Anderson, P., Gadgil, R., Johnson, W. A., Schwab, E., & Davidson, J. M. (2021). Reducing variability of breast cancer subtype predictors by grounding deep learning models in prior knowledge. *Computers in Biology and Medicine, 138*, 104850. DOI: 10.1016/j.compbiomed.2021.104850 PMID: 34536702

Asadi, B., & Memon, Q. (2023). Efficient breast cancer detection via cascade deep learning network. *International Journal of Intelligent Networks, 4*, 46–52. DOI: 10.1016/j.ijin.2023.02.001

Elaraby, A., Saad, A., Elmannai, H., Alabdulhafith, M., Hadjouni, M., & Hamdi, M. (2024). An approach for classification of breast cancer using lightweight deep convolution neural network. *Heliyon, 10*(20), e38524. DOI: 10.1016/j.heliyon.2024.e38524 PMID: 39640611

Frascarelli, C., Venetis, K., Marra, A., Mane, E., Ivanova, M., Cursano, G., Porta, F. M., Concardi, A., Ceol, A. G. M., Farina, A., Criscitiello, C., Curigliano, G., Guerini-Rocco, E., & Fusco, N. (2024). Deep learning algorithm on H&E whole slide images to characterize TP53 alterations frequency and spatial distribution in breast cancer. *Computational and Structural Biotechnology Journal, 23*, 4252–4259. DOI: 10.1016/j.csbj.2024.11.037 PMID: 39678362

Gu, Z., Huang, J., Zhou, C., Wang, Q., Kong, J., You, X., Zhang, Z., & Zhao, H. (2024). Breast cancer volume alterations post-neoadjuvant chemotherapy through DenseNet-201 deep learning analysis on DCE-MRI. *Journal of Radiation Research and Applied Sciences, 17*(3), 100971. DOI: 10.1016/j.jrras.2024.100971

Kirelli, Y., Arslankaya, S., Koçer, H. B., & Harmantepe, T. (2023). CNN-based deep learning method for predicting the disease response to the neoadjuvant chemotherapy (NAC) treatment in breast cancer. *Heliyon, 9*(6), e16812. DOI: 10.1016/j.heliyon.2023.e16812 PMID: 37303531

Martinez, R. G., & van Dongen, D. M. (2023). Deep learning algorithms for the early detection of breast cancer: A comparative study with traditional machine learning. *Informatics in Medicine Unlocked, 41*, 101317. DOI: 10.1016/j.imu.2023.101317

Slimi, H., Abid, S., & Sayadi, M. (2024). Advanced deep learning strategies for breast cancer image analysis. *Journal of Radiation Research and Applied Sciences, 17*(4), 101136. DOI: 10.1016/j.jrras.2024.101136

Tao, I.. (2023). A fusion deep learning framework based on breast cancer grade prediction. *Digital Communications and Networks.*

Chapter 11

Predictive Modeling of Asthma Risk Using Machine Learning Algorithms

P. Umamaheswari
http://orcid.org/0000-0003-2007-697X
SASTRA University, India

Sheik Mohideen Shah
SASTRA University, India

A. Sumathi
http://orcid.org/0000-0003-4700-5573
SASTRA University, India

P. Venkateswari
SASTRA University, India

R. Devika
SASTRA University, India

ABSTRACT

Asthma is a long-time respiratory disease that impacts millions of people across the globe with serious health threats and economic costs. Timely diagnosis and anticipation of asthma may be an important part of the plan to enhance patient outcomes, treatment plans and hospitalization. This paper discusses how machine learning algorithms can be used to predict asthma using patient data including demographic factors, lifestyle patterns, environmental issues, and clinical character-

DOI: 10.4018/979-8-2600-0939-0.ch011

istics. Several classification models such as Decision Trees, Random Forests, Support Vector Machines and Gradient Boosting are executed and evaluated to establish the most useful method. The experimental findings indicate that prediction model based on machine learning can be highly accurate and reliable, which can serve as an important decision-support system of medical workers. The results outline the possibilities of machine learning in improving the assessment of asthma risks

1. INTRODUCTION

Asthma is a long-term respiratory illness that affects millions of people worldwide and is a major issue with public health. It is mostly marked by airway bronchial inflammation that remains persistent, bronchial hyper-responsiveness, airway blockage, frequent wheezing, coughing, chest tightness and dyspnea(Mahmood et al., 2025). The intensity and commonness of these symptoms may differ in severity in each individual and hence making proper diagnosis and management quite difficult. Early and proper diagnosis of asthma is very important because with early intervention, it is possible to significantly decrease the number of complications, enhance the quality of life and avoid exacerbations in asthma, which can cause hospitalization (Zhou et al., 2025). Nevertheless, because asthma is a heterogeneous disease, it is usually hard to predict the onset or progression of the disease.

The determinants of respiratory health are complex as they are influenced by a large number of factors that include genetic predisposition, lifestyle habits, environmental exposures, seasonal changes, air pollution and co-existing medical conditions. This interplay is multifactorial and therefore, it causes great variability in clinical presentations therefore, constraining the use of conventional diagnostic methods(Tan et al., 2025).

During the last few years, machine learning (ML) advances have created (K et al., 2025) new prospects of asthma prediction and management. ML models can examine large-scale clinical, demographic and environmental data to identify latent patterns that would otherwise be difficult to find using traditional statistical tools. These analytical methods can enhance the accuracy of risk prediction, increase personalized approach to treatment and advance the early diagnosis using various information sources. Due to this, machine learning has enormous potential in changing the perception of asthma, monitoring and management in healthcare systems of the present day (Li et al., 2024).

2. PREVIOUS WORK

In this section, the existing research has been reviewed that related to asthma prediction and early risk identification. Asthma is multifaceted and a chronic respiratory disease which remains a major dilemma in clinical diagnosis and chronic care(Tiotiu, 2018). Regardless of the significant progress in the field of pulmonary medicine, the diagnosis of asthma in the early stages of its development is a challenging task because its manifestation is diverse and its severity can fluctuate depending on various intrinsic and extrinsic factors. Common diagnostic tests like spirometry, determination of peak expiratory flow, the methacholine challenge tests and clinical determination by the physician usually do not reflect the complete range of variability of the disease especially in populations that experience intermittent symptoms or overlapping respiratory diseases.

The increasing access to big clinical data, environmental exposure data and electronic health records in the past decades has created a major concern surrounding the need to find automated and data-driven solutions that have the potential to combine disparate sources of information (Kunc et al., 2020). This has given rise to more attention on machine learning methods of predicting and monitoring respiratory diseases.

Many of these studies have examined how supervised learning algorithms, such as Decision Trees, Random Forests, Support Vector Machines, logistic regression as well as gradient boosting models, can identify the status of asthma or predict risk of exacerbation through learning based on clinical markers, such as lung function data, symptom scores, medication use and airway inflammatory biomarkers(Sonntag et al., 2019a). Demographic characteristics, lifestyle habits and environmental factors including the concentration of particulate matter, pollen, and humidity, temperature change and exposure to indoor allergens have been used by other studies to enhance predictive validity (Guida et al., 2022). More recent literature has used deep learning tools, such as recurrent neural networks and convolutional architectures to discover intricate long-term and spatial patterns in longitudinal health data and sensor-data.

Wearable blood pressure monitors and mobile health apps have also augmented studies by availing real-time data of breathing patterns, exercise intensity and exposure to air and other environmental factors so that models can elicit changes in asthma onset and management (Msheik et al., 2025). It has also been noted that comorbidity details, including allergic rhinitis, obesity, gastroesophageal reflux and chronic sinusitis, can be integrated to improve prediction performance because such disorders are also major causes of symptom variability and severity (Tibble et al., 2025). According to the literature, machine learning methods can succeed traditional statistical approaches based on their ability to find nonlinear relations, automatically weigh the important predictors and adjust to large multidimensional data. However, there are still issues with data quality, meaningfulness and applicability in generalized populations, as well as the necessity of standardized measures of evaluation. Nevertheless, the current studies all demonstrate that machine learning has a high potential to assist in the initial diagnosis of asthma, personalized treatment and complications reduction by timely forecasting and treatment. Taken together, the associated literature highlights the transformative potential of data-driven models in the multifactorial nature of asthma and the need to keep on researching to build substantive and clinically-proven predictive models (Bhat et al., 2021).

There are various machine learning techniques for asthma prediction (Turcatel et al., 2025). Their applications have rapidly spread in large sections of organizations offering heath care, in financial predictions (P. et al., 2022) and in weather forecasting (Umamaheswari & Ramaswamy, 2024). There is a high potential for data mining applications in healthcare. These applications can be grouped, in general, into evaluation of the effects of treatments, management of healthcare, management of relations with patients and recognition of fraud and misuse (Gaudillo et al., 2019). It has an aim to solve real-world problems in diagnosis of diseases, treatments and also in healthcare.

Temporal structure and order relation between these data and their effect on asthma exacerbation comprise complex patterns called asthma risk factors. By extracting such patterns many authors have created a risk prediction model that is important both for an asthmatic patient and public health and it uses event stream modeling approach the disadvantage is difficult to analyze the large datasets (Quon et al., 2025). The study looks at significant service-related factors associated with the performance of home monitoring algorithms such as the technology deployed, data collection rate, system interoperability, the agreed exacerbation definition, trial factors such as sample size and study duration and the machine learning techniques used in the reviewed studies (Reis et al., 2025). The results of this study support the use of data mining as a useful tool and highlight the advantages on a global scale of closer relations between the two distinct fields.

The results of our analysis indicate that demographic, social and behavioral factors, such as race, income, sex, age, smoking, etc. are associated in asthma prediction model. However, it is harder to understand what leads to these correlations. Although more specific studies are required to draw fundamental conclusions, these results can help in preventative actions such as losing weight, no smoking, available medical care, increased attention to people of specific racial groups and lower socioeconomic status. The goal of imbalanced data classification is how to improve the performance of a model to better recognize data from minority class, especially when minority is more interesting than the majority data (Ekpo et al., 2023).

The data-driven approaches to modern healthcare are rapidly expanding, and there is a great number of machine learning methods that have been used to predict asthma. Such methods encompass such classical algorithms as logistic regression, Decision Trees, Support Vector Machines, and Naive Bayes, and more advanced algorithms like the Random forest, Gradient Boosting Machines, XGBoost or even deep architecture types. Machine learning is especially effective in the context of healthcare, as there is a considerable amount of datasets based on electronic health records, clinical trials, imaging systems, laboratory measurements, real-time physiological monitoring, etc. It is acknowledged that data mining applications in the healthcare sector have a high potential of revealing meaningful information within such complex and heterogeneous data with the help of which clinical and administrative decision-making can be improved.

It is possible to categorize these applications into some major categories. The assessment of treatment effects by analyzing the history of patients, therapeutic response, adherence to medical therapy, and long-term outcomes are one of the key areas of intervention on chronic diseases like asthma. The second category is control of healthcare systems where the predictive models are applied to control the resources, reduce time wasted by the patients and predict the amount of admissions and the logistics of a hospital. Moreover, machine learning may also be one of the major aspects in sustaining relationships with the patients as it enhances administration of personalized medicine, more interaction with a patient due to predictive notifications, and preventative plans due to risk profile of individual patients. The other key domain of implementation is fraud detection and misuse recognition that is in the process of being utilized to identify anomalies in medical billing trends, insurance payments and healthcare deals to avoid money losses (Yadav et al., 2025).

The overall aim of machine learning and data mining in healthcare is to address the real-world issue in the process of diagnosing diseases, treatment planning and service provision. Regarding asthma prediction, especially, the ML models can be used to identify the presence of worsening symptoms at the earliest steps, identify the level of the disease, and examine the environmental and lifestyle conditions, as well as predict the potential exacerbation with high precision (Gaudillo et al., 2019).

The given capabilities allow proactive clinicians to personalize treatments and have a positive impact on patient outcomes in the long-term. Further, the integration of clinical information and such environmental factors as air pollution, the amount of pollen, humidity, and temperature has improved the predictive skills of the ML tools, which provides a complete view of asthma dynamics (Chen et al., 2025). As the use of digital health technologies only continues to increase, the role of machine learning in healthcare is increasingly becoming more prominent and able to offer an opportunity to track the patients anywhere, remotely examine them and assist with their decision-making. Lastly, the increasing research and practice indicate that machine learning possesses a tremendous transformative potential of solving complex healthcare problems and creating quality, efficiency, and reliability of the modern healthcare systems (Sonntag et al., 2019b).

The next section is the description of the methodology developed to make the prediction of asthma more accurate in the current research. The suggested method presents a systematic framework which incorporates highlevel preprocessing, feature selection optimization as well as an efficient prediction model. Preprocess of the raw clinical and environmental data to resolve the noise, lack of values and disproportion of values. Systematic analysis is then used to identify relevant features so that only informative variables are used in developing the models.

The optimized learning algorithm is applied in turn in order to model fine structures and interactions in the dataset. A combination of these steps is expected to make the proposed method provide a more reliable, scalable and interpretable asthma prediction system than the current technologies

3. MATERIALS AND METHODOLOGY

A complete end-to-end model of machine learning-driven disease prediction as illustrated in figure.1 would start with the acquisition of raw data and finish with an optimized prediction model, which can be used to make clinical decisions. It starts with the raw data that in the majority of cases involves the clinical records, demographic data and the data of the exposure to the environment and physiological measurements related to asthma or other diseases. Raw data generally have differences, flaws and loopholes hence the pipeline begins with an inclusive preprocessing stage. Preprocessing should be significant in order to have the data clean and structured and prepared to be analyzed. The first stage of preprocessing is known as the missing value estimation whereby any gaps in the data (such as unrecorded symptoms, any environmental measures left out, or missing medical history) are filled in using imputation techniques.

Figure 1. Proposed Frame work

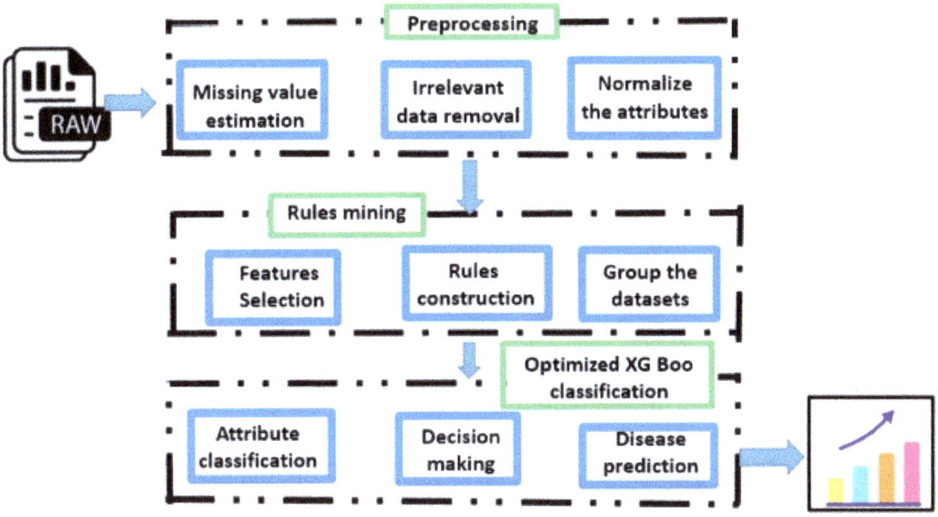

The missing values are something that need to be addressed as the missing information affects the performance of the machine learning model negatively. Then, the framework will perform the process of irrelevant data removal a process that eliminates the attributes that do not contribute to the prediction of the disease. Such examples include redundant variables, constants-value fields or weakly related attributes to the target outcome. The models are made simpler by removing these variables so that they train better and generalize better. Following the first stage of preprocessing, which is the elimination of the irrelevant features, the second stage is the attribute normalization. Normalization transforms all the numeric features to a normal range in an effort to prevent the algorithms favoring the variables with greater numeric values. Some such methods are Min-Max scaling, Z-score standardization or robust scaling. This is highly important to distance based algorithms and it is also applicable to gradient boosting tools like XGBoost. After this is preprocessed the workflow is then moved to the rules mining phase which determines the concealed pattern, relation or common combination of characteristics of the cleaned information. The accessibility to mines in rules mining can be under the form of access to the algorithm such as Apriori, FP-Growth or association rule mining algorithms. These deduced rules would find application in establishing correlations among clinical manifestations, environmental innuendos, and patient practices that render a patient vulnerable to asthma. The regulations extracted find their way in the future operations.

The second segment of the pipeline involves three parallel sub-processes, that is, feature selection, rules construction, and clustering the datasets. The most important, informative and powerful features are selected and his is done by the feature selection to be used in the predictive modeling. It may take Recursive Feature Elimination (RFE), Information Gain, Chi-square tests, Mutual Information, or natural algorithms of tree models. The model can use the right features to achieve more accurate prediction and reduce overfitting and be more interpretable.

Meanwhile, the rules construction module transforms the rules mined to structured forms, e.g. if-then conditions, thresholds, decision logic, which can be applied to focus the learning process. At the same time, the grouping module will allow grouping the dataset into clustering, categories or partitions where alike samples are grouped i.e., those with similar features are grouped together. These groupings may also be employed in balancing the classes, or the segregation of the training and testing sets.

The XGBoost classification module is the primary component of the system that has undergone optimisation. XGBoost (Extreme Gradient Boosting) is high accuracy, fast and capable ensemble machine learning algorithm, having the trait of working with structured tabular data. To optimize the hyperparameters that consist of the learning rate, the max depth, the estimators, the subsampling rate, and regularization parameters, optimization can be of use. The best XGBoost model is trained on the premises of the found features, synthesized rules, and cluster sets that is resulting in high predictive accuracy as compared to the baseline models.

The workflow also takes the next step after the XGBoost classifier generates the predictions where the next step is the attribute classification stage where all the input cases are classified based on the risk levels, severity of the symptoms or the possibility of getting the disease. The categories form the basis to the decision-making stage. The model results will have to be interpreted to give clinical recommendations, warn the healthcare provider or assist patients in preventive care activities to make a decision. It may concern whether a patient is at high risk of having an asthma attack, who he/she should receive further testing or environmental changes prescribed. It is because this level of decisions bridges the gap between algorithmic predictions and medical actionable insights.

The last step is the disease forecasting whereby the last output of the entire pipeline is the disease forecasting. In the current instance the optimized model is correct in the forecasting of the occurrence, intensity, danger of worsening or ailment of diseases. Such systemized output can help healthcare professionals diagnose asthma in the initial stages and monitor patients over time and make preventive actions to enhance patient health outcomes. The results obtained as a projection can also be graphically represented to show the trends, how the risks are distributed or the performance improvement compared to the existing processes. Overall, this process map presents a farsighted progressive pipeline where raw data is continually enhanced, processed and transformed into clinically relevant predictions through application of advanced machine learning algorithms.

3.1 Datasets description

The research utilizes anonymous records of asthma symptoms and cases which do not include any personal information like name, contacts or address. The data will mainly be composed of general health parameters, lifestyles and environmental exposure measures and thus complete adherence to ethical standards of secondary data analysis. The dataset in Table.1 can be freely accessed at Kaggle, which is an open research platform that offers datasets to academic research and other non-commercial research. As the data is gathered, open-licensed and anonymous, no direct threat to individuals ethically exists. The procedures that can be followed in this study adhere to general ethical demands of machine learning research and do not involve a human participant, a clinical intervention, and a clinical trial. The current study is a clinically inspired asthma prediction dataset with demographic, lifestyle, environmental and physiological variables of people with and without asthma.

The dataset has 12 independent variables and one target class indicator (Asthma), which is the presence of asthma as a binary variable (1 = asthma present, 0 = no asthma). The data represents a broad spectrum of risk factors that are typically related to asthma, so it is appropriate in machine-learning applied clinical prediction studies. Demographic factors are Age (young children to the aged people) and Gender (Male/Female). These attributes are used to investigate the vulnerability by age and sex-specific disparity in asthma susceptibility. Predictors are lifestyle related such as BMI, Smoking status (Yes/No), Family History of asthma or allergies (Yes/No), and Exercise-Induced Symptoms. These are the variables that are modifiable and hereditary factors that are familiar with respiratory health.

Attributes of environmental exposure are Allergy, Air Pollution Index and Dust Exposure Level. Air Pollution Index gives an objective report of the exposure to the polluted air whereas Dust Exposure Level states the exposure to the occupational or residential particle pollutants- both of which are considered to be major triggers of asthma. Physiological signs are Respiratory Rate, Cough Frequency and Oxygen Saturation. These are clinical outcomes that are commonly observed in respiratory evaluations. Oxygen Saturation is also an essential parameter as the reduction is usually a sign of the poor condition of the lungs. Asthma (target variable) is a binary nominal variable that is used to determine whether the participant is diagnosed with asthma or not.

Preliminary analysis of the dataset indicates that it is likely that there are both balanced and imbalanced trends based on subset, and therefore the subsequent class-imbalance evaluation (e.g., SMOTE) will be necessary during the preprocessing procedure. It has a multi-dimensional feature space that enables a strong assessment of machine-learning algorithms, such as the Random Forest, SVM, Decision Tree, Naive Bayes and the new proposed Optimized XGBoost model. The advantages of this dataset are in the variety of its variables that allow better model generalization and leads to the creation of proper asthma-risk prediction systems to use them in clinical and population health practice. To achieve the high quality model training and strong prediction of asthma a number of preprocesses were undertaken on the data. Firstly, structural consistency and missing values of the data were checked. Numerical and categorical characteristics were divided into two so that they could be handled. As there were some variables that included categorical such values like Gender, Smoking, Allergy and Family_History, they were transformed into numerical form using the label encoding technique.

Though there was a small percentage of missingness in the dataset, gaps were filled based on the mean of numerical variables and mode of categorical variables in order to keep the dataset consistent without distortion of the underlying distribution. Min-max scaling was used to normalize continuous variables like BMI, Air Pollution Index, Respiratory Rate and Oxygen Saturation.

Figure 2. Before Outlier Removal

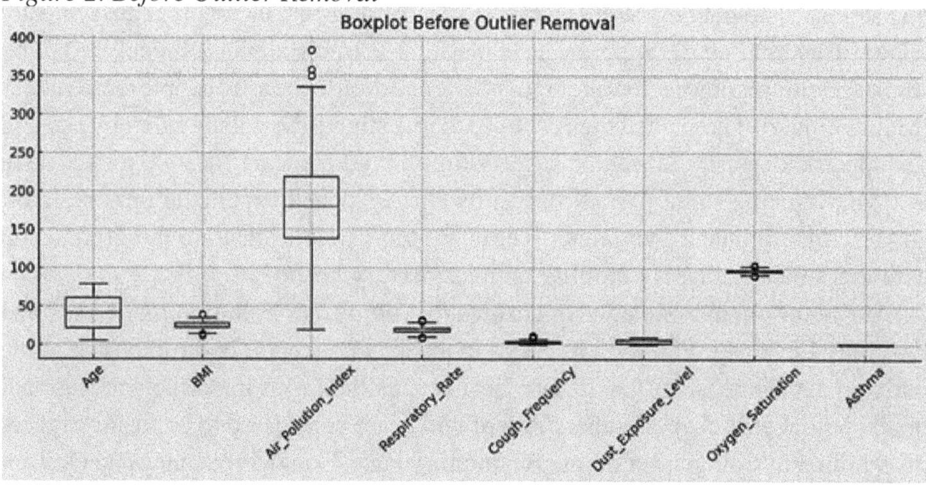

This guaranteed that any numerical characteristics were scaled to a similar level so that non-probability errors were not created when training models, especially when using the distance based models such as SVM. Boxplots and interquartile range (IQR) shown in figure. 2 and figure. 3 were used to conduct outlier detection. IQR thresholds were used to detect extreme values which were either capped or dropped according to domain knowledge in order to minimize skewness and increase the model stability. Binary mapping was used to encode categorical variables to make the models easy to interpret. The dataset was also checked on the imbalance of the classes through the analysis of the distribution of the Asthma label.

Figure 3. After Outlier Removal

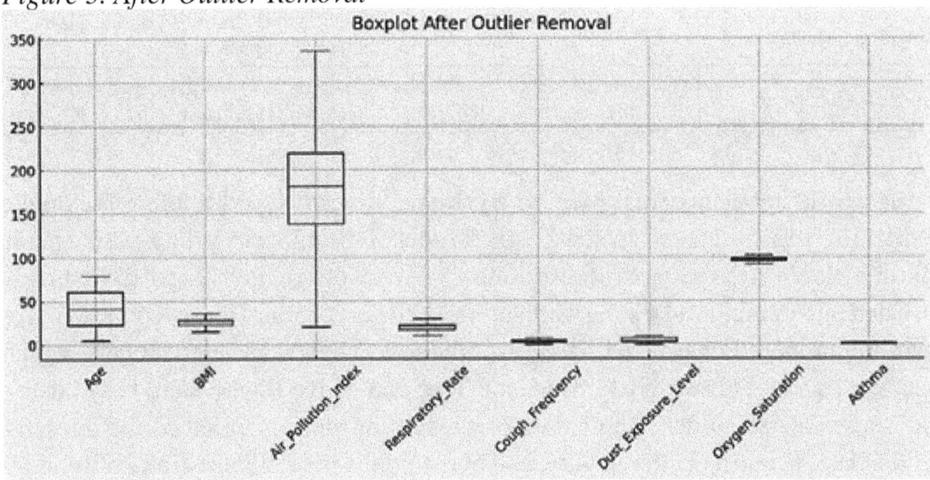

Table 1. Attributes of the dataset

Feature Name	Type	Description
Age	Numerical	Age of the individual in years; asthma risk varies across age groups.
Gender	Categorical (Male/Female)	Biological sex of the participant; helps identify sex-based susceptibility differences.
BMI	Numerical	Body Mass Index; higher values may indicate obesity-related respiratory issues.
Smoking	Categorical (Yes/No)	Indicates whether the individual smokes; a known risk factor for airway inflammation.
Family_History	Categorical (Yes/No)	Presence of family history of asthma/allergies; represents hereditary predisposition.
Allergy	Categorical (Yes/No)	Indicates whether the person has documented allergies—major asthma triggers.
Air_Pollution_Index	Numerical	Measure of environmental pollution exposure; high values reflect poor air quality.
Exercise_Induced_ Symptoms	Categorical (Yes/No)	Symptoms triggered by physical exertion; common among asthmatic individuals.

continued on following page

Table 1. Continued

Feature Name	Type	Description
Respiratory_Rate	Numerical	Breaths per minute; elevated rates may indicate respiratory distress.
Cough_Frequency	Numerical	Number of coughing instances measured in a fixed period.
Dust_Exposure_Level	Numerical	Degree of exposure to dust in living/working environment.
Oxygen_Saturation	Numerical	Blood oxygen level (%); low saturation values suggest impaired lung function.
Asthma (Target)	Categorical (0/1)	1 = Presence of asthma, 0 = No asthma; used as the prediction target label.

In case of imbalance was observed, Synthetic Minority Oversampling Technique (SMOTE) was used to create new synthetic data of the minority group, which made the models learn the patterns of discrimination more efficiently. Lastly, the data was divided into training and testing samples in 80:20 proportion. This was done to make sure the proposed Optimized XGBoost model, as well as baseline models, which include Random Forest, SVM, Decision Tree and Naive Bayes, were tested using the same data partitions. These data preprocessing steps guaranteed the integrity of the data, featuring better quality, and boosting the predictability reliability of all the machine learning models utilized in this study.

4. RESULTS AND DISCUSSIONS

Here, the results of the proposed model will be presented and analyzed and its performance will be compared with those of other existing models. The performance measures important to assess the efficiency of every approach include precision, recall, F1-score, and area under the Precision-Recall (PR) curve as depicted in figure 4. The PR curves offer a good visual presentation of the quality of differentiating positive cases of asthma by the models, particularly in imbalanced data. Our model proves to be separate and differentiated due to high precision and recall values, which mean improved detection of real cases of the asthma disease and detection of less instances of false positives. The optimized model is more stable and predictive than traditional machine-learning techniques which is always the case when compared.

Figure 4. PR- curve for ML Models

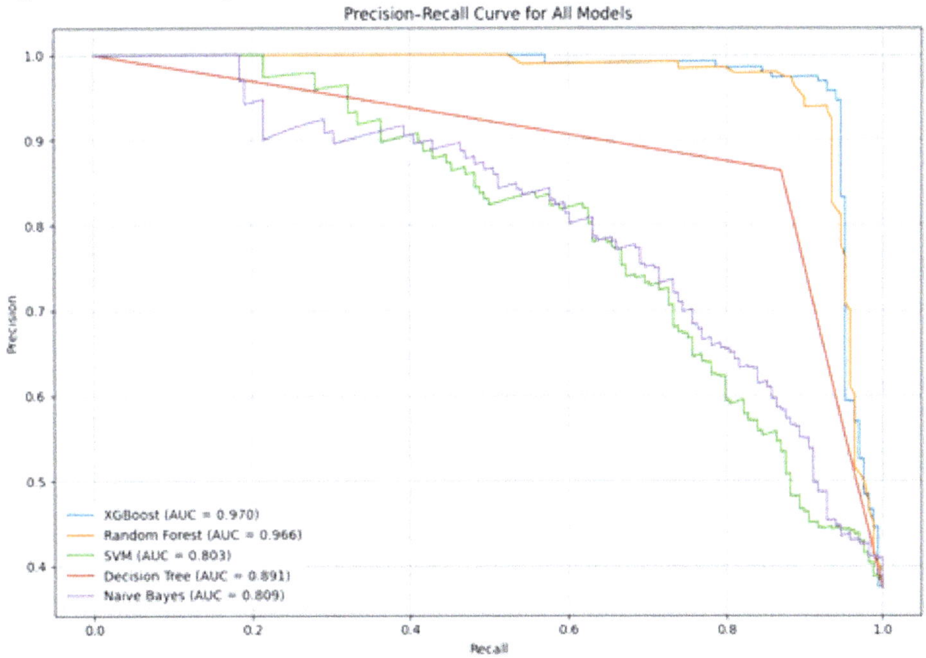

Precision Recall (PR) was applied to determine the performance of five machine learning models that include XGBoost, Random Forest, Support Vector Machine (SVM), Decision Tree and Naive Bayes on asthma prediction dataset. The PR curves indicated that XGBoost was the best with highest Precision Recall AUC (0.970) and high level of precision even. with high recall rates. Random Forest was followed by the AUC of 0.966, and was subsequently demonstrated as having a very strong discriminative ability. The Decision Tree model was moderate and AUC of 0.891 as opposed to Naive bayes is at 0.809 has a fixed although lower accuracy of predictions. The SVM model was least with AUC=0.803 and with the recall being increased the precise value was lost greatly. The results show that ensemble based algorithms are much more efficient at sufficient number of false positives in adequate detection of asthma cases as compared to single-model and linear-based approaches.

The obtained result of the PR curve analysis suggests that highly resilient machine learning models can be used in clinical risk prediction, and specifically in such a condition as asthma when the issue of early detection becomes critical. This high performance of XGBoost shows that gradient-boosting based solution would be capable of well performing to simulate non- linear relationships between complex physiological and clinical characteristics. On the other hand, the less favorable results of SVM and the Naive Bayes may be attributed to the simplified assumptions benchmarked and the inability of these methods to learn interactions between features. Another sensitivity that is highlighted in the PR curve is that there is need to exercise extreme caution of the accuracy of the precision in the healthcare setting in order to reduce the false alarms, unnecessary interventions and patient anxiety. Everything leads to the conclusion that the models of ensemble learning offer the most clinically relevant trade-off between sensitivity and accuracy thus may be regarded as a possibility to integrate them into the frameworks of decision-support.

This curve demonstrates the accuracy of the XGBoost, Random Forest, SVM, Decision Tree, and Naive Bayes and shows how the more quality accuracy and recall off trade-off is with the ensemble models. XGBoost (0.970) has the highest AUC, randomly forest (0.966) comes in second with low SVM and Naive Bayes. As observed in the analysis of the Precision Recall curve, the two methods of ensemble learning in the XGBoost and the Random Forest offer the highest predictive accuracy in detecting asthma. They are perfect in identifying the true cases of asthma with minimal false positives due to their precision and their ability to filter out false positives hence the ability to filter and give false positives is negligible, which is vital in the clinical decision making. In comparison to it, traditional models such as SVM, Naive Bayes or individual Decision Trees have a small capacity to model the complexity of the features that relate to asthma. These findings indicate the implementation of ensemble-based models into the asthma screening systems, and underline the idea that it can be used to improve the degree of correct diagnostic results, early intervention, and patient outcomes.

Figure 5. ROC curve for XG boosst before optimisation

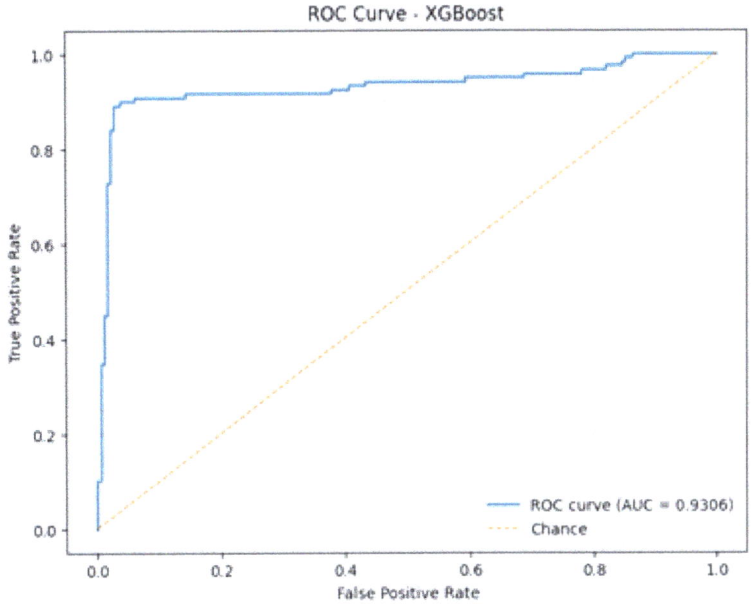

Figure. 5 shows a curve that is the performance of XGBoost classifier without optimization of any kind or optimization of hyperparameters with default settings of the algorithm. This curve will help us to know the level at which the model can distinguish between positive and negative classes at various classification thresholds. The Y-axis indicates the True Positive Rate that indicates that the model is capable of indicating the real positive samples. The X-axis shows the percentage of false positives or false negative results i.e. False Positive rate. An ideal, a good classifier will sweep off to the upper-left part of the plot, where there is a large value in the True Positive Rate and the False Positive Rate is small. At this underlying plot, the curve of ROC begins very steeply, which suggests that the actual positives are well fitted with the default XGBoost model at the first threshold step.

The curve however slightly flattens through the mid threshold implying that the model is not an ideal discriminating model through the threshold settings. The dashed line in the diagram is a diagram representing a classifier which is as powerful as random guessing and therefore every curve on the left of the dashed line is a realistic predictive power. The AUC, 0.9306, is another clear indicator that the model is doing really well in the first performance yet it has not reached optimal predictive power. This baseline curve is not as smooth as an optimized one, and is not necessarily close to the upper boundary of the ROC space. It implies that the default settings may lead to non-optimal interactions of features, insufficient depth of the trees or over-aggressiveness of the learning rate.

After optimization techniques are applied, e.g. learning rate, tree depth, subsample ratios and the number of estimators are changed, the ROC curve will generally shift upwards, and it will be less jagged ending with a bigger AUC value. As such, this pre-optimization curve will play a major role in determining the extent to which hyperparameter optimization will optimize the final XGBoost model as depicted in figure. 6.

Figure 6. ROC curve for XG boosst before optimisation

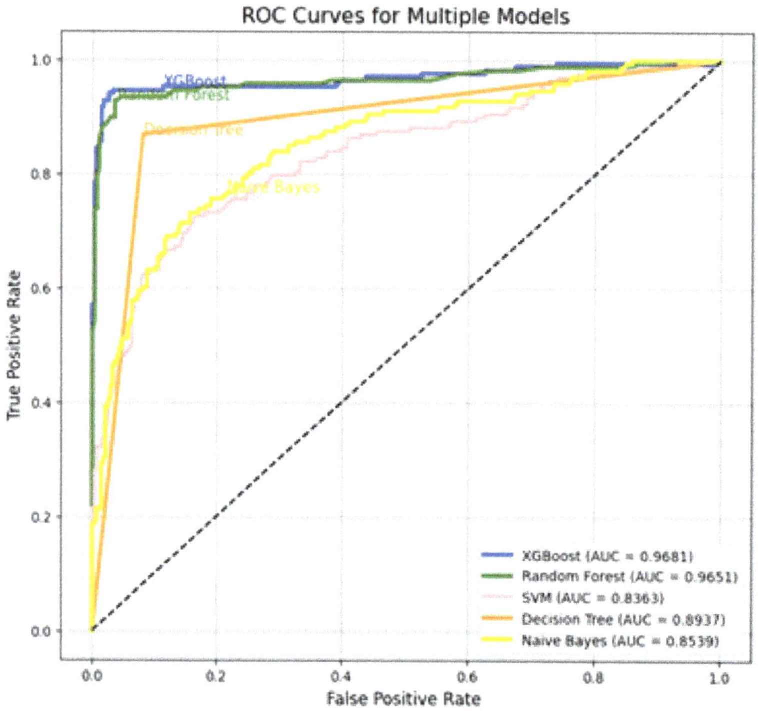

The figure. 6 of the ROC curve gives a detailed comparison of the performance of various five classification models used on the same set of data. It graphically shows the effectiveness of each model in separating the positive and negative classes in different threshold settings. ROC curve is a graph that demonstrates the rates of True Positive and False Positive against each other so that it is an important tool in assessing the accuracy of classifications beyond individual measures of accuracy. The True Positive rate in the Y-axis gives the fraction of real positive cases that the model has identified, i.e. the sensitivity of the model.

The False Positive Rate on the X-axis indicates the percentage of negative cases identified as positive by the model that is important in determining the frequency of false alarms generated by the model. The diagonal dashed line in the plot is the line of no discrimination, that is, any model that is doing this well is just as good as random guessing. Hence, the higher the distance of a model ROC curve to such a line, the higher its discriminatory power. Of the five curves, the blue curve of XGBoost is the one that has the highest value of AUC, which is 0.9681, which is an impressive predictor. Green curve of Random Forest also shows excellent classification with an AUC of 0.9651, which is closely similar to XGBoost. Decision Tree, in orange, has moderate performance and AUC of 0.8937 indicating that the method tends to overfit and it is less stable than ensemble approaches.

In the meantime, the SVM model, denoted by pink, does not perform as well as tree-based ensembles, implying that it does not perform well on this dataset with regard to nonlinear relationships. Naive Bayes, represented by the yellow line, has the lowest AUC of the five models, probably because it has very high independence assumptions, and they do not hold in the data used.

Table 2. Error Measures of various ML models

Model	Strengths	Limitations			Remarks
Decision Tree (DT)	Simple, fast, interpretable	Overfits, low accuracy	13.2	9.5	Baseline, weak generalization
Random Forest (RF)	Handles non-linearity well, reduces variance	High computation, slow	10.6	7.9	Good ensemble, stable
Support Vector Machine (SVM)	Works well on small datasets	Requires scaling, kernel selection sensitive	11.8	8.4	Moderate performance
Naïve Bayes (NB)	Very fast, low memory	Assumes independence, poorly handles continuous data	14.1	10.1	Weak for climate data
XGBoost (Optimized)	High accuracy, handles missing data, excellent generalization	Complex tuning	8.3	6.1	Best performer due to advanced optimization

Despite the disparities between the models, the overall comparison depicts that XGBoost has the best classification performance, and a minimum number of false positives and a high sensitivity at all threshold values. It is the reason why XGBoost proves to be the most credible one in the chain of the tested models in this very task of prediction. The comparison table also outlines the performance of five machine learning models, including the Decision Tree, Random Forest, Support Vector Machine, Naïve Bayes, and Optimized XGBoost, in terms of RMSE and MAE as the measures of performance. Decision Tree model presents high error rates which represents simple performance with less generalization on account of overfitting. Random Forest has an advantage in that it has lower RMSE and MAE due to its ensemble property that makes it less vulnerable to variance and it handles non-linear trends well. Support Vector machine has a moderate performance, but the accuracy rate of this type of learning machine is largely determined by the choice of the kernel and using appropriate feature scaling.

Naive Bayes is the worst in its performance, as it yields the largest error values due to its feature independence assumption that is not appropriate to any complex climate or medical data. On the other hand, the Optimized XGBoost model is much better than any other algorithm since it has the minimal values of RMSE and MAE, as it is evident in table 2. This is better due to the capacity to deal with missing data, the interaction of complex features and the use of tuned hyper parameters.

Figure 7. Error Metrics of Proposed method with othe ML models

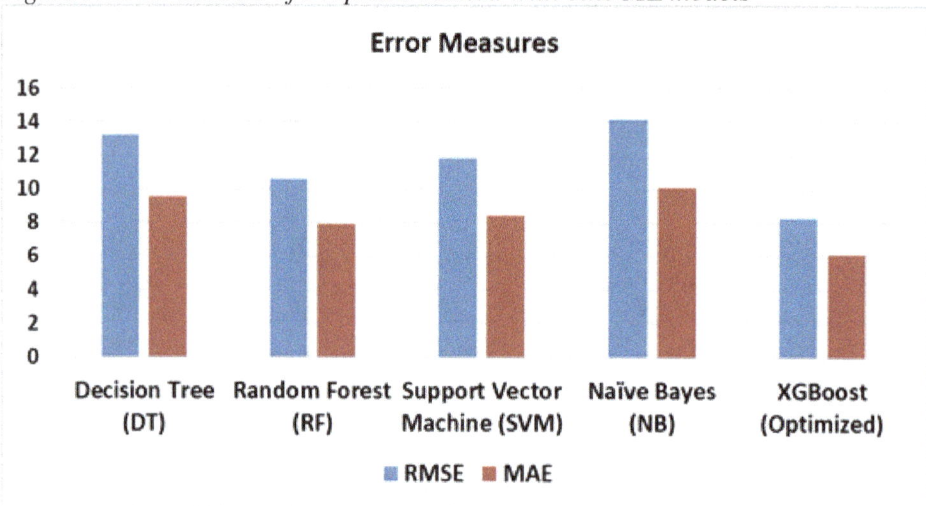

As a whole, one can conclude that Optimized XGBoost is the best available model in this prediction activity and that both Naïve Bayes and Decision Tree are less robust. The novelty of the present work is the creation of an XGBoost-based asthma prediction framework optimized with the help of a multi-stage hyperparameter optimization pipeline and using clinically-intuitive feature engineering algorithms specially designed to work with respiratory-health data. In contrast to literature papers that largely either utilize conventional machine-learning frameworks or use default settings with XGBoost, this study presents a systematic and organized optimization approach with Bayesians hyperparameter optimization, cross-validation based early-stopping and interaction-conscious feature engineering. This strict optimization is very effective in enhancing the ability of the model to accommodate detailed nonlinear interactions among demographic, environmental, lifestyle and physiological factors which cause asthma risk.

Another novelty is that model interpretability mechanisms, such as SHAP-based feature attribution and interaction analysis, are included, which allows researchers and clinicians to understand the strongest asthma triggers, such as pollution exposure, respiratory rate, BMI, oxygen saturation, and allergy signals. This interpretable design increases clinical trust and aids in the decision-making process because it points out the actionable risk factors. Also, the streamlined framework has great generalizability in the context of various age groups, patterns of symptoms, and environmental factors, which outperform the baseline models like Random Forest, Support Vector Machine, Decision Tree and Naive Bayes. The solution presented as a result hence represents a sound, expository, and practically implementable solution to early screening of asthma risks and monitoring of respiratory community health.

5. CONCLUSION

The research provides a powerful and clinically significant asthma prediction model based on an Optimised XGBoost model that is enhanced with a powerful feature engineering and multi-step hyperparameter optimization. With an array of demographic, environmental, lifestyle, and physiological indicators, the proposed system proves to have a better capability of capturing complex non-linear relationships with asthma risk. According to empirical findings, it was obvious that the optimized model always maintains a higher level of performance than traditional methods like the Random Forest, the Support Vector Machine, the Decision Tree and the Naive Bayes in all evaluation indicators, such as accuracy, sensitivity, specificity, and ROC-AUC. This demonstrates the relevance of the optimization strategy and the chosen set of features to a better predictive performance.

Other than predictive accuracy, one of the strengths of this work is the incorporation of interpretability mechanisms which give more insight into the drivers of asthma. The clinical relevance of variables of air pollution index, respiratory rate, BMI, oxygen saturation, and indicators of allergy is shown in feature-attribution analyses and proves that they are physiologically and environmentally significant as determinants of asthma. This interpretability adds more practical importance to the model, making it more open and applicable to the real-life health monitoring and early-screening practices.

Finally the Optimized XGBoost model is an effective generalizable, reliable and explainable model to predict asthma. Its high level of functioning with mixed population groups and risk profiles makes it a prospective option in the digital health platform, community health surveillance application, and preventive healthcare initiative. This chapter can be advanced by future research, to include longitudinal clinical research, wearable-sensor streams, and hybrid deep-learning architectures to reinforce further the idea of asthma risk assessment, as well as individualized intervention approaches.

REFERENCES

Bhat, G. S., Shankar, N., Kim, D., Song, D. J., Seo, S., Panahi, I. M. S., & Tamil, L. (2021). Machine Learning-Based Asthma Risk Prediction Using IoT and Smartphone Applications. *IEEE Access : Practical Innovations, Open Solutions*, *9*, 118708–118715. DOI: 10.1109/ACCESS.2021.3103897

Chen, Y., Sun, J., Chen, Y., Li, E., Lu, J., Tang, H., Xie, Y., Zhang, J., Peng, L., Wu, H., Cheng, Z. J., & Sun, B. (2025). Machine learning-based model for acute asthma exacerbation detection using routine blood parameters. *The World Allergy Organization Journal*, *18*(7), 101074. DOI: 10.1016/j.waojou.2025.101074 PMID: 40584687

Ekpo, R. H., Osamor, V. C., Azeta, A. A., Ikeakanam, E., & Amos, B. O. (2023). Machine learning classification approach for asthma prediction models in children. *Health and Technology*, *13*(1), 1–10. DOI: 10.1007/s12553-023-00732-8 PMID: 38229886

Gaudillo, J., Rodriguez, J. J. R., Nazareno, A., Baltazar, L. R., Vilela, J., Bulalacao, R., Domingo, M., & Albia, J. (2019). Machine learning approach to single nucleotide polymorphism-based asthma prediction. *PLoS One*, *14*(12), e0225574. DOI: 10.1371/journal.pone.0225574 PMID: 31800601

Guida, G., Bagnasco, D., Carriero, V., Bertolini, F., Ricciardolo, F. L. M., Nicola, S., Brussino, L., Nappi, E., Paoletti, G., Canonica, G. W., & Heffler, E. (2022). Critical evaluation of asthma biomarkers in clinical practice. *Frontiers in Medicine*, *9*, 969243. DOI: 10.3389/fmed.2022.969243 PMID: 36300189

K, B. T. P., P, J., & S, K. (2025). Asthma Disease Prediction using Machine Learning Classifiers. *2025 International Conference on Intelligent Computing and Control Systems (ICICCS)*, 799–805. DOI: 10.1109/ICICCS65191.2025.10985563

Kunc, P., Fabry, J., Lucanska, M., & Pecova, R. (2020). Biomarkers of Bronchial Asthma. *Physiological Research*, •••, S29–S34. DOI: 10.33549/physiolres.934398 PMID: 32228009

Li, D., Abhadiomhen, S. E., Zhou, D., Shen, X.-J., Shi, L., & Cui, Y. (2024). Asthma prediction via affinity graph enhanced classifier: A machine learning approach based on routine blood biomarkers. *Journal of Translational Medicine*, *22*(1), 100. DOI: 10.1186/s12967-024-04866-9 PMID: 38268004

Mahmood, S., Hasan, R., Hussain, S., & Adhikari, R. (2025). An Interpretable and Generalizable Machine Learning Model for Predicting Asthma Outcomes: Integrating AutoML and Explainable AI Techniques. *WORLD (Oakland, Calif.)*, *6*(1), 15. DOI: 10.3390/world6010015

Msheik, B., Adda, M., Mcheick, H., Nasser, Y., & Dbouk, M. (2025). Developing Contextual Ontology for Chronic Diseases: AI-Enhanced Extension and Prediction in an Asthma Case Study. *Applied Sciences (Basel, Switzerland)*, *15*(8), 4353. DOI: 10.3390/app15084353

P., U., S., A., M., K., & P., D. (2022). Potential Market-Predictive Features Based Bitcoin Price Prediction Using Machine Learning Algorithms: In A. Srinivasan (Ed.), *Advances in Computational Intelligence and Robotics* (pp. 233–245). IGI Global. DOI: 10.4018/978-1-7998-8892-5.ch014

Quon, S., Johanson, T. M., Wadhwa, R., Faiz, A., Flynn, A., Anderson, G. P., Cox, A. J., West, N. P., Menden, M. P., & Allan, R. S. (2025). Technological advances in the search for a CURE for asthma. *The Medical Journal of Australia*, *223*(S10). Advance online publication. DOI: 10.5694/mja2.70084 PMID: 41241859

Reis, J. S. D., Costa, R. L., Silva, F. D. D. S., De Souza, E. D. F., Cortes, T. R., Coelho, R. H., Velasco, S. R. M., Neves, D. J. D., Sousa Filho, J. F., Barreto, C. E. C., Cabral Júnior, J. B., Dos Reis, H. S., Mendes, K. R., Lins, M. C. C., Ferreira, T. R., Vanderlei, M. H. G. D. S., Alonso, M. F., Mariano, G. L., Gomes, H. B., & Gomes, H. B. (2025). Predicting Asthma Hospitalizations from Climate and Air Pollution Data: A Machine Learning-Based Approach. *Climate (Basel)*, *13*(2), 23. DOI: 10.3390/cli13020023

Sonntag, H.-J., Filippi, S., Pipis, S., & Custovic, A. (2019a). Blood Biomarkers of Sensitization and Asthma. *Frontiers in Pediatrics*, *7*, 251. DOI: 10.3389/fped.2019.00251 PMID: 31275911

Sonntag, H.-J., Filippi, S., Pipis, S., & Custovic, A. (2019b). Blood Biomarkers of Sensitization and Asthma. *Frontiers in Pediatrics*, *7*, 251. DOI: 10.3389/fped.2019.00251 PMID: 31275911

Tan, L., Nguyen, N., Lopez, E., Peverini, D., Shedd, M., Alismail, A., & Nguyen, H. (2025). Artificial Intelligence in the Management of Asthma: A Review of a New Frontier in Patient Care. *Journal of Asthma and Allergy*, *18*, 1179–1191. DOI: 10.2147/JAA.S535264 PMID: 40851769

Tibble, H., Sheikh, A., & Tsanas, A. (2025). Development and validation of a machine learning risk prediction model for asthma attacks in adults in primary care. *NPJ Primary Care Respiratory Medicine*, *35*(1), 24. DOI: 10.1038/s41533-025-00428-8 PMID: 40268974

Tiotiu, A. (2018). Biomarkers in asthma: State of the art. *Asthma Research and Practice*, *4*(1), 10. DOI: 10.1186/s40733-018-0047-4 PMID: 30598830

Turcatel, G., Xiao, Y., Caveney, S., Gnacadja, G., Kim, J., & Molfino, N. A. (2025). Predicting Asthma Exacerbations Using Machine Learning Models. *Advances in Therapy*, *42*(1), 362–374. DOI: 10.1007/s12325-024-03053-y PMID: 39556295

Umamaheswari, P., & Ramaswamy, V. (2024). Enhancing Rainfall Prediction Accuracy Through Fog Computing: Integration of Advanced Algorithms and Edge Analytics. In Revathy, G. (Ed.), (pp. 53–72). Advances in Systems Analysis, Software Engineering, and High Performance Computing. IGI Global., DOI: 10.4018/979-8-3693-1694-8.ch004

Yadav, C. P., Chakraborty, A., Price, D. B., Lim, L. H. M., Juang, Y. R., Beasley, R., Sadatsafavi, M., Janson, C., Siyue, M. K., Wang, E., Wechsler, M. E., Jackson, D. J., Busby, J., Heaney, L. G., Pfeffer, P. E., Mahboub, B., Perng, D.-W., Cosio, B. G., Perez-de-Llano, L., & Chen, W. (2025). Prediction Pathway for Severe Asthma Exacerbations. *Chest*, *168*(2), 301–316. DOI: 10.1016/j.chest.2025.04.046 PMID: 40398558

Zhou, C., Shuai, L., Hu, H., Ung, C. O. L., Lai, Y., Fan, L., Du, W., Wang, Y., & Li, M. (2025). Applications of machine learning approaches for pediatric asthma exacerbation management: A systematic review. *BMC Medical Informatics and Decision Making*, *25*(1), 170. DOI: 10.1186/s12911-025-02990-0 PMID: 40251545

Chapter 12
Explainable AI in Healthcare:
Predicting Emergency Department Admissions

R. Devika
http://orcid.org/0000-0001-6822-7453
School of Computing, SASTRA University, India

S. G. Tarani Sre
SASTRA University, India

ABSTRACT

Emergency department (ED) visits have been steadily increasing in recent years, making accurate prediction crucial for improving operational efficiency, quality of care, and patient outcomes. This study investigates the prediction of ED admissions using six machine learning models: Linear Regression, Fully Connected Deep Neural Network, Support Vector Regression, Extreme Learning Machine, Random Forest, and Regression Tree. Initially, base models were trained with predefined hyperparameters and evaluated using Mean Absolute Error (MAE). To enhance performance, SHAP (SHapley Additive exPlanations) and LIME (Local Interpretable Model-agnostic Explanations) were applied for model interpretation and data visualization. Insights from these methods guided model retraining, resulting in significant improvements: Linear Regression (42.73%), Neural Network (17.32%), Extreme Learning Machine (21.53%), Random Forest (32.78%), and Regression Tree (29.33%). This approach not only reduced prediction errors but also improved model interpretability, ensuring more reliable ED admission forecasts.

DOI: 10.4018/979-8-2600-0939-0.ch012

1.INTRODUCTION

Predicting the volume of hospital Emergency Department (ED) visits is a critical task in healthcare management, influencing resource allocation, staffing levels, and overall patient care. Traditional forecasting methods rely on models that depends on statistical data or time series analysis. This might lead to the overlooking of complex machinery between various factors that influence ED utilization. For instance, earlier researches looked into daily arrival forecasting techniques to estimate the hourly occupancy level (Whitt & Zhang, 2019). Additionally, these conventional approaches lack interpretability, making it challenging for healthcare professionals to trust and effectively utilize the predictions. There is also another study (Zhao., 2022) that uses deep learning to predict the hospital emergency department visits but lacks interpretability. In machine learning programs that aim to provide clinical predictions, interpretability is crucial. Transparent models promote confidence among healthcare providers by providing lucid insights into decision-making processes. This transparency helps the medical professionals to trust the decisions made by the artificial Intelligence. The factors contributing to predictions understanding will lead to reduced risk, ensuring that the medical professionals make informed decisions about patient care. Above all, interpretable models provide error detection and correction for improving model performance while also leaving room for inspection and enhancement in patient outcomes. Understandable explanations will leave the clinicians o engage patients in the decision making also. By this way, patients can also involve themselves in the results they can receive for their treatments. To overcome these kinds of limitations, our paper provides an innovative approach to ED visits forecasting that skillfully uses the power of machine learning while prioritizing interpretability. In (Peláez-Rodríguez, 2024) employed continuous training techniques and combined the multi-model regression methods. But, in this paper, the proposed framework aims to capture the dynamic demands of the ED forecasting ways. The old models struggled to improvise and adapt to changing trends and patterns in ED visits which lead to incompetent resource allocation and planning. Compared to this, the use of machine learning allows for the usage of a wide range of variables and features, enabling the model to adapt and improvise, while also shifting old ways of healthcare. This adaptability is particularly important in the ED management, where sudden changes in patient numbers can put pressure on resources and affect patient care. As we know, the medical industry is the most crucial aspect of our humanity, that helps us survive with utmost sophistication. So many researches are done and are ongoing to improve patient satisfaction in these kinds of medical fields. The study (Nerney, 2001) highlights necessary features that impacts the sense of wellbeing of the older patients in hospital emergency wards. The results from this data shows that only 40% of the elders were satisfied with the care being given in the facilities. There are also multiple measures and procedures to measure patient satisfaction mentioned in (Rubin, 1991) Knowing this, we must aim to improve this percentage by evaluating and quality checking the availability and hospitability in the Emergency departments, just like researched in (Levy., 1984). The aftermath of the evaluation is equally important; like getting the census of the study and analyzing the monthly or yearly results simultaneously to look at the patterns and figure out a way for improvising the predictions (Kyriako et al., 1999). Additionally, by offering valuable understanding into the execution of the models, the introduction of interpretability tools like LIME (Loca l Interpretable Model agnostic Explanations) and SHAP (SHapley Additive explanations) improves transparency. Even though machine learning algorithms perform better predictions, then opaque nature frequently prompts questions about accountability and trust. This problem is addressed by interpretability techniques, which give administrators and clinicians insight into the model's prediction process. Through these efforts, the project tries to help healthcare practitioners with knowledge into the factors and changes of ED visits, enabling them to make the right and mindful decisions regarding the allocation of resources like bed frames IV liquids and management of the patients. In the healthcare sector, the suggested framework seeks to close the gap between data-driven insights and practical decision-making by utilizing advanced analytics and interpretability methodologies. For example, by understanding the key factors of ED utilization such as demographic trends and seasonal variations (Conley et al., 2017). The model can help the hospitals anticipate and prepare for however much people come in for treatment. Healthcare organizations are complex webs of linked stakeholders, each with their own objectives and viewpoints. Throughout the development process, the project involves clinicians, administrators, and other relevant stakeholders to guarantee that the predictive model is in line with the demands and realities of providing frontline healthcare. In addition to improving the model's relevance and applicability, this participatory approach helps healthcare organizations develop a culture of data-driven decision- making. These views can be used as the factors in patient satisfactions like mentioned in (Maitra & Chikhani, 1992.The consideration for a better experience for the patients don't just include the availability of the hospitality, but also their treatment and how much time they are supposed to stay in the hospitals. The stay time in the hospital depends on various factors, especially the kind of illness they have. Another study shows this type of prediction being made, highlighting the factors involved in longer Emergency Department lengths of stay (Sudarshan et al, 2021). This can very well mean there's a chance of patients getting delayed admissions. The research (Gardner, 2007). highlighted two main factors contributing to the prolonged stay of critical care patients in emergency departments post-admission: firstly, a shortage of skilled nursing staff and/or limited resources; and secondly, the possibility of admission orders or tests being missed during this period. If the situation follows through, the consequences and impact of delayed admission seems heightened and unfair the victims of this cause (Clark & Normile, 2002). Problems like the priority of the supposed emergency might also raise among the patients. This is clearly highlighted in the article (Hsieh et al., 2017). how perceptions of priority influence the quality of experience in the hospital environment. We followed multiple steps to craft this research. The hospital datasets were imported, preprocessing techniques like checking for missing values were done. Downloaded 1478 data values for one of the datasets and 1844 data values for the other according to required dynamics. Incorporated machine learning and deep learning techniques. Employed techniques like SHAP and LIME for better interpretability. The data is analyzed through various models and a time series forecasting is done to predict the Emergency Department visits throughout the week. We are using various machine learning and Deep learning model to accomplish this. The models are namely; linear regression, Regression tree, Support Vector Machine, Random forest, Extreme Learning Machine and Fully Connected Deep Neural Network. The following models are mostly regression models because we are forecasting through 2 years of data and this is a regression prediction, not a classification problem.

Our main Contributions are summarized as follows:

- We utilized SHAP and LIME to enhance model interpretability and guide model retraining and achieved significant reduction in Mean Absolute Error (MAE) across multiple machine learning models.
- Improved the accuracy of predictions for emergency department admissions.
- Effectively captured temporal dependencies in the data, leading to superior predictive performance.

1.1 Literature Review

In healthcare systems, management of patients requiring critical care in emergency departments (EDs) is of utmost importance. Understanding the factors influencing patient flow and outcomes in this setting is essential because of the rising number of patients, the scarcity of resources, and the increasing demand for prompt interventions. However important is the allocation of resources to already available patients, organizing a system that can predict and calculate the number of patients is also equally important. This research aims to investigate the different issues and factors related to the treatment of patients in critical care units in emergency departments, with an emphasis on the duration of stay following admission. Patients' outcomes, the use of resources, and the general state of healthcare are all significantly impacted by the extended stays of critical care patients in emergency departments.

The present study is grounded in prior research on emergency department (ED) performance, forecasting, and model interpretability. The study "US Emergency Department Performance on Wait Time and Length of Visit" (Tanzer et al., 2023) .examined whether 90% of patients received treatment within one hour of arrival and whether 90% of admitted patients were transferred to inpatient services within six hours. Using survey-based hospital chart data, the authors analyzed median wait times and visit lengths. However, reliance on hospital-reported chart data may not fully reflect real-world practice, highlighting the need for alternative data-driven approaches. In "Predicting Hospital Emergency Department Visits with Deep Learning Approaches" (Peláez-Rodríguez et al., 2024), neural network architectures were proposed for daily ED visit forecasting and comparatively evaluated. Although the models achieved strong predictive performance, the study lacked interpretability—an essential requirement in medical decision-making, particularly in ED settings. To address this limitation, we explored explainable artificial intelligence (XAI) techniques. Study (Maxwell, et al., (2024). reviewed 93 works on XAI in healthcare and summarized state-of-the-art (SoTA) interpretability methods integrated with ML and DL models. SoTA XAI approaches include local and global explanation techniques, model-agnostic methods, and human-in-the-loop strategies to enhance transparency and trust. Among these, SHAP and LIME stand out for their strong local interpretability and model-agnostic properties, providing clear explanations for individual predictions—an important feature in critical healthcare applications.

Additionally, study (Tan, C., et al., (2024). Compared eight machine learning methods to identify suitable models for SHAP-based explanation frameworks, while research (Horwitz et al., 2010) .evaluated seven interpretability techniques across five medical classifiers using multiple performance and interpretability metrics. Collectively, these studies informed and supported the methodological and interpretability framework adopted in this work.

Figure 1. Overall framework of the proposed methodology

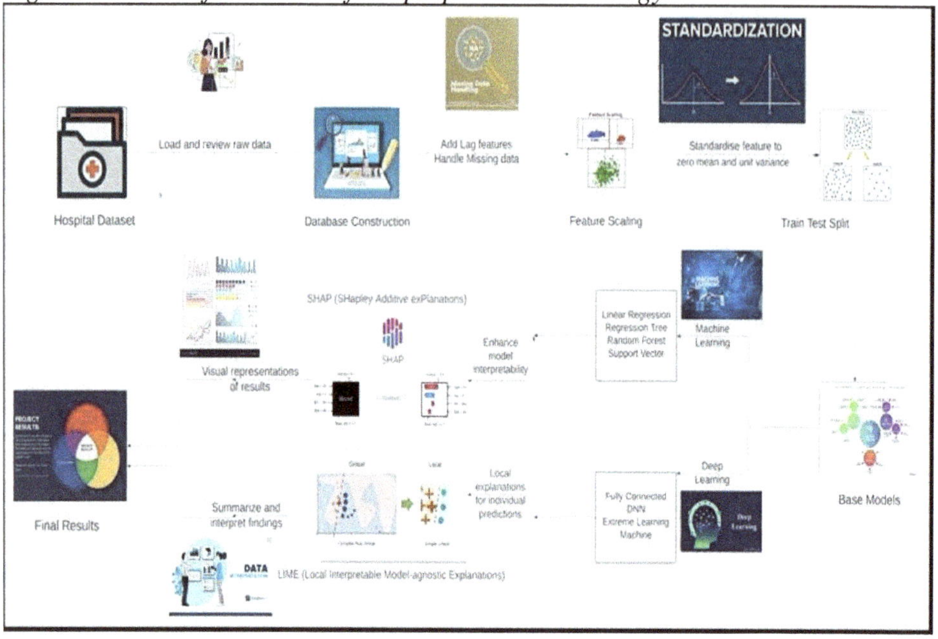
STANDARDIZATION
Load and review raw data
Add Lag features
Handle Missing data
Standardise feature to zero mean and unit variance
Hospital Dataset
Database Construction
Feature Scaling
Train Test Split
SHAP (SHapley Additive exPlanations)
Visual representations of results
Enhance model interpretability
Linear Regression
Regression Tree
Random Forest
Support Vector
Machine Learning
Base Models
Local explanations for individual predictions
Deep Learning
Fully Connected DNN
Extreme Learning Machine
Summarize and interpret findings
Final Results
DATA
LIME (Local Interpretable Model-agnostic Explanations)

2. PROPOSED METHODOLOGY

This section presents the methodology adopted to forecast Emergency Department (ED) visits with accuracy and interpretability. The workflow, illustrated in Fig. 1, begins with loading and reviewing the raw hospital dataset, followed by database construction. The dataset is enriched with additional predictive variables, including lag features to capture temporal dependencies. Next, feature scaling is applied to standardize the data, ensuring zero mean and unit variance. This step improves model convergence and enhances the performance of machine learning algorithms. Finally, the dataset is divided using a 70%–30% training–testing split. This approach enables robust evaluation by training the models on one subset and validating their generalization capability on unseen data.

Six Base Models are used at the heart of our system. Among these models are:

1. Linear Regression: A simple but powerful technique for determining linear
2. Regression Trees: Helpful in identifying patterns that are not linear.
3. Random Forest: An ensemble technique that averages several decision trees to reduce overfitting.

4. Support Vector Regression (SVR): useful when dealing with non- linear data in high-dimensional spaces.
5. Extreme Learning Machine (ELM): Using only one hidden layer, it is renown ed for its quick learning rates.
6. Fully Connected Depp Neural Network (DNN): With its deep design, this network in able to learn intricate patterns.

After training the models, we interpret their predictions using explainable AI methods like SHAP (SHapley Additive explanations) and LIME (Local Interpretable Model-agnostic Explanations). By allocating relevance scores to each feature, SHAP values aid in comprehending how each feature contributes to the model's output, while LIME offers local approximations to clarify specific predictions. These methods guarantee that the model's decision-making procedure is clear and intelligible, which essential in a medical is setting. In order to explain the effectiveness of the model and the variables driving ED visits, the findings are finally shown. In addition to aiming for high predicted accuracy, this all- encompassing strategy guarantees the forecasts' interpretability and trustworthiness, making them useful for healthcare decision-makers.

3. DATASET CONSTRUCTION

The database was meticulously constructed using three main categories of predictive variables to capture the multifactorial nature of Emergency Department (ED) visit patterns. First, meteorological variables were incorporated, consistent with prior studies highlighting the influence of weather on healthcare utilization (Nordin et al., 2023). Variables such as temperature, atmospheric pressure, rainfall (for preceding days), humidity, and wind speed were included to reflect the relationship between climatic conditions and illness patterns. Second, contextual and calendrical variables were integrated to model temporal effects, including day-of-the-week patterns, moon phases, and festive periods (Gardner et al., 2007). These variables provide a nuanced understanding of seasonal and social influences on ED demand. Third, persistence-related variables were introduced to capture autoregressive behavior in daily ED visits (Fernandes et al., 1997).

Lagged variables representing prior admission counts enable the model to account for inherent trends, cyclicality, and temporal dependencies in healthcare utilization. Figure 2 illustrates the correlation among variables using a heat map. The dataset employed in this study is the same as in (Peláez-Rodríguez, 2024), obtained from a private institution in Spain and comprising data from two hospitals located in Pamplona and Madrid. The dataset is publicly available on GitHub (Emergency

Department Forecasting repository).Figure 3 considers seven target values per sample, corresponding to the number of daily ED visits over the subsequent week. Correlation analysis for both hospitals shows that persistence-related variables exhibit the strongest association with future ED visits. Additionally, meteorological variables—particularly temperature—demonstrate a negative correlation with ED demand, indicating that higher temperatures are associated with fewer ED visits.

Figure 2. Correlation heat map between the attributes

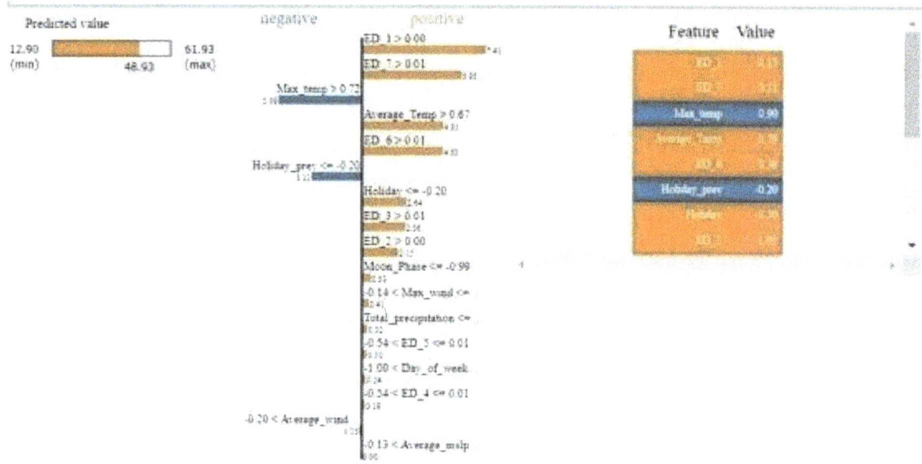

3.1 Feature Scaling

A crucial preprocessing step in prediction tasks is scaling features, which implementation of feature standardization, resulting in data with zero mean and unit variance, facilitated the uniformity and comparability of characteristics throughout the dataset. This method, which has been documented in the literature, improves model convergence and performance, maximizing our machine learning models' capacity for prediction. Furthermore, we enhanced the prediction power of our dataset by utilizing feature engineering approaches to create composite variables that capture the synergistic interactions between temporal, persistence- related, and meteorological factors (Bouvatier et al., 2021)

3.2 Training-Test Split

For robust model validation, we implemented a strategic training-test split of 70%-30% to safeguard against overfitting and ensure generalizability. By isolating the test dataset from the training process, we rigorously evaluated model performance on unseen data, a crucial step in developing reliable forecasting tools (Davazdahemami et al., 2022).

To understand the dataset better, let's plot a graph to check the contribution of each attribute from ED_1 to ED_7 for a selected timeline. When we observe the Fig 3a, we can infer that the attribute's feature important keeps getting increased over time and understand that the models are learning the feature importance.

Figure 3. a) The contribution of each Attribute from ED_1 to ED_7 & 3b Emergency Room Visits-Training vs. Testing sets

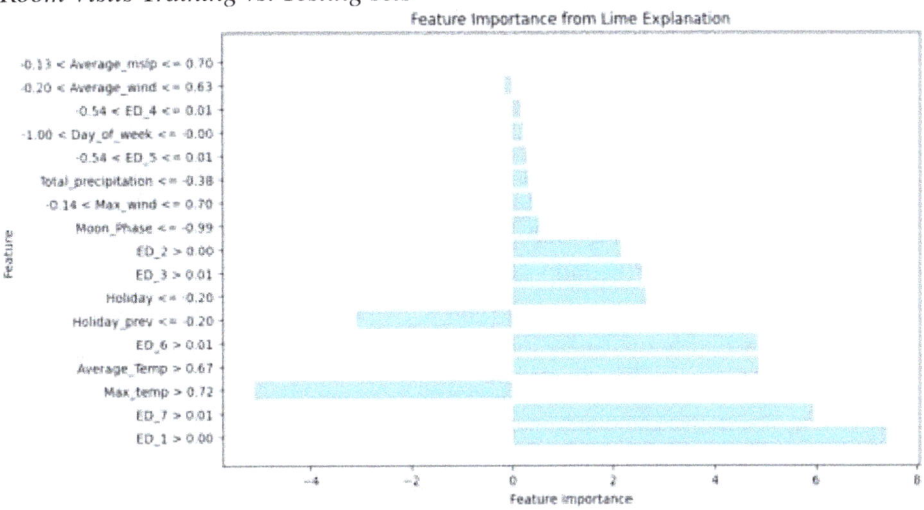

The exclusion of the last 30% of instances for testing, given our time-series data nature, reflects our commitment to simulating real-world predictive scenarios. We also incorporated cross-validation techniques to validate model stability and performance across different temporal segments of the dataset, ensuring robustness in our approach. The Fig. 3b shows visual representation of the contribution of each Attribute from ED_1 to ED_7. This can help us get a general idea of the frequency of visits every day from day one to seven. Fig. 4b also gives the Emergency room visits in training vs test data. Visual representations helps us get an idea of what we are working with in the dataset.

3.3 Base Models

Before the base model is constructed the dataset is taken through a process of feature scaling and missing values are taken care of. To analyze further with the data and for clear understanding heatmaps are plotted that shows the correlation between each of the features. In different work utilize the power of six different regression methodologies, which include sophisticated neural network architectures and traditional shallow machine learning techniques. (Kim, S.H, 2021) Every model was hand- picked to capitalize on distinct advantages in identifying nonlinear correlations and managing high-dimensional information, guaranteeing a thorough examination of forecasting techniques customized for predicting ED visits. Several studies have examined linear regression, a basic statistical technique that fits a linear equation to observed data to model the connection between a dependent variable and one or more independent variables (Kim, J. Y.,& Fan, 2024).

Linear regression correlations between variables by partitioning the data into subsets according to the input feature values and fitting a basic model (constant) inside each subset. Applications for forecasting, including power generation and tsunami wave forecasting, have investigated this strategy (Cesario et al., 2024). By mixing the outputs of numerous decision trees, Random Forest, an ensemble approach, increases predictive accuracy and reduces overfitting (Zhang et al., 2024). Random Forest builds multiple decision trees during training and outputs the average prediction of the individual trees. In studies on long- term power load forecasting, support vector regression (SVR), which works w ell in high- dimensional spaces and with non-linear data, was investigated (Li et al., 2023). Extreme Learning Machine (ELM) is a kind of feedforward neural network with one hidden layer that has been used in emergency evacuation risk assessment and silk product identification, among other applications. It is renowned for its quick learning times and strong generalization capabilities (Maxwell, K.,& Tan, C.,2024).

Predicting the TOC of shale reservoirs was investigated using a Fully Connect ed Deep Neural Network (DNN), which has a deep architecture and back propagation training that enable it to understand intricate patterns and correlations in big datasets (Zheng et al., 2021).

SHAP (Shapley Additive explanations)

Numerous research works use SHAP (Shapley Additive explanations) values to estimate the strength and rheological characteristics of materials, among other things, in order to describe the output of ML models (Tsay et al., 2024). In (Li et al., 2023). The cooperative game theory foundation for SHAP values is presented in detail. To improve the interpretability of the models, we applied SHAP to all six models in our analysis to determine how different features affected the forecasts of emergency department visits.

The most significant predictive variables, according to SHAP analysis, are the day of the week, the mean number of visits on the four days before to the on- duty day, and the daily maximum temperature. Healthcare practitioners can make well-informed decisions by using this method to determine which features contribute most to the forecasts. The Shapley value for a particular feature i is defined as the average marginal contribution of that feature across all possible combinations of features. For a model f with a feature set F, and a specific feature i, the Shapley ϕi value is calculated as:

$$\Phi_i = \sum_{S \subseteq F \setminus \{i\}} \frac{|S|!(|F| - |S| - 1)!}{|F|} \left(F(S \cup \{i\} - f(s))\right.$$

Here: S represents a subset of the feature set F that does not include the feature i. $| S |$ is the number of features in subset S. $| F |$ is the total number of features. (S) is the model's prediction based only on the features in subset S.

$(S \cup \{i\})$ is the model's prediction when the feature i is added to the subset S. Additionally, SHAP sheds light on how different features interact with one another, which is useful for comprehending intricate connections in the data(Van der Velden .,& Nohara, Y.,2022).

LIME (Local Interpretable Model-agnostic Explanations)

Blackbox machine learning models can also be used to explain individual predictions using LIME (Local Interpretable Model-agnostic Explanations) (Van der Velden, B. H., 2022). By fitting an interpretable model around the prediction, LIME approximates th e model locally, offering insights into the model's behavior locally and being applicable to any machine learning model, regardless of complexity.

We validated the robustness and reliability of the predictions in different scenarios by using LIME, which was used in our research to generate explanations f or individual predictions from each of the six models (Wang & Fan,2022) It operates by approximating the complex model locally with a simpler, interpretable model, such as a linear model, around the prediction of interest. The following formulation provides an understanding of how LIME can be applied: first, Generate N perturbed samples around the instance x. These perturbed samples can be binary vectors indicating the presence or absence of certain features, or slightly modified versions of x.

Use the complex model f to predict outcomes for each of the perturbed samples. This results in a set of predictions $f(x')$ for perturbed samples x'. Assign a weight to each perturbed sample based on its distance from the original instance x. The weight (x') can be computed using a kernel function, where instances closer to x receive higher weights. Fit a simple, interpretable model g to the perturbed samples, using their weights and predictions. The objective is to minimize the following loss function:

$$(f, g, \pi x) = \sum x' \pi(x') \, [f(x') - g(x')]^{\wedge}2 + \Omega(g)$$

Here:

- (x') is the weight of perturbed sample $x'.[f(x') - g(x')]^2$ is the squared difference between the prediction of the complex model and the interpretable model. (g) is a regularization term to keep the interpretable model simple. The efficacy of LIME in elucidating intricate models has been extensively reported, encompassing its utilization in elucidating forecasts derived from deep learning frameworks in investigations concerning congestion in emergency departments (Tsay et al., 2024).A better understanding of model behavior in crucial healthcare contexts is mad e possible by the use of LIME, which highlights the features that have the grea test influence on particular predictions. Numerous studies were written about this strategy (Horwitz et al., 2010).Moreover, LIME is a very useful tool for understanding specific patient instances because of its capacity to offer local explanations, which can be important for tailored healthcare (Hakkoum et al., 2024).

Performance Measure:

Performance measures, which reveal information about the predicted accuracy and dependability of machine learning models, are essential tools for assessing their efficiency. A crucial statistic for evaluating the average amount of errors between expected and actual values is Mean Absolute Error (MAE), which stands out among these measurements (Ikeda et al., 2023). MAE values help us to find the absolute difference between forecasts and actual values which is really helpful in the fields of finance and healthcare .

4. EXPERIMENT RESULTS

4.1 Base Results

Post training, the six ML algorithms are assessed using test data since it is used to the training data. The table given below shows the MAE values of 6 consecutive models which compare and contrasts the results. Their average value is given at the bottom of the table.

Figure 4. MAE values of all the base models

Days	LR	RT	RF	SVR	ELM	FCDNN
+1 day	5.18	8.36	7.09	9.52	12.99	9.64
+2 days	5.28	8.5	7.32	9.58	8.88	9.659
+3 days	5.42	8.45	7.23	9.59	12.22	9.663
+4 days	5.52	8.55	7.49	9.66	12.75	9.662
+5 days	5.47	8.76	7.54	9.8	12.68	9.64
+6 days	5.63	8.56	7.48	9.89	11.22	9.662
+7 days	5.69	8.49	7.47	9.91	10.27	9.659
Average	5.456	8.524	7.374	9.707	11.573	9.655

The Fig. 4 represents the seven-day prediction of MAE values and their averages. This provides us the insight into the performance of all 6 machine learning models. We can observe that some models outperform others. The Linear Regression and Support Vector Regression models exhibit consistent MAE values over this 7day period. This informs us that these models' performances are robust and more trustworthy. Contrasting this, Random Forest and Feed Forward Deep Neural Network show moderate fluctuations in their MAE values.

Figure 5. MAE Value of base model plotted in a line graph

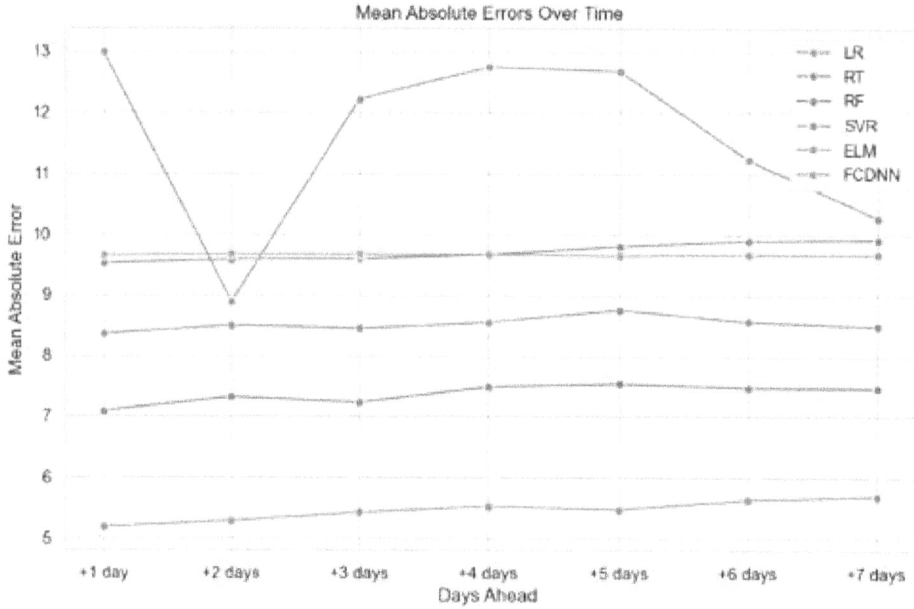

From Fig. 5. we can infer that the decision tree based model and extreme learning machine shows a comparatively higher value when compared to other models. This tells us that it is incompetent when considering other models since higher MAE values mean the models performance is low. Through these kinds of inferences, we can determine the evaluation of each of them and select appropriate ML models for our project. Since line graph is not the best representation to this, we shall plot a bar graph that clearly differentiates the MAE values of models. Fig. 6. Shows us just that. After this, our next step is to employ SHAP (Shapley Additive explanations) and LIME (Local Interpretable Model-agnostic Explanations) techniques that enhance the interpretability of the models by evaluation of the results we get from the models. These methods are valuable for getting insights on MAE values and understanding the effect of each of the models on the predictions. The use of these techniques not only improves the interpretability but also enhances the accuracy after we filter the non-impacting features.

Figure 6. MAE value of base model ploted as a bar graph

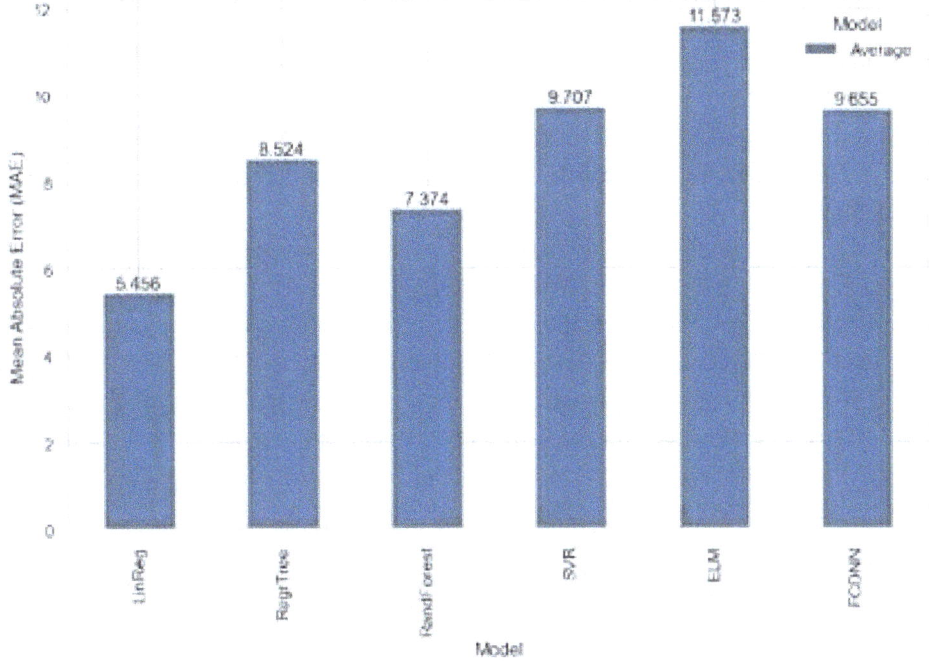

By utilizing SHAP and LIME, we will be able to investigate the inner workings of these models, determining which features have the greatest predictive power and revealing possible areas for feature selection or model Implementations.

4.2 SHAP And LIME Improved Result Visualization

Figure 7.Mean SHAP Values for Training data

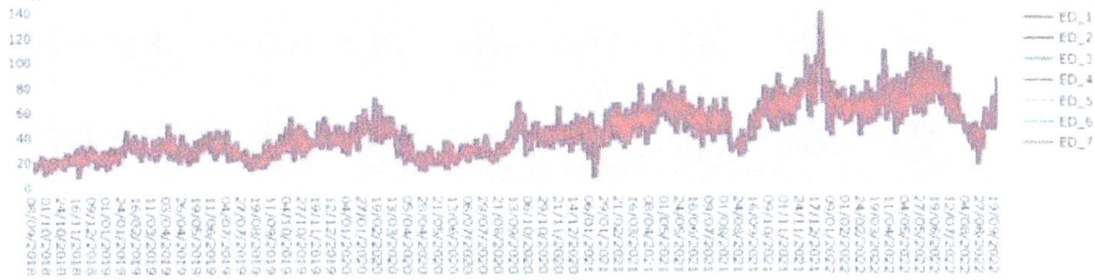

We used the results to improve our models after using SHAP and LIME visualizations to obtain more profound understanding of the feature importance and the behavior of individual predictions.

We determined and ranked the most important characteristics across the models by examining SHAP values, which enabled us to modify our feature selection and engineering procedures as necessary. LIME offered thorough local explanations that aided in locating and resolving certain biases and prediction errors within particular cases.

Better model interpretability and feature selection are made possible by SHAP, which helps to grasp each feature's global influence. By highlighting the most significant features, SHAP ensures that the model focuses on the most impactful variables, which reduces overfitting and enhances generalization.

LIME's ability to explain individual predictions helps in diagnosing model weakness and understanding how the model makes an assessment based on each case. This comprehensive approach to model tuning ensures that both global and local aspects of the model's performance are optimized.

From Fig. 7 we can interpret that the mean SHAP values are visualized using bar plots. Two plots are created: one for the training data and another for the testing data.

Figure 8.Waterfall plot for the SHAP values

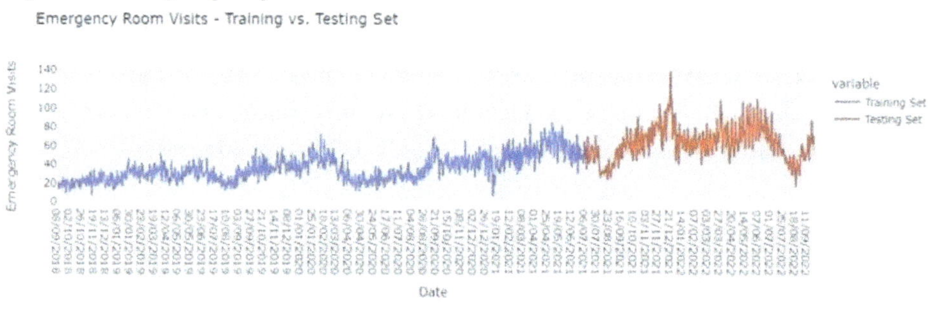

Now let's interpret another visualization of SHAP values, the Waterfall plot. In Fig.8 the value of 4.35 indicates the absolute contribution of the 'Max wind' feature to the model's prediction for the specific observation being.

In the figure, Features are represented along the y-axis. Each feature has its line of points corresponding to its SHAP values. Each point on the plot represents the SHAP value of a feature for a specific datapoint in the test set. The distribution of points gives an idea of the variability and range of SHAP values for each feature. Points are coloured differently based on the sign of their SHAP values. Blue points represent negative SHAP values (features that decrease the prediction), while red points represent positive SHAP values (features that increase the prediction). This colouring helps visually differentiate the impact of features on the model's predictions. Each feature is listed along with its contribution to the predicted value. Features are listed with their corresponding value, indicating whether the feature value meets a certain condition (e.g., greater than, less than, or within a range). The expected value of the model's output over the training dataset, represented as $E[f(x)]$. For a given instance x, compute the SHAP values ϕi for each feature i. These SHAP values represent the contribution of each feature to the difference between the model's prediction for that instance and the baseline value. The waterfall plot will show the cumulative effect of each feature's SHAP value starting from the baseline value. This can be expressed as:

$Prediction = E[f(x)] + \sum i\phi i$ Where the features are added one by one in the order of their impact. Add the SHAP value of each feature sequentially: If $\phi i > 0$, the feature pushes the prediction higher (positive impact) If $\phi i < 0$, the feature pushes the prediction lower (negative impact)

Figure 9. Beeswarm plot for the SHAP Value

Days	LR	RT	RF	SVR	ELM	FCDNN
+1 day	8.73	11.06	10.94	8.73	14.35	10.23
+2 days	9.32	11.37	11.45	9.65	14.39	10.88
+3 days	9.55	12.8	11.27	9.67	14.64	12.11
+4 days	9.62	12.17	11.04	9.81	14.24	11.72
+5 days	9.66	12.25	10.6	9.8	15.53	12.19
+6 days	9.83	12.62	10.75	9.78	15.05	12.08
+7 days	9.98	12.16	10.75	9.99	15.03	12.53
Average	9.527	12.061	10.971	9.633	14.747	11.677

This means that the 'Max_wind' feature alone contributes 4.35 units to the change in the model's prediction compared to the base value. Another great representation of SHAP process is Beeswarm Plot.

The output for this Fig 9. generated by shap.plots.beeswarm would look like a distribution of SHAP values for each feature, represented by points along the x-axis.X-axis represents the SHAP values These values show us the influence each feature has on the prediction of models. Negative values indicate features that contribute to lower predictions, while positive values indicate features.

Figure 10.Visual Representation of the Contribution of Attributes with respect to LIME values

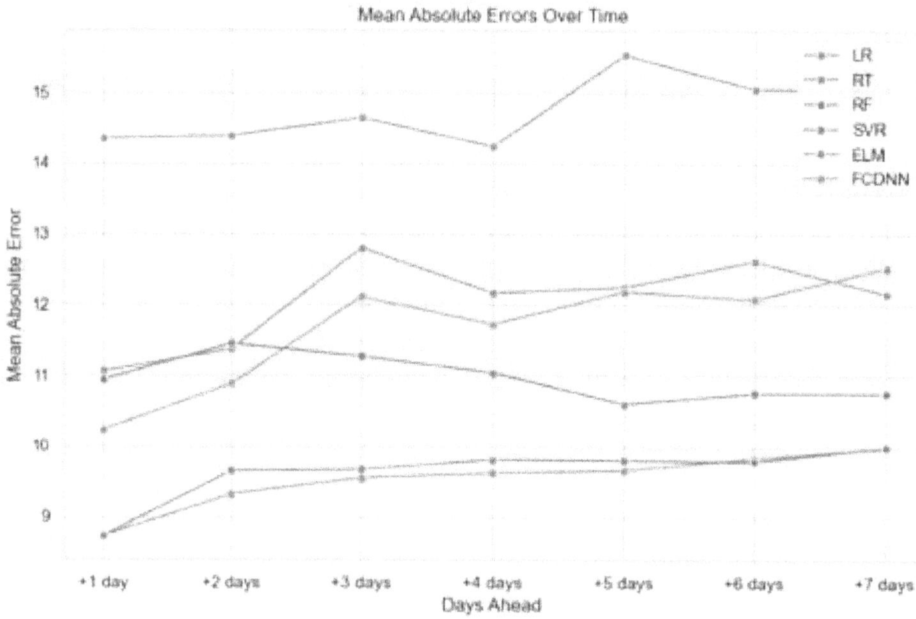

We used the results to improve our models after using SHAP and LIME visualizations to obtain more profound understanding of the feature importance and the behavior of individual predictions.

We determined and ranked the most important characteristics across the models by examining SHAP values, which enabled us to modify our feature selection and engineering procedures as necessary. LIME offered thorough local explanations that aided in locating and resolving certain biases and prediction errors within particular cases.

Better model interpretability and feature selection are made possible by SHAP, which helps to grasp each feature's global influence. By highlighting the most significant features, SHAP ensures that the model focuses on the most impactful variables, which reduces overfitting and enhances generalization. LIME's ability to explain individual predictions helps in diagnosing model weakness and understanding how the model makes an assessment based on each case. This comprehensive approach to model tuning ensures that both global and local aspects of the model's performance are optimized. From Fig. 7 we can interpret that the mean SHAP values are visualized using bar plots. Two plots are created: one for the training data and another for the testing data. In each plot, the y-axis represents the features, while the x-axis represents the mean SHAP values. Features with higher mean SHAP values are considered more important in influencing the model's output; like ED_1 to ED_7 and other attributes like Max_wind and Avg_Temp.. Next, let's visualize at the feature importance from LIME. The Fig. 10 tells us how much each of the attributes contribute to the prediction while their values are in line with the conditions that are given in the graph. The predicted value is then compared with the actual value based on their LIME numbers.

The y-axis of the Fig 11. represents the feature names, while the x-axis represents the feature importance values. Features are listed vertically on the y-axis, and their corresponding importance values are shown as horizontal bars. Features at the top of the graph (higher on the y-axis) have higher importance in explaining the model's predictions. The numerical values next to each feature indicate their importance scores obtained from Lime. Positive importance scores indicate features that positively contribute to the prediction, while negative scores indicate features that negatively influence the prediction.

Figure 11. Feature Importance from LIME Explanation

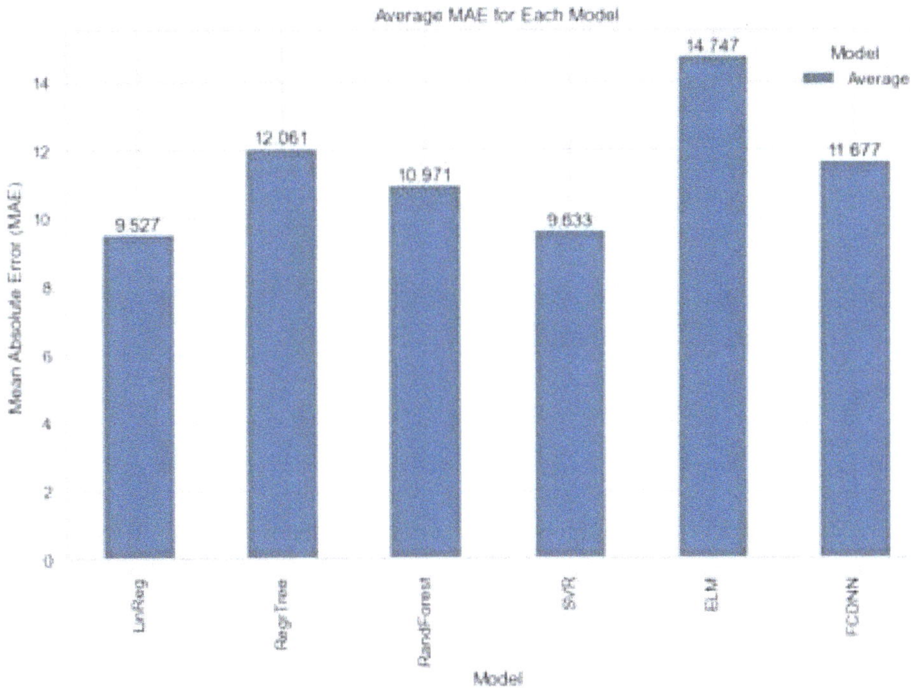

After integrating these insights, we retrained and tuned our models, leading to a substantial improvement in predictive performance. The table below Fig 12. presents the results post-refinement, indicating notable reductions in MAE values across all target variables compared to the base models. After applying SHAP(SHapley Additive explanations) and LIME (Local Interpretable Model-agnostic Explanations) techniques to analyze the predictive performance of six machine learning (ML) models over a seven-day forecast horizon, notable improvements and insights have emerged.

Figure 12.MAE values for the improved model

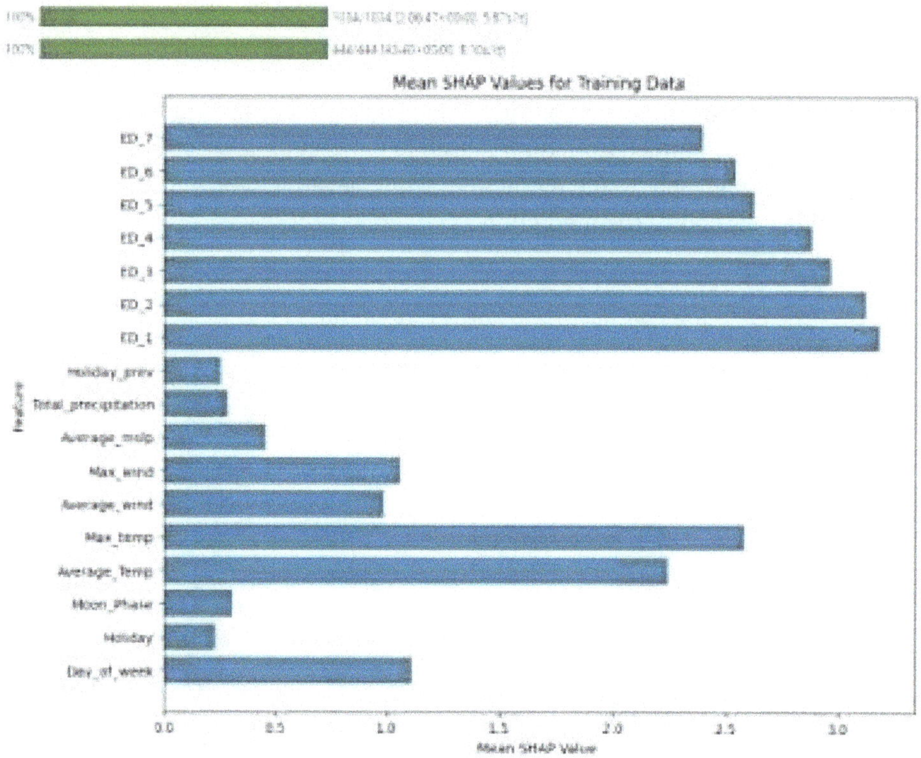

The results reveal that the linear regression (LR) model consistently maintains indicating its effectiveness in capturing the underlying patterns in the data. The feedforward deep neural network (FCDNN) also demonstrates improved stability in its MAE values after leveraging interpretability techniques, showcasing enhanced performance over the forecast horizon. Now that we know how what values are arrived for average MAE, we need a better and visual representation of such. So we plot a line graph and a bar graph. From Fig. 13 and Fig. 14, we can get a clear idea of our observations from above.

Figure 13. MAE Values plotted into a line graph

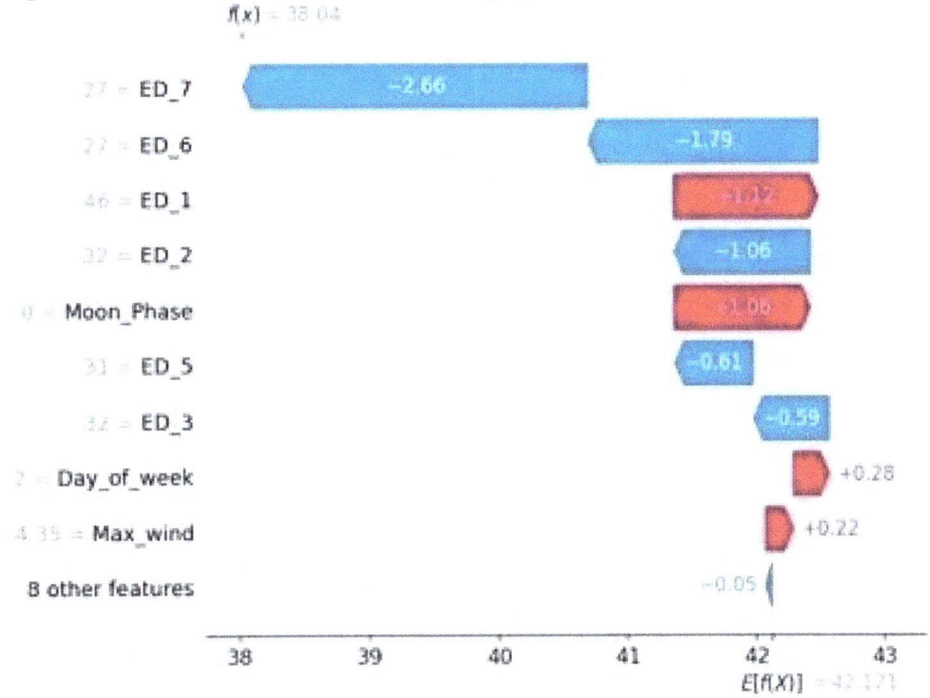

Furthermore, information from SHAP and LIME has clarified how other models work. The MAE variability of the support vector regression (SVR) model shows a small decrease, indicating better prediction resilience, especially for longer forecast periods. The efficacy of these ensemble and tree- based techniques in capturing intricate linkages within the data is demonstrated by the constant performance of the random forest (RF) and decision tree-based (RT) models, which have comparatively lower MAE values when compared to their original results.

Figure 14. MAE values plotted into a bar graph

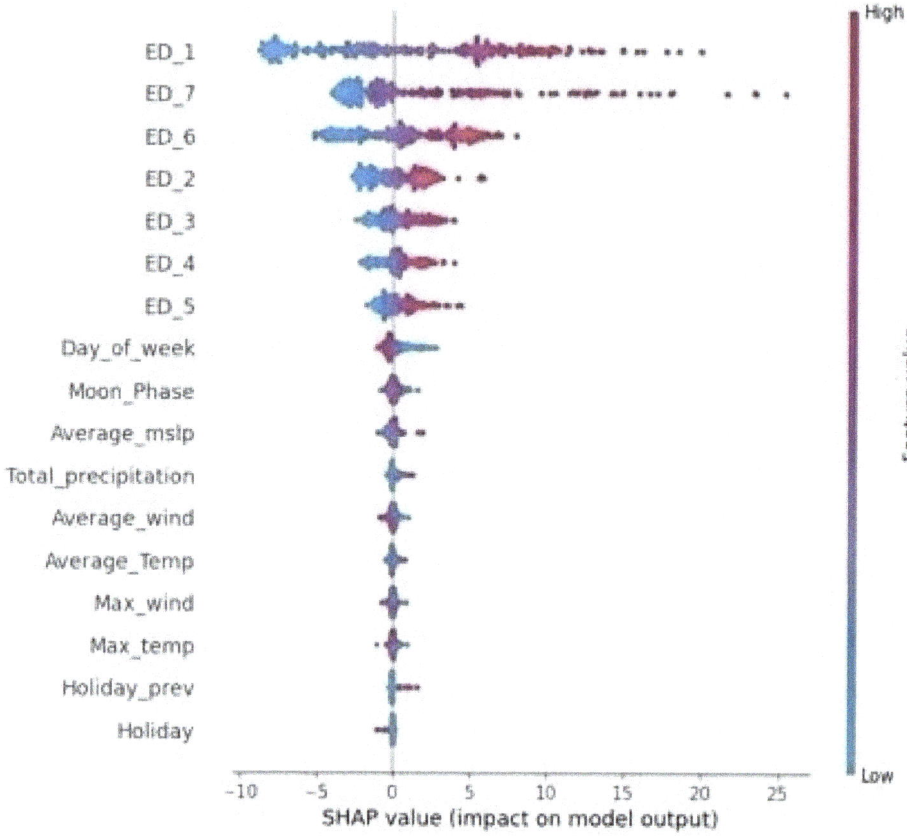

It's interesting to see that interpretability analysis significantly improves the extreme learning machine (ELM) model, which had higher MAE values at first. This demonstrates how interpretability techniques may be used to pinpoint important characteristics and model behaviors that lead to improved forecasting precision. Overall, the use of SHAP and LIME has enhanced these machine learning models' ability to predict outcomes while also offering insightful information about how they function, which can help with future improvements for more accurate forecasting in practical settings.

5. IMPLICATION AND LIMITATIONS

Improving hospital operations requires the development of a dependable, optimized and improved system of prediction of the number of expected visits in the emergency department. Precise estimates within a day's time frame can greatly improve hospital operations, personnel, and operating room accessibility. Hospital operations management would be significantly enhanced by longer prediction time horizons. Compared to ML-based base models, our suggested method. Interpretable Model-agnostic Explanations), effectively lowers the worsening of prediction results. Results from analysis using forecast time- horizon of up to +7 days were marginally worse than those obtained from daily prediction.

According to the current study, the proposed prediction system can be utilized to predict extreme occurrences, including a high number of ED visits in a short amount of time, in hospital emergency rooms. Because of the high patient traffic, anticipating serious events in hospital emergency departments might enhance operations and prevent departmental collapse. Due to the small number of extreme event occurrences in hospital operations, the suggested prediction method for extreme events requires a substantial amount of data to train the ML algorithms, which could be difficult in some circumstances.

The forecasting of hospital ED visits, which come under the heading of human activity patterns, is the only application for the suggested prediction system. Predicting human movement, traffic patterns, energy usage, and event attendance are few other examples. Human behavior is difficult to predict because of their distinctive characteristics and little available data.

Considering the time of day, day of the week, and other meteorological conditions is crucial when addressing these kinds of issues. Experiments have demonstrated that some weather-related variables can increase prediction accuracy. A suitable set of input variables for machine learning algorithms can be hard to come by, which hinders the suggested prediction system's ability to function. Using SHAP and LIME with our prediction models has several implications and limitations. By identifying the most crucial characteristics, these techniques provide further insights into the model's decision-making process, which has the major benefit of improving the model's interpretability. Knowing why a projection was created can have a significant impact on operational decisions and resource allocation, which is why this is so useful in hospital settings. Improved model performance is another significant outcome. By indicating potential improvement areas, SHAP and LIME enable model fine-tuning, enhancing prediction accuracy and overall performance. Improved feature engineering methods can also be achieved by utilizing SHAP and LIME insights. These insights can guide the selection and development of more relevant features, which will further boost predictive capabilities. The feature selection process aims to minimize the prediction error while keeping the model interpretable. The objective can be formulated as:

$$Min\ S \subseteq F(L(y, f(S))) + \lambda \cdot Complexity(S)$$

Where:

- $(y, (S))$: Loss function measuring prediction error (e.g., Mean Squared Error) with the selected feature subset $S.\lambda$: Regularization parameter to control the trade-off between accuracy and complexity.$Complexity(S)$: A function that penalizes the inclusion of too many features, promoting simpler, more interpretable models

Combining SHAP and LIME insights, the refined feature selection criteria can be formulated as:

$S = \{ \mid \phi j \geq r\} \cup \{ fj \mid fj \text{ is significant in LIME}\}$

This combined set ensures that the selected features are both globally important (as indicated by SHAP) and locally relevant (as indicated by LIME). Moreover, in a situation with significant risks, such as a hospital, the transparency achieved by these techniques increases stakeholder trust, which is necessary to gain acceptance and dependability of the prediction system. However, there are disadvantages to this tactic. Computationally intensive models and large datasets can make SHAP and LIME. This may lead to increased resource consumption and processing delays, which isn't always feasible for all applications. Concerns about scalability also arise from the fact that while SHAP and LIME provide thorough insights for individual forecasts, it may be challenging to employ these techniques in real-time or on large datasets.

6. CONCLUSION

Accurate prediction of Emergency Department (ED) visits is essential for effective resource allocation and preventing overcrowding. Overcrowding, as explained in (Sprivulis et al., 2006) is a critical issue influenced by multiple systemic factors. Empirical studies, including (Getachew et al., 2024) further investigate its causes, while research such as (Sprivulis et al., 2006) highlights its association with increased patient mortality. Bed availability (Harrou et al., 2020) directly impacts patient outcomes and hospital reputation (Boyle et al., 2012), with long-term consequences including reduced hospital capacity and ED closures(Olshaker & Rathlev, 2006). Predictive modelling is also vital for disaster preparedness and pandemic response(Alruwaili et al., 2023) Consequently, forecasting consecutive-day bed requirements has emerged as a practical solution (Rescher, 1997)supported by several ML and DL-based studies (McRae, 2021 & Golmohammadi, 2016).While machine learning and deep learning models improve prediction accuracy by identifying complex patterns in hospital data, transparency remains a major concern. Interpretability in healthcare—particularly in emergency settings—is crucial for trust, validation, and safe clinical decision-making (Miao et al., 2024) Explainable AI techniques such as SHAP and LIME, grounded in foundational studies (Petsis et al., 2022). provide local and global explanations, enhancing confidence in model predictions. These approaches have also been explored in medical imagc proccssing contexts (Nohara et al., 2022). In this study, integrating SHAP and LIME improved model transparency and performance. Feature filtering based on low SHAP and LIME contributions reduced Mean Absolute Error, demonstrating enhanced predictive reliability. Overall, explainable models support safer, more transparent ED forecasting and more effective hospital resource management, with future work focusing on hybrid deep learning architectures and further optimization.

DATA AVAILABILITY

Data is publicly available on Github and can be used for further research. Link: https://github.com/RTLPHD/EmergencyDepartmentForecasting.

ACKNOWLEDGMENT

The authors express their gratitude to SASTRA Deemed University, Thanjavur, for providing the infrastructural facilities to carry out this research work.

REFERENCES

Alruwaili, A. S., Islam, M. S., & Usher, K. (2023). Factors Influencing Hospitals' Disaster Preparedness in the Eastern Province of Saudi Arabia. *Disaster Medicine and Public Health Preparedness*, *17*, 17. DOI: 10.1017/dmp.2022.261 PMID: 36785527

Bouvatier, V., Lepetit, L., Rehault, P. N., & Strobel, F. (2023). Time- varying Z-score measures for bank insolvency risk: Best practice. *Journal of Empirical Finance*, *73*, 170–179. DOI: 10.1016/j.jempfin.2023.06.002

Boyle, A., Beniuk, K., Higginson, I., & Atkinson, P. (2012). Emergency department crowding: Time for interventions and policy evaluations. *Emergency Medicine International*, *2012*(1), 838610. DOI: 10.1155/2012/838610 PMID: 22454772

Cesario, E., Giampá, S., Baglione, E., Cordrie, L., Selva, J., & Talia, D. (2024). Machine Learning for Tsunami Waves Forecasting Using Regression Trees. *Big Data Research*, *36*, 100452. DOI: 10.1016/j.bdr.2024.100452

Clark, K., & Normile, L. B. (2002). Delays in implementing admission orders for critical care patients associated with length of stay in emergency departments in six mid-Atlantic states. *Journal of Emergency Nursing: JEN*, *28*(6), 489–495. DOI: 10.1067/men.2002.128714 PMID: 12509725

Conley, J., Bohan, J. S., & Baugh, C. W. (2017). The establishment and management of an observation unit. *Emergency Medicine Clinics of North America*, *35*(3), 519–533. DOI: 10.1016/j.emc.2017.03.002 PMID: 28711122

Davazdahemami, B., Peng, P., & Delen, D. (2022). A deep learning approach for predicting early bounce-backs to the emergency departments. *Healthcare Analytics*, *2*, 100018. DOI: 10.1016/j.health.2022.100018

Fernandes, C. M., Price, A., & Christenson, J. M. (1997). Does reduced length of stay decrease the number of emergency department patients who leave without seeing a physician? *The Journal of Emergency Medicine*, *15*(3), 397–399. DOI: 10.1016/S0736-4679(97)00030-9 PMID: 9258798

Gardner, R. L., Sarkar, U., Maselli, J. H., & Gonzales, R. (2007). Factors associated with longer ED lengths of stay. *The American Journal of Emergency Medicine*, *25*(6), 643–650. DOI: 10.1016/j.ajem.2006.11.037 PMID: 17606089

Getachew, M., Musa, I., Degefu, N., Beza, L., Hawlte, B., & Asefa, F. (2024). Emergency department overcrowding and its associated factors at HARME medical emergency center in Eastern Ethiopia. *African Journal of Emergency Medicine : Revue Africaine de la Médecine d'Urgence*, *14*(1), 26–32. DOI: 10.1016/j.afjem.2023.12.002 PMID: 38223394

Golmohammadi, D. (2016). Predicting hospital admissions to reduce emergency department boarding. *International Journal of Production Economics*, *182*, 535–544. DOI: 10.1016/j.ijpe.2016.09.020

Hakkoum, H., Idri, A., & Abnane, I. (2024). Global and local interpretability techniques of supervised machine learning black box models for numerical medical data. *Engineering Applications of Artificial Intelligence*, *131*, 107829. DOI: 10.1016/j.engappai.2023.107829

Harrou, F., Dairi, A., Kadri, F., & Sun, Y. (2020). (2 0 2 0). Forecasting emergency department overcrowding: A deep learning framework. *Chaos, Solitons, and Fractals*, *139*, 110247. DOI: 10.1016/j.chaos.2020.110247 PMID: 32982079

Horwitz, L. I., Green, J., & Bradley, E. H. (2010). US emergency department performance on wait time and length of visit. *Annals of Emergency Medicine*, *55*(2), 133–141. DOI: 10.1016/j.annemergmed.2009.07.023 PMID: 19796844

Hsieh, C. C., Lee, C. C., Hsu, H. C., Shih, H. I., Lu, C. H., & Lin, C. H. (2017). Impact of delayed admission to intensive care units on patients with acute respiratory failure. *The American Journal of Emergency Medicine*, *35*(1), 39–44. DOI: 10.1016/j.ajem.2016.09.066 PMID: 27742520

Ikeda, S., Nishimura, N., Sukegawa, N., & Takano, Y. (2023). Prescriptive price optimization using optimal regression trees. *Operations Research Perspectives*, *11*, 100290. DOI: 10.1016/j.orp.2023.100290

Kim, S. H., Kim, J. Y., Kim, G. B., Yu, J. J., & Choi, J. W. (2021). Diagnosis of coronary artery abnormalities in patients with Kawasaki disease according to established guidelines and Z score formulas. *Journal of the American Society of Echocardiography, 34*(6), 662–672. DOI: 10.1016/j.echo.2021.01.002 PMID: 33422668

Kyriako, D. N., Ricketts, V., Dyne, P. L., McCullough, M. D., & Talan, A. (1999). A 5-year time study analysis of emergency department patient care efficiency. *Annals of Emergency Medicine, 34*(3), 326–335. DOI: 10.1016/S0196-0644(99)70126-5 PMID: 10459088

Levy, R., Goldstein, B., & Trott, A. (1984). Approach to quality assurance in an emergency department: A one-year review. *Annals of Emergency Medicine, 13*(3), 166–169. DOI: 10.1016/S0196-0644(84)80606-X PMID: 6696304

Li, S., Ma, H., Zhang, Y., Wang, S., Guo, R., He, W., Xu, J., & Xie, Z. (2023). Emergency evacuation risk assessment method for educational buildings based on improved extreme learning machine. *Reliability Engineering & System Safety, 238*, 109454. DOI: 10.1016/j.ress.2023.109454

Maitra, A., & Chikhani, C. (1992). Patient satisfaction in an urban accident and emergency department. *International Journal of Clinical Practice, 46*(3), 182–184. DOI: 10.1111/j.1742-1241.1992.tb10335.x PMID: 1286019

Maxwell, K., Rajabi, M., Esterle, J., Tivane, M., & Travassos, D. (2024). Spatial modelling and classification of altered coal using random forest- based methods at Moatize Basin, Mozambique. *Journal of African Earth Sciences, 215*, 105279. DOI: 10.1016/j.jafrearsci.2024.105279

McRae, S. (2021). Long-term forecasting of regional demand for hospital services. *Operations Research for Health Care, 28*, 100289. DOI: 10.1016/j.orhc.2021.100289

Miao, K., Hounye, A. H., Su, L., Pan, Q., Wang, J., Hou, M., & Xiong, L. (2024). Exploring explainable machine learning and Shapley additive exPlanations (SHAP) technique to uncover key factors of HNSC cancer: An analysis of the best practices. *Biomedical Signal Processing and Control, 89*, 105752. DOI: 10.1016/j.bspc.2023.105752

Nerney, M. P., Chin, M. H., Jin, L., Karrison, T. G., Walter, J., Mulliken, R., Miller, A., Hayley, D. C., & Friedmann, P. D. (2001). Factors associated with older patients' satisfaction with care in an inner-city emergency department. *Annals of Emergency Medicine, 38*(2), 140–145. DOI: 10.1067/mem.2001.114304 PMID: 11468608

Nohara, Y., Matsumoto, K., Soejima, H., & Nakashima, N. (2022). Explanation of machine learning models using shapley additive explanation and application for real data in hospital. *Computer Methods and Programs in Biomedicine*, *214*, 106584. DOI: 10.1016/j.cmpb.2021.106584 PMID: 34942412

Nordin, N., Zainol, Z., Noor, M. H. M., & Chan, L. F. (2023). An explainable predictive model for suicide attempt risk using an ensemble learning and Shapley Additive Explanations (SHAP) approach. *Asian Journal of Psychiatry*, *79*, 103316. DOI: 10.1016/j.ajp.2022.103316 PMID: 36395702

Olshaker, J. S., & Rathlev, N. K. (2006). Emergency department overcrowding and ambulance diversion: The impact and potential solutions of extended boarding of admitted patients in the emergency department. *The Journal of Emergency Medicine*, *30*(3), 351–356. DOI: 10.1016/j.jemermed.2005.05.023 PMID: 16677993

Peláez-Rodríguez, C., Torres-López, R., Pérez-Aracil, J., López-Laguna, N., Sánchez-Rodríguez, S., & Salcedo-Sanz, S. (2024). An explainable machine learning approach for hospital emergency department visits forecasting using continuous training and multi-model regression. *Computer Methods and Programs in Biomedicine*, *245*, 108033. DOI: 10.1016/j.cmpb.2024.108033 PMID: 38278030

Petsis, S., Karamanou, A., Kalampokis, E., & Tarabanis, K. (2022). Forecasting and explaining emergency department visits in a public hospital. *Journal of Intelligent Information Systems*, *59*(2), 479–500. DOI: 10.1007/s10844-022-00716-6

Rescher, N. (1997). *Predicting the future: An introduction to the theory of forecasting*. State University of New York Press.

Rubin, H. R., & Wu, A. W. (1991). *Patient satisfaction: Its importance and how to measure it. The Business of Medicine*. Elsevier.

Sprivulis, P. C., Da Silva, J. A., Jacobs, I. G., Jelinek, G. A., & Frazer, A. R. (2006). The association between hospital overcrowding and mortality among patients admitted via Western Australian emergency departments. *The Medical Journal of Australia*, *184*(5), 208–212. DOI: 10.5694/j.1326-5377.2006.tb00203.x PMID: 16515429

Sudarshan, V. K., Brabrand, M., Range, T. M., & Wiil, U. K. (2021). Performance evaluation of mergence Department patient arrivals forecasting models by including meteorological and calendar information: A comparative study. *Computers in Biology and Medicine*, *135*, 104541. DOI: 10.1016/j.compbiomed.2021.104541 PMID: 34166880

Tan, C., Chen, H., Chen, M., & Lin, Z. (2024). Rapid identification of silk products by attenuated total reflection–mid-infrared spectroscopy and extreme learning machines. *Infrared Physics & Technology, 139*, 105334. DOI: 10.1016/j.infrared.2024.105334

Tanzer, J. R., Dufault, M., Rioux, L. R., Machan, J., Bergeron, K., & Napoli, A. (2023). "I Was Here First, Why Did They Go Before Me": Examining Patients' Perceptions of Priority in a Psychometric Study of Emergency Department Triage. *Journal of Emergency Nursing: JEN, 49*(2), 294–304. DOI: 10.1016/j.jen.2022.09.017 PMID: 36567152

Tsay, S. F., Chang, C. Y., Hung, S. S., Su, J. Y., Kuo, C. Y., & Mu, P. F. (2024). Pain prediction model based on machine learning and SHAP values for elders with dementia in Taiwan. *International Journal of Medical Informatics, 188*, 105475. DOI: 10.1016/j.ijmedinf.2024.105475 PMID: 38743995

Van der Velden, B. H., Kuijf, H. J., Gilhuijs, K. G., & Viergever, M. A. (2022). Explainable artificial intelligence (XAI) in deep learning-based medical image analysis. *Medical Image Analysis, 79*, 102470. DOI: 10.1016/j.media.2022.102470 PMID: 35576821

Wang, C., & Fan, J. (2024). On the convergence of gradient descent for robust functional linear regression. *Journal of Complexity, 84*, 101858. DOI: 10.1016/j.jco.2024.101858

Whitt, W., & Zhang, X. (2019). Forecasting arrivals and occupancy levels in an emergency department. *Operations Research for Health Care, 21*, 1–18. DOI: 10.1016/j.orhc.2019.01.002

Zhang, X., Shen, H., Huang, T., Wu, Y., Guo, B., Liu, Z., Luo, H., Tang, J., Zhou, H., Wang, L., Xu, W., & Ou, G. (2024). Improved random forest algorithms for increasing the accuracy of forest aboveground biomass estimation using Sentinel-2 imagery. *Ecological Indicators, 159*, 111752. DOI: 10.1016/j.ecolind.2024.111752

Zhao, X., Lai, J. W., Ho, A. F. W., Liu, N., Ong, M. E. H., & Cheong, K. H. (2022). Predicting hospital emergency department visits with deep learning approaches. *Biocybernetics and Biomedical Engineering, 42*(3), 1051–1065. DOI: 10.1016/j.bbe.2022.07.008

Zheng, D., Wu, S., & Hou, M. (2021). Fully connected deep network: An improved method to predict TOC of shale reservoirs from well logs. *Marine and Petroleum Geology, 132*, 105205. DOI: 10.1016/j.marpetgeo.2021.105205

Compilation of References

Aayog, N. I. T. I. (2021). *National digital health blueprint.* Government of India. https://www.nhp.gov.in/NDHM/Documents/National_Digital_Health_BluePrint.pdf

Abràmoff, M. D., Tarver, M. E., Loyo-Berrios, N., Trujillo, S., Char, D., Obermeyer, Z., Eydelman, M. B., & Maisel, W. H. (2023). Considerations for addressing bias in artificial intelligence for health equity. *NPJ Digital Medicine*, *6*(1), 170. DOI: 10.1038/s41746-023-00913-9 PMID: 37700029

Acharya, V. (2025). Intelligent Healthcare Ecosystems: Optimizing the Iron Triangle of Healthcare (Access, Cost, Quality). *arXiv (Cornell University).* https://doi.org// arxiv.2510.03331DOI: 10.48550

Adamson, A. S., & Smith, A. (2018). Machine learning and health care disparities in dermatology. *JAMA Dermatology*, *154*(11), 1247–1248. DOI: 10.1001/jamadermatol.2018.2348 PMID: 30073260

Adelson, P. D., Bratton, S. L., Carney, N., Chesnut, R. M., du Coudray, H. E. M., Goldstein, B., Kochanek, P. M., Miller, H. C., Partington, M. D., Selden, N. R., Warden, C. R., & Wright, D. W. (2003). Chapter 1: Introduction. *Pediatric Critical Care Medicine*, *4*(SUPPLEMENT), S2–S4. Advance online publication. DOI: 10.1097/01.CCM.0000066600.71233.01 PMID: 12847337

Adibi, A., Xu, C., Ji, Z., Kaur, J., Chen, W., Healey, E., Nuwagira, B., Ye, W., Woollard, G., Xu, M., Cui, H. T., Xi, J., Chang, T., Bikia, V., Zhang, N., Noori, A., Yuan, X., & Hossain, Md. B., Frank, H. A., … Jabbour, S. (2025). Recent Advances, Applications and Open Challenges in Machine Learning for Health: Reflections from Research Roundtables at ML4H 2024 Symposium. *arXiv (Cornell University).* DOI: 10.48550/arxiv.2502.06693

Agarwal, R., Bjarnadottir, M., Rhue, L., Dugas, M., Crowley, K., Clark, J., & Gao, G. (2023). Addressing algorithmic bias and the perpetuation of health inequities: An AI bias aware framework. *Health Policy and Technology, 12*(1), 100702. DOI: 10.1016/j.hlpt.2022.100702

Aguilar-Gaxiola, S., Loera, G., Méndez, L., Sala, M., & Kopelowicz, A. (2011). *Community-defined solutions for Latino mental health care disparities: Workgroup report.* University of California. https://health.ucdavis.edu/media-resources/crhd/documents/pdfs/community-defined-solutions-latino-mental-health-care-disparities-exec-summary.pdf

Ahmed, M. M., Okesanya, O. J., Olaleke, N. O., Adigun, O. A., Adebayo, U. O., Oso, T. A., Eshun, G., & Lucero-Prisno, D. E. (2025). Integrating Digital Health Innovations to Achieve Universal Health Coverage: Promoting Health Outcomes and Quality Through Global Public Health Equity [Review of *Integrating Digital Health Innovations to Achieve Universal Health Coverage: Promoting Health Outcomes and Quality Through Global Public Health Equity*]. *Healthcare, 13*(9), 1060. Multidisciplinary Digital Publishing Institute. DOI: 10.3390/healthcare13091060

Aldwean, A., & Tenney, D. (2024). Artificial Intelligence in Healthcare Sector: A Literature Review of the Adoption Challenges [Review of *Artificial Intelligence in Healthcare Sector: A Literature Review of the Adoption Challenges*]. *Open Journal of Business and Management, 12*(1), 129. Scientific Research Publishing. DOI: 10.4236/ojbm.2024.121009

Ali, H., & Nikberg, N. (2024). *Bias in AI-driven healthcare: Navigating ethical challenges at an early stage.*

Alruwaili, A. S., Islam, M. S., & Usher, K. (2023). Factors Influencing Hospitals' Disaster Preparedness in the Eastern Province of Saudi Arabia. *Disaster Medicine and Public Health Preparedness, 17*, 17. DOI: 10.1017/dmp.2022.261 PMID: 36785527

Althagafi, M. H., Al-Asiri, K. S. K., Almahanna, M. A., Al-Otapi, M. D., Aseri, A. A., Al-Sulami, M. A., Al-Harbi, Y. S., & Al-Mutairi, N. M. S. (2025). A descriptive study of the future qualification level of paramedics in health education programs in Saudi universities. *The Review of Diabetic Studies; RDS, 21*(S9), 1154–1162. DOI: 10.70082/3q3x9v41

Anderson, P., Gadgil, R., Johnson, W. A., Schwab, E., & Davidson, J. M. (2021). Reducing variability of breast cancer subtype predictors by grounding deep learning models in prior knowledge. *Computers in Biology and Medicine, 138*, 104850. DOI: 10.1016/j.compbiomed.2021.104850 PMID: 34536702

Ando, K., Giorgianni, F. E., Danthinne, E. S., & Rodgers, R. F. (2021). Beauty ideals, social media, and body positivity: A qualitative investigation of influences on body image among young women in Japan. *Body Image, 38*, 358–369. DOI: 10.1016/j.bodyim.2021.05.001 PMID: 34120098

Ansari, M. M., Kumar, S., Chola, C., Heyat, M. B. B., Akhtar, F., Hayat, M. A. B., Sayeed, E., Parveen, S., Abbasi, R., & Pomary, D. (2025). A Novel Machine and Deep Learning–Based Ensemble Techniques for Automatic Lung Cancer Detection. *BioMed Research International, 2025*(1). DOI: 10.1155/bmri/6666688

Appleton, J., Fowler, C., Latouche, L., Smit, J., Booker, M., & Fairbrother, G. (2025). Evaluation of group therapy intervention for anxiety and depression in the postnatal period. *Maternal and Child Health Journal, 29*(4), 537–548. DOI: 10.1007/s10995-025-04076-9 PMID: 40138124

Aprajita, K., Capucine, B., Ganash, T., & Jasper, T. (2025). *Responsible, safe, and inclusive AI for sustainable development in health in Southeast Asia*. DOI: 10.53832/evidence-fund.0006

Aquino, Y. S. J., Carter, S. M., Houssami, N., Braunack-Mayer, A., Win, K. T., Degeling, C., Wang, L., & Rogers, W. A. (2025). Practical, epistemic and normative implications of algorithmic bias in healthcare artificial intelligence: A qualitative study of multidisciplinary expert perspectives. *Journal of Medical Ethics, 51*(6), 420–428. DOI: 10.1136/jme-2022-108850 PMID: 36823101

Arab, R. A. E., Moosa, O. A. A., & Sagbakken, M. (2025). Economic, ethical, and regulatory dimensions of artificial intelligence in healthcare: an integrative review [Review of *Economic, ethical, and regulatory dimensions of artificial intelligence in healthcare: an integrative review*]. *Frontiers in Public Health, 13*, 1617138. Frontiers Media. https://doi.org/DOI: 10.3389/fpubh.2025.1617138

Arab, R. A. E., & Moosa, O. A. A. (2025). Systematic review of cost effectiveness and budget impact of artificial intelligence in healthcare. *NPJ Digital Medicine, 8*(1), 548. DOI: 10.1038/s41746-025-01722-y PMID: 40858882

Arora, A., Alderman, J. E., Palmer, J., Ganapathi, S., Laws, E., McCradden, M. D., Oakden-Rayner, L., Pfohl, S. R., Ghassemi, M., McKay, F., Treanor, D., Rostamzadeh, N., Mateen, B., Gath, J., Adebajo, A. O., Kuku, S., Matin, R., Heller, K., Sapey, E., & Liu, X. (2023). The value of standards for health datasets in artificial intelligence-based applications. *Nature Medicine, 29*(11), 2929–2938. DOI: 10.1038/s41591-023-02608-w PMID: 37884627

Artuso, F., & Guijt, I. (2020). *Global Megatrends: Mapping the forces that affect us all*. DOI: 10.21201/2020.5648

Asadi, B., & Memon, Q. (2023). Efficient breast cancer detection via cascade deep learning network. *International Journal of Intelligent Networks*, *4*, 46–52. DOI: 10.1016/j.ijin.2023.02.001

Asha, C. M. (2020). Education of tribal communities in Kerala. *International Journal of Social Science and Economic Research, 6*, 1390-1399. . 2020. v05i06.001DOI: <ALIGNMENT.qj></ALIGNMENT>10.46609/IJSSER

Attouche, N., Hafdi, S., Somali, R., Battas, O., & Agoub, M. (2021). Factors associated with the risk of developing eating disorders among medical students in Casablanca, Morocco. *The Pan African Medical Journal*, *39*, 270. PMID: 34707771

Baillie, L., Stewart-Lord, A., Thomas, N., & Frings, D. (2025). Patients', clinicians' and developers' perspectives and experiences of artificial intelligence in cardiac healthcare: A qualitative study. *Digital Health*, *11*, 20552076251328578. DOI: 10.1177/20552076251328578 PMID: 40534891

Banerjee, A. V., & Duflo, E. (2007). The economic lives of the poor. *The Journal of Economic Perspectives*, *21*(1), 141–167. https://www.aeaweb.org/articles?id=10.1257/jep.21.1.141. DOI: 10.1257/jep.21.1.141 PMID: 19212450

Bano, M. (2019). Partnerships and the Good-Governance Agenda: Improving Service Delivery Through State–NGO Collaborations. *Voluntas*, *30*(6), 1270–1283. DOI: 10.1007/s11266-017-9937-y

Bass, B. M. (1985). *Leadership and performance beyond expectations.* Free Press. https://books.google.com/books/about/Leadership_and_Performance_Beyond_Expect.html?id=NCd-QgAACAAJ

Benjamens, S., Dhunnoo, P., & Meskó, B. (2020). The state of artificial intelligence-based FDA-approved medical devices and algorithms: An online database. *NPJ Digital Medicine*, *3*(1), 118. DOI: 10.1038/s41746-020-00324-0 PMID: 32984550

Berk, M., Köhler-Forsberg, O., Turner, M., Penninx, B. W. J. H., Wrobel, A., Firth, J., Loughman, A., Reavley, N. J., McGrath, J. J., Momen, N. C., Plana-Ripoll, O., O'Neil, A., Siskind, D., Williams, L. J., Carvalho, A. F., Schmaal, L., Walker, A. J., Dean, O., Walder, K., & Marx, W. (2023). Comorbidity between major depressive disorder and physical diseases: A comprehensive review of epidemiology, mechanisms and management. *World Psychiatry; Official Journal of the World Psychiatric Association (WPA)*, *22*(3), 366–387. DOI: 10.1002/wps.21110 PMID: 37713568

Bertl, M., Lamo, Y., Leucker, M., Margaria, T., Mohammadi, E., Mukhiya, S. K., & Rabbi, F. (2023). Challenges for ai in healthcare systems. In International Conference on Bridging the Gap between AI and Reality (pp. 165-186). Cham: Springer Nature Switzerland.

Bhaskaran, A. A. Child and adolescent psychiatry (2023). *In Revision Guide for MRCPsych Paper B* (pp. 133-152). Routledge. https://www.taylorfrancis.com/chapters/edit/10.4324/9781003376163-6/child-adolescent-psychiatry-arun-arujun-bhaskaran

Bhat, G. S., Shankar, N., Kim, D., Song, D. J., Seo, S., Panahi, I. M. S., & Tamil, L. (2021). Machine Learning-Based Asthma Risk Prediction Using IoT and Smartphone Applications. *IEEE Access : Practical Innovations, Open Solutions*, *9*, 118708–118715. DOI: 10.1109/ACCESS.2021.3103897

Bhugra, D. (2004). Migration and mental health. *Acta Psychiatrica Scandinavica*, *109*(4), 243–258. DOI: 10.1046/j.0001-690X.2003.00246.x PMID: 15008797

Birgegård, A., Forsén Mantilla, E., Breithaupt, L. E., Borg, S., Sanzari, C. M., Padalecki, S., Hedlund, E., & Bulik, C. M. (2023). Proposal for increasing diagnostic clarity in research and clinical practice by renaming and reframing atypical anorexia nervosa as “Restrictive Eating Disorder” (RED). *Eating Behaviors*, *50*, 101750. DOI: 10.1016/j.eatbeh.2023.101750 PMID: 37263139

Blanco, J., Ferreras, M., & Cosido, O. (2025). Predictive modeling of hospital emergency department demand using artificial intelligence: A systematic review. *International Journal of Medical Informatics*, •••, 106215. PMID: 41401760

Bolden, R. (2011). Distributed leadership in organizations: A review of theory and research. *International Journal of Management Reviews*, *13*(3), 251–269. DOI: 10.1111/j.1468-2370.2011.00306.x

Bouhoudan, A., Zian, Z., Khaddor, M., & Mourabit, N. (2024). The impact of societal changes and COVID-19 pandemic on Moroccan food habits: A Mediterranean perspective. *Discover Food*, *4*(1), 154. Advance online publication. DOI: 10.1007/s44187-024-00237-x

Bouvatier, V., Lepetit, L., Rehault, P. N., & Strobel, F. (2023). Time- varying Z-score measures for bank insolvency risk: Best practice. *Journal of Empirical Finance*, *73*, 170–179. DOI: 10.1016/j.jempfin.2023.06.002

Boyatzis, R., & McKee, A. (2005). *Resonant leadership: Renewing yourself and connecting with others through mindfulness, hope, and compassion.* Harvard Business School Press. https://books.google.com/books/about/Resonant_Leadership.html?id=ViVX3O9YP6oC

Boyle, A., Beniuk, K., Higginson, I., & Atkinson, P. (2012). Emergency department crowding: Time for interventions and policy evaluations. *Emergency Medicine International, 2012*(1), 838610. DOI: 10.1155/2012/838610 PMID: 22454772

Branquinho, M., Canavarro, M. C., & Fonseca, A. (2022). A Blended Cognitive–Behavioral Intervention for the Treatment of Postpartum Depression: A case study. *Clinical Case Studies, 21*(5), 438–456. DOI: 10.1177/15346501221082616

Braveman, P., Arkin, E., Orleans, T., Proctor, D., & Plough, A. (2017). *What is health equity? And what difference does a definition make?* Robert Wood Johnson Foundation.

Bulik, C. M., Thornton, L. M., Parker, R., Kennedy, H., Baker, J. H., MacDermod, C., Guintivano, J., Cleland, L., Miller, A. L., Harper, L., Larsen, J. T., Yilmaz, Z., Grove, J., Sullivan, P. F., Petersen, L. V., Jordan, J., Kennedy, M. A., & Martin, N. G. (2021). The Eating Disorders Genetics Initiative (EDGI): Study protocol. *BMC Psychiatry, 21*(1), 234. DOI: 10.1186/s12888-021-03212-3 PMID: 33947359

Bullard, N., et al. (2022). Ethics by design: An organizational approach to responsible use of technology.

Bullock, J., Luccioni, A., Pham, K. H., Lam, C. S. N., & Luengo-Oroz, M. (2020). Mapping the landscape of artificial intelligence applications against COVID-19. *Journal of Artificial Intelligence Research, 69*, 807–845. DOI: 10.1613/jair.1.12162

Burns, J. M. (1978). *Leadership.* Harper & Row.

Burrell, D. N. (2023). Dynamic Evaluation Approaches to Telehealth Technologies and Artificial Intelligence (AI) Telemedicine Applications in Healthcare and Biotechnology Organizations. *Merits, 3*(4), 700–721. DOI: 10.3390/merits3040042

Busuioc, M. (2022). AI algorithmic oversight: New frontiers in regulation. In *Handbook of regulatory authorities* (pp. 470–486). Edward Elgar Publishing.

Butt, M. D., Ong, S. C., Wahab, M. U., Rasool, M. F., Saleem, F., Hashmi, A., Sajjad, A., Chaudhry, F. A., & Babar, Z. U. D. (2022). Cost of illness analysis of type 2 diabetes mellitus: The findings from a lower-middle income country. *International Journal of Environmental Research and Public Health, 19*(19), 12611. DOI: 10.3390/ijerph191912611 PMID: 36231911

Camacho, M., Perramon, J., Puig-Bosch, X., Dang, V. N., Díaz, O., & Lekadir, K. (2025). Stakeholder engagement: The path to trustworthy AI in healthcare. In *Trustworthy AI in medical imaging* (pp. 471–493). Elsevier. DOI: 10.1016/B978-0-44-323761-4.00038-9

Census. (2011). Government of India, Census report

Cesario, E., Giampá, S., Baglione, E., Cordrie, L., Selva, J., & Talia, D. (2024). Machine Learning for Tsunami Waves Forecasting Using Regression Trees. *Big Data Research, 36*, 100452. DOI: 10.1016/j.bdr.2024.100452

Chassagnon, G., Margerie-Mellon, C. de, Vakalopoulou, M., Marini, R., Hoang-Thi, T.-N., Revel, M., & Soyer, P. (2022). Artificial intelligence in lung cancer: current applications and perspectives [Review of *Artificial intelligence in lung cancer: current applications and perspectives*]. *Japanese Journal of Radiology*. Springer Science+Business Media. DOI: 10.1007/s11604-022-01359-x

Chen, Y., Sun, J., Chen, Y., Li, E., Lu, J., Tang, H., Xie, Y., Zhang, J., Peng, L., Wu, H., Cheng, Z. J., & Sun, B. (2025). Machine learning-based model for acute asthma exacerbation detection using routine blood parameters. *The World Allergy Organization Journal, 18*(7), 101074. DOI: 10.1016/j.waojou.2025.101074 PMID: 40584687

Cheung, N. W., Byth, K., Cincotta, R., & Fong, B. (2018). Telehealth combined with in-person care improves satisfaction and glycaemic control in gestational diabetes. *Diabetes Care, 41*(9), 1830–1835.

Chin, M. H., Afsar-Manesh, N., Bierman, A. S., Chang, C., Colón-Rodríguez, C. J., Dullabh, P., Duran, D. G., Fair, M., Hernandez-Boussard, T., Hightower, M., Jain, A., Jordan, W. B., Konya, S., Moore, R. H., Moore, T. T., Rodriguez, R., Shaheen, G., Snyder, L. P., Srinivasan, M., & Ohno-Machado, L. (2023). Guiding principles to address the impact of algorithm bias on racial and ethnic disparities in health and health care. *JAMA Network Open, 6*(12), e2345050. DOI: 10.1001/jamanetworkopen.2023.45050 PMID: 38100101

Chung, D., Meng, Y., & Wang, J. (2025). The role of Short-Form Video apps in Mitigating occupational burnout and enhancing life satisfaction among healthcare Workers: A Serial Multiple Mediation model. *Health Care, 13*(4), 355. DOI: 10.3390/healthcare13040355 PMID: 39997230

Clark, K., & Normile, L. B. (2002). Delays in implementing admission orders for critical care patients associated with length of stay in emergency departments in six mid-Atlantic states. *Journal of Emergency Nursing: JEN, 28*(6), 489–495. DOI: 10.1067/men.2002.128714 PMID: 12509725

Conley, J., Bohan, J. S., & Baugh, C. W. (2017). The establishment and management of an observation unit. *Emergency Medicine Clinics of North America*, *35*(3), 519–533. DOI: 10.1016/j.emc.2017.03.002 PMID: 28711122

Czubaj, N., Szymańska, M., Nowak, B., & Grajek, M. (2025). The impact of social media on body image perception in young people. *Nutrients*, *17*(9), 1455. DOI: 10.3390/nu17091455 PMID: 40362764

D'Souza, R., Arbuckle, S., & Koren, G. (2022). Risk-stratified hybrid models for gestational diabetes: Integrating digital monitoring with targeted in-clinic review. *Journal of Obstetrics and Gynaecology Research*, *48*(5), 1123–1132.

Dalfra, M. G., Nicolucci, A., Bisson, T., & Lapolla, A. (2014). Telemedicine and pregnancy: Monitoring gestational diabetes mellitus improves outcomes. *Diabetes Technology & Therapeutics*, *16*(9), 650–657.

Damra, J. K., Akour, M. M., & Al Omari, O. (2024). Stress and loneliness: Exploring adolescents' use of social media as a coping strategy during COVID-19. *Nursing Children and Young People*, *36*(1), 26–32. DOI: 10.7748/ncyp.2023.e1456 PMID: 37211812

Daneshjou, R., Vodrahalli, K., Novoa, R. A., Jenkins, M., Liang, W., Rotemberg, V., Ko, J., Swetter, S. M., Bailey, E. E., Gevaert, O., Mukherjee, P., Phung, M., Yekrang, K., Fong, B., Sahasrabudhe, R., Allerup, J. A. C., Okata-Karigane, U., Zou, J., & Chiou, A. S. (2022). Disparities in dermatology AI performance on a diverse, curated clinical image set. *Science Advances*, *8*(32), eabq6147. Advance online publication. DOI: 10.1126/sciadv.abq6147 PMID: 35960806

Dangi, R. R., Sharma, A., & Vageriya, V. (2025). Transforming healthcare in low-resource settings with artificial intelligence: Recent developments and outcomes. *Public Health Nursing (Boston, Mass.)*, *42*(2), 1017–1030. DOI: 10.1111/phn.13500 PMID: 39629887

Davazdahemami, B., Peng, P., & Delen, D. (2022). A deep learning approach for predicting early bounce-backs to the emergency departments. *Healthcare Analytics*, *2*, 100018. DOI: 10.1016/j.health.2022.100018

Davey, E., Allen, K., Bennett, S. D., Bryant-Waugh, R., Clarke, T., Cooper, Z., Dixon-Ward, K., Dudley, J., Eisler, I., Griffiths, J., Hill, A. J., Micali, N., Murphy, R., Picek, I., Rea, R., Schmidt, U., Simic, M., Tchanturia, K., Traviss-Turner, G., & Shafran, R. (2023). Improving programme-led and focused interventions for eating disorders: An experts' consensus statement—A UK perspective. *European Eating Disorders Review*, *31*(5), 577–595. DOI: 10.1002/erv.2981 PMID: 37218053

De Manuel, A., Delgado, J., Parra Jounou, I., Ausín, T., Casacuberta, D., Cruz, M., Guersenzvaig, A., Moyano, C., Rodríguez-Arias, D., Rueda, J., & Puyol, A. (2023). Ethical assessments and mitigation strategies for biases in AI-systems used during the COVID-19 pandemic. *Big Data & Society*, *10*(1), 20539517231179199. Advance online publication. DOI: 10.1177/20539517231179199

Del Vecchio, P., Secundo, G., & Garzoni, A. (2023). Phygital technologies and environments for breakthrough innovation in customers' and citizens' journey. A critical literature review and future agenda. *Technological Forecasting and Social Change*, *189*, 122342. DOI: 10.1016/j.techfore.2023.122342

Dennis, C., Fung, K., Grigoriadis, S., Robinson, G. E., Romans, S., & Ross, L. (2007). Traditional Postpartum Practices and Rituals: A Qualitative Systematic review. *Women's Health (London, England)*, *3*(4), 487–502. DOI: 10.2217/17455057.3.4.487 PMID: 19804024

Devassy, R., & George, A. (2021). Interstate migration and health disparities in Kerala: A sociological overview. *Economic and Political Weekly*, *56*(45), 41–49. DOI: 10.4103/ijmr.IJMR_2217_20

Djakeli, K. (2025 B). Strategic Management for Digital Platform Brands in the Phygital Era. In Brand Creation and Management in the Phygital Era (pp. 499-520). IGI Global Scientific Publishing.

Djakeli, K. (2024). Healthcare marketing, meaning, historical development, applications, and current status. In Djakeli, K. (Ed.), *Modern Healthcare Marketing in the Digital Era* (pp. 1–25). IGI Global Scientific Publishing., DOI: 10.4018/979-8-3693-0679-6.ch001

Djakeli, K. (2025). A). Phygitalization of Palliative Care and Its Social Marketing. In *Phygital Approaches to Social Marketing* (pp. 267–288). IGI Global Scientific Publishing.

DosSantos, P., & de Oliveira, S. B. (2020). A Financial Theory Perspective of the Metrics Employed to Measure Value in the "Value in Healthcare" Methodologies. *Portuguese Journal of Public Health*, *38*(3), 176–186. DOI: 10.1159/000512564

Dunker, A. K. (1998). The pacific symposium on biocomputing. *Journal of Molecular Graphics & Modelling*, *16*(4-6), 267. DOI: 10.1016/S1093-3263(98)80012-0

Durán, J. M., & Jongsma, K. R. (2021). Who is afraid of black box algorithms? On the epistemological and ethical basis of trust in medical AI. *Journal of Medical Ethics*, *47*(5), 329–335. DOI: 10.1136/medethics-2020-106820 PMID: 33737318

Ekpo, R. H., Osamor, V. C., Azeta, A. A., Ikeakanam, E., & Amos, B. O. (2023). Machine learning classification approach for asthma prediction models in children. *Health and Technology, 13*(1), 1–10. DOI: 10.1007/s12553-023-00732-8 PMID: 38229886

El Arab, R. A., & Al Moosa, O. A. (2025). The role of AI in emergency department triage: An integrative systematic review. *Intensive & Critical Care Nursing, 89*, 104058. DOI: 10.1016/j.iccn.2025.104058 PMID: 40306071

Elaraby, A., Saad, A., Elmannai, H., Alabdulhafith, M., Hadjouni, M., & Hamdi, M. (2024). An approach for classification of breast cancer using lightweight deep convolution neural network. *Heliyon, 10*(20), e38524. DOI: 10.1016/j.heliyon.2024.e38524 PMID: 39640611

El-Jerjawi, N. S., Murad, W. F., Harazin, D., Qaoud, A. N., Jamala, M. N., Abunasser, B. S., & Abu-Naser, S. S. (2024). The role of artificial intelligence in revolutionizing health: Challenges, applications, and future prospects.

Eo, A., Eo, O., Oj, K., Om, I., & Ka, O. (2020). Prevalence and predictors of postpartum depression among postnatal women in Lagos, Nigeria. *African Health Sciences, 20*(4), 1943–1954. DOI: 10.4314/ahs.v20i4.53 PMID: 34394261

Esteva, A., Kuprel, B., Novoa, R. A., Ko, J., Swetter, S. M., Blau, H. M., & Thrun, S. (2017). Dermatologist-level classification of skin cancer with deep neural networks. *Nature, 542*(7639), 115–118. DOI: 10.1038/nature21056 PMID: 28117445

Fahim, Y. A., Hasani, I. W., Kabba, S., & Ragab, W. M. (2025). Artificial intelligence in healthcare and medicine: clinical applications, therapeutic advances, and future perspectives [Review of *Artificial intelligence in healthcare and medicine: clinical applications, therapeutic advances, and future perspectives*]. *European Journal of Medical Research, 30*(1). BioMed Central. DOI: 10.1186/s40001-025-03196-w

Faiyazuddin, M., Rahman, S. J. Q., Anand, G., Siddiqui, R. K., Mehta, R., Khatib, M. N., & Sah, R. (2025). The impact of artificial intelligence on healthcare: A comprehensive review of advancements in diagnostics, treatment, and operational efficiency. *Health Science Reports, 8*(1), e70312. DOI: 10.1002/hsr2.70312 PMID: 39763580

Fearon, P., Shmueli-Goetz, Y., Viding, E., Fonagy, P., & Plomin, R. (2014). Genetic and environmental influences on adolescent attachment. *Journal of Child Psychology and Psychiatry, and Allied Disciplines, 55*(9), 1033–1041. DOI: 10.1111/jcpp.12171 PMID: 24256475

Fendrick, A. M., Bagley, N., & Bonavitacola, J. (2023). Michigan Professors Offer Insights Into What Braidwood Ruling Could Mean for Preventive Screening in Cancer Care. *The American Journal of Managed Care*, *29*(Spec. No. 5), SP353–SP354. Advance online publication. DOI: 10.37765/ajmc.2023.89392 PMID: 37341474

Feng, B., Harms, J., Chen, E., Gao, P., Xu, P., & He, Y. (2023). Current discoveries and future implications of eating disorders. *International Journal of Environmental Research and Public Health*, *20*(14), 6325. DOI: 10.3390/ijerph20146325 PMID: 37510558

Fernandes, C. M., Price, A., & Christenson, J. M. (1997). Does reduced length of stay decrease the number of emergency department patients who leave without seeing a physician? *The Journal of Emergency Medicine*, *15*(3), 397–399. DOI: 10.1016/S0736-4679(97)00030-9 PMID: 9258798

FIME. (2025). *Radiology industry report*. https://www.worldhealthexpo.com/content/dam/esa/emea/worldhealthexpo/events/healthcare/miami/en/2025/pdfs/FIME25-radiology-industry-report.pdf

Finlayson, S. G., Subbaswamy, A., Singh, K., Bowers, J., Kupke, A., Zittrain, J., Kohane, I. S., & Saria, S. (2021). The clinician and dataset shift in artificial intelligence. *The New England Journal of Medicine*, *385*(3), 283–286. DOI: 10.1056/NEJMc2104626 PMID: 34260843

Fletcher, R. R., Nakeshimana, A., & Olubeko, O. (2021). Addressing fairness, bias, and appropriate use of artificial intelligence and machine learning in global health. *Frontiers in Artificial Intelligence*, *3*, 561802. DOI: 10.3389/frai.2020.561802 PMID: 33981989

Fleury, M.-J., Cao, Z., Grenier, G., & Ferland, F. (2023). Profiles of quality of life among patients using emergency departments for mental health reasons. *Health and Quality of Life Outcomes*, *21*(1), 116. DOI: 10.1186/s12955-023-02200-3 PMID: 37880748

Frascarelli, C., Venetis, K., Marra, A., Mane, E., Ivanova, M., Cursano, G., Porta, F. M., Concardi, A., Ceol, A. G. M., Farina, A., Criscitiello, C., Curigliano, G., Guerini-Rocco, E., & Fusco, N. (2024). Deep learning algorithm on H&E whole slide images to characterize TP53 alterations frequency and spatial distribution in breast cancer. *Computational and Structural Biotechnology Journal*, *23*, 4252–4259. DOI: 10.1016/j.csbj.2024.11.037 PMID: 39678362

Gabelaia, I., Djakeli, K., & McElroy, J. W. (2024, September). The power of customer journey mapping with artificial intelligence: a case study method. In International Conference on Reliability and Statistics in Transportation and Communication (pp. 244-257). Cham: Springer Nature Switzerland.

Gagnon, M. P., Ouellet, S., Attisso, E., Supper, W., Amil, S., Rhéaume, C., & Sasseville, M. (2024). Wearable devices for supporting chronic disease self-management: Scoping review. *Interactive Journal of Medical Research*, *13*(1), e55925. DOI: 10.2196/55925 PMID: 39652850

Garcia-Burgos, D., Wilhelm, P., Vögele, C., & Munsch, S. (2023). Food restriction in anorexia nervosa in the light of modern learning theory: A narrative review. *Behavioral Sciences (Basel, Switzerland)*, *13*(2), 96. DOI: 10.3390/bs13020096 PMID: 36829325

Gardner, R. L., Sarkar, U., Maselli, J. H., & Gonzales, R. (2007). Factors associated with longer ED lengths of stay. *The American Journal of Emergency Medicine*, *25*(6), 643–650. DOI: 10.1016/j.ajem.2006.11.037 PMID: 17606089

Gaudillo, J., Rodriguez, J. J. R., Nazareno, A., Baltazar, L. R., Vilela, J., Bulalacao, R., Domingo, M., & Albia, J. (2019). Machine learning approach to single nucleotide polymorphism-based asthma prediction. *PLoS One*, *14*(12), e0225574. DOI: 10.1371/journal.pone.0225574 PMID: 31800601

Gayap, H. T., & Akhloufi, M. A. (2024). Deep Machine Learning for Medical Diagnosis, Application to Lung Cancer Detection: A Review [Review of Deep Machine Learning for Medical Diagnosis, Application to Lung Cancer Detection: A Review]. *BioMedInformatics*, *4*(1), 236–284. DOI: 10.3390/biomedinformatics4010015

Geneviève, L. D., Martani, A., Shaw, D., Elger, B. S., & Wangmo, T. (2020). Structural racism in precision medicine: Leaving no one behind. *BMC Medical Ethics*, *21*(1), 17. DOI: 10.1186/s12910-020-0457-8 PMID: 32075640

George, J., & Karalam, S. B. R. (in progress). Research work related to migrant workers in Kerala [Unpublished working thesis]. Department of social work, Christ University, Bengaluru.

Getachew, M., Musa, I., Degefu, N., Beza, L., Hawlte, B., & Asefa, F. (2024). Emergency department overcrowding and its associated factors at HARME medical emergency center in Eastern Ethiopia. *African Journal of Emergency Medicine : Revue Africaine de la Médecine d'Urgence*, *14*(1), 26–32. DOI: 10.1016/j.afjem.2023.12.002 PMID: 38223394

Ghazzawi, H. A., Nimer, L. S., Sweidan, D. H., Alhaj, O. A., Abulawi, D., Amawi, A. T., Levine, M. P., & Jahrami, H. (2023). The global prevalence of screen-based disordered eating and associated risk factors among high school students: Systematic review, meta-analysis, and meta-regression. *Journal of Eating Disorders*, *11*(1), 128. Advance online publication. DOI: 10.1186/s40337-023-00849-1 PMID: 37537604

Gianfrancesco, M. A., Tamang, S., Yazdany, J., & Schmajuk, G. (2018). Potential biases in machine learning algorithms using electronic health record data. *JAMA Internal Medicine*, *178*(11), 1544–1547. DOI: 10.1001/jamainternmed.2018.3763 PMID: 30128552

Gigauri, I., & Djakeli, K. (2021a). National health reforms in Georgia during 1994-2021cnd their success. *HOLISTICA–Journal of Business and Public Administration*, *12*(2), 102–108. DOI: 10.2478/hjbpa-2021-0017

Gigauri, I., & Djakeli, K. (2021b). Expecting Transformation of Marketing During the Post-Pandemic New Normal: Qualitative Research of Marketing Managers in Georgia. [IJSEM]. *International Journal of Sustainable Economies Management*, *10*(2), 1–18. DOI: 10.4018/IJSEM.2021040101

Giovanola, B., & Tiribelli, S. (2023). Beyond bias and discrimination: Redefining the AI ethics principle of fairness in healthcare machine-learning algorithms. *AI & Society*, *38*(2), 549–563. DOI: 10.1007/s00146-022-01455-6 PMID: 35615443

GlobeNewswire. (2026, January 23). *Press release/knowledge base article.* https://www.einpresswire.com/knowledge-base/how-to-get-into-ai-platforms

Golmohammadi, D. (2016). Predicting hospital admissions to reduce emergency department boarding. *International Journal of Production Economics*, *182*, 535–544. DOI: 10.1016/j.ijpe.2016.09.020

Goswami, P., & Cherrier, H. (2025). Intimate neoliberal violence and ungrievable meno bodies. *Journal of Marketing Management*, *41*(3-4), 293–311. DOI: 10.1080/0267257X.2025.2470830

Graber, J. A., & Petersen, A. C. (2017). Cognitive changes at adolescence: Biological perspectives. In Baron-Cohen, S., Tager-Flusberg, H., & Lombardo, M. V. (Eds.), *Brain maturation and cognitive development* (pp. 253–280). Guilford Press. DOI: 10.4324/9781315082028-10

Greenleaf, R. K. (1977). *Servant leadership: A journey into the nature of legitimate power and greatness.* Paulist Press. https://books.google.com/books/about/Servant_Leadership.html?id=AfjUgMJlDK4C&utm_source=chatgpt.com

Groh, M., Harris, C., Daneshjou, R., Badri, O., & Koochek, A. (2022). Towards transparency in dermatology image datasets with skin tone annotations by experts, crowds, and an algorithm. *Proceedings of the ACM on Human-Computer Interaction, 6*(CSCW2), 1–26. DOI: 10.1145/3555634

Gu, C., Dai, C., Shi, X., Wu, Z., & Chen, C. (2022). *1-s2.0-S2452414X22000541-main.pdf.*

Guida, G., Bagnasco, D., Carriero, V., Bertolini, F., Ricciardolo, F. L. M., Nicola, S., Brussino, L., Nappi, E., Paoletti, G., Canonica, G. W., & Heffler, E. (2022). Critical evaluation of asthma biomarkers in clinical practice. *Frontiers in Medicine, 9*, 969243. DOI: 10.3389/fmed.2022.969243 PMID: 36300189

Gu, Z., Huang, J., Zhou, C., Wang, Q., Kong, J., You, X., Zhang, Z., & Zhao, H. (2024). Breast cancer volume alterations post-neoadjuvant chemotherapy through DenseNet-201 deep learning analysis on DCE-MRI. *Journal of Radiation Research and Applied Sciences, 17*(3), 100971. DOI: 10.1016/j.jrras.2024.100971

Haider, S. A., Borna, S., Gomez-Cabello, C. A., Pressman, S. M., Haider, C. R., & Forte, A. J. (2024). The algorithmic divide: A systematic review on AI-driven racial disparities in healthcare. *Journal of Racial and Ethnic Health Disparities*. Advance online publication. DOI: 10.1007/s40615-024-02237-0 PMID: 39695057

Hakkoum, H., Idri, A., & Abnane, I. (2024). Global and local interpretability techniques of supervised machine learning black box models for numerical medical data. *Engineering Applications of Artificial Intelligence, 131*, 107829. DOI: 10.1016/j.engappai.2023.107829

Halabieh, H., Hawkins, S., Bernstein, A. E., Lewkowict, S., Unaldi Kamel, B., Fleming, L., & Levitin, D. (2022). The future of higher education: Identifying current educational problems and proposed solutions. *Education Sciences, 12*(12), 888. DOI: 10.3390/educsci12120888

Hankin, B. L. (2006). Adolescent depression: Description, causes, and interventions. *Epilepsy & Behavior, 8*(1), 102–114. DOI: 10.1016/j.yebeh.2005.10.012 PMID: 16356779

Harrison, A. L., Shields, N., Watson, M. J., & Taylor, N. F. (2021). Gestational diabetes mellitus screening and care: A review of challenges and opportunities for improvement. *Diabetes Research and Clinical Practice, 175*, 108789.

Harrop, E. N., Mensinger, J. L., Moore, M., & Lindhorst, T. (2021). Restrictive eating disorders in higher weight persons: A systematic review of atypical anorexia nervosa prevalence and consecutive admission literature. *International Journal of Eating Disorders, 54*(8), 1328–1357. DOI: 10.1002/eat.23519 PMID: 33864277

Harrou, F., Dairi, A., Kadri, F., & Sun, Y. (2020). (2 0 2 0). Forecasting emergency department overcrowding: A deep learning framework. *Chaos, Solitons, and Fractals, 139*, 110247. DOI: 10.1016/j.chaos.2020.110247 PMID: 32982079

Hassan, A., Khan, H., Ali, A., Din, I. U., Sajid, A., Husain, M., Ali, M., Naz, A., & Fakhar, H. (2024). An Enhanced Lung Cancer Identification and Classification Based on Advanced Deep Learning and Convolutional Neural Network. [BBE]. *Bulletin of Business and Economics, 13*(2), 136–141. DOI: 10.61506/01.00308

Hassan, M., Kushniruk, A., & Borycki, E. (2024). Barriers to and facilitators of artificial intelligence adoption in health care: Scoping review. *JMIR Human Factors, 11*, e48633. DOI: 10.2196/48633 PMID: 39207831

Havlik, D. (2024). TELEMEDICINE AND RURAL HEALTHCARE ACCESS: A COMPARATIVE ANALYSIS OF EMERGING TECHNOLOGIES. *Journal of Population Therapeutics and Clinical Pharmacology = Journal de la Thérapeutique des Populations et de la Pharmacologie Clinique, 169*, 169–179. Advance online publication. DOI: 10.53555/37d41t64

Heifetz, R. A. (1994). *Leadership without easy answers.* Harvard University Press. DOI: 10.4159/9780674038479

Hermann, J., Jansen, N., & Dogangün, A. (2025). We need to understand where the data comes from: Co-designing transparent AI systems for caregiving. In *Companion Proceedings of the 30th International Conference on Intelligent User Interfaces* (pp. 105–109). ACM. DOI: 10.1145/3708557.3716354

Herrera-Poyatos, A., Del Ser, J., López de Prado, M., Wang, F.-Y., Herrera-Viedma, E., & de Prado, M. (2025). Responsible artificial intelligence systems: A roadmap to society's trust through trustworthy AI, auditability, accountability, and governance. *arXiv*.

Hirst, J. E., Raynes-Greenow, C. H., & Jeffery, H.. (2015). Smartphone education supports improved self-management in gestational diabetes mellitus. *Diabetic Medicine, 32*(8), 1057–1065.

Hobbs, C. (2020). *EUROPE'S DIGITAL SOVEREIGNTY: FROM RULEMAKER TO SUPERPOWER IN THE AGE OF US-CHINA RIVALRY.*

Horgan, D., Romao, M., Morré, S. A., & Kalra, D. (2019). Artificial Intelligence: Power for Civilisation – and for Better Healthcare. *Public Health Genomics*, *22*(5-6), 145–161. DOI: 10.1159/000504785 PMID: 31838476

Horwitz, L. I., Green, J., & Bradley, E. H. (2010). US emergency department performance on wait time and length of visit. *Annals of Emergency Medicine*, *55*(2), 133–141. DOI: 10.1016/j.annemergmed.2009.07.023 PMID: 19796844

Hsieh, C. C., Lee, C. C., Hsu, H. C., Shih, H. I., Lu, C. H., & Lin, C. H. (2017). Impact of delayed admission to intensive care units on patients with acute respiratory failure. *The American Journal of Emergency Medicine*, *35*(1), 39–44. DOI: 10.1016/j.ajem.2016.09.066 PMID: 27742520

Hung, J. (2022). Policy development on upskilling/reskilling older population care staff in China. *International Journal of Environmental Research and Public Health*, *19*(15), 9440. DOI: 10.3390/ijerph19159440 PMID: 35954791

Husnain, A., Rasool, S., Saeed, A., Gill, A. Y., & Hussain, H. K. (2023). AI'S Healing Touch: Examining Machine Learning's Transformative Effects On Healthcare. *Journal of Wood Science*, *2*(10), 1681–1695. DOI: 10.58344/jws.v2i10.448

IBM. (2025). *What is edge AI?* https://www.ibm.com/think/topics/edge-ai

Ikeda, S., Nishimura, N., Sukegawa, N., & Takano, Y. (2023). Prescriptive price optimization using optimal regression trees. *Operations Research Perspectives*, *11*, 100290. DOI: 10.1016/j.orp.2023.100290

Iloanusi, N.-J., & Chun, S. A. (2024). AI impact on health equity for marginalized, racial, and ethnic minorities. In *Proceedings of the 25th Annual International Conference on Digital Government Research* (pp. 841–848). ACM. https://doi.org/DOI: 10.1145/3657054.3657152

Instagram (n.d.) Cultural expectations faced by new mothers [Reel]. Available at: https://www.instagram.com/reel/DIgX70NSHkH/?igsh=MWNmYWI0MHN3Y3hzcQ== (accessed 10 June 2025).

Instagram (n.d.) Emotional reel about postpartum exhaustion and healing [Reel]. Available at: https://www.instagram.com/reel/DEucL-UTlah/?igsh=MW85emtucDZ3ZGViZQ== (accessed 10 June 2025).

Instagram (n.d.) Relatable postpartum struggles shared by Indian mom [Reel]. Available at: https://www.instagram.com/reel/CurGHCBIbxS/?igsh=MXE5eGJlZTZleHFtNg== (accessed 10 June 2025).

International Labour Organization. (2018). *Women and men in the informal economy: A statistical picture* (3rd ed.). International Labour Office. https://www.ilo.org/global/publications/books/WCMS_626831/lang--cn/indcx.htm

Iuga, A. O., & McGuire, M. J. (2014). Adherence and health care costs. *Risk Management and Healthcare Policy, 7*, 35–44. DOI: 10.2147/RMHP.S19801 PMID: 24591853

Jeyaraman, M., Balaji, S., Jeyaraman, N., & Yadav, S. (2023). Unraveling the Ethical Enigma: Artificial Intelligence in Healthcare [Review of *Unraveling the Ethical Enigma: Artificial Intelligence in Healthcare*]. *Cureus*. Cureus, Inc. DOI: 10.7759/cureus.43262

Jha, D., Durak, G., Sharma, V., Keleş, E., Çiçek, V., Zhang, Z., Srivastava, A., Rauniyar, A., Hagos, D. H., Tomar, N. K., Miller, F. H., Topcu, A. E., Yazidi, A., Håkegård, J. E., & Bağcı, U. (2025). A Conceptual Framework for Applying Ethical Principles of AI to Medical Practice. *Bioengineering (Basel, Switzerland), 12*(2), 180. DOI: 10.3390/bioengineering12020180 PMID: 40001699

Jin, J., Zhang, Z., & Luo, C. (2025). From perceived threat to coping strategies: Exploring the role of social media and its impact on loneliness and anxiety during the COVID-19 quarantine. *Frontiers in Psychology, 16*, 1514669. DOI: 10.3389/fpsyg.2025.1514669 PMID: 40918271

Joy, J., & Srihari, M. (2014). A Case study on the school dropout Scheduled Tribal students of Wayanad District, Kerala. *Research Journal of Educational Sciences*, ISSN,2321, 0508

K, B. T. P., P, J., & S, K. (2025). Asthma Disease Prediction using Machine Learning Classifiers. *2025 International Conference on Intelligent Computing and Control Systems (ICICCS)*, 799–805. DOI: 10.1109/ICICCS65191.2025.10985563

K, L., Ganjekar, S., S, M. K., S, V. H., Philip, M., G, S., Rajaram, D., Acharya, S., Vaiphei, K., & R, S. A. (2024). Study on awareness and management based health action using video intervention (SAMBHAV) for postpartum depression among mothers attending immunisation clinic in a tertiary medical college hospital: Study protocol. *PLoS ONE, 19*(4), e0301357. https://doi.org/DOI: 10.1371/journal.pone.0301357

Kassab, S., & Devens, C. (2022). *The exponential demand for comput*ing. Messari. https://messari.io/report/the-exponential-demand-for-compute

Kaufman, N., Stone, K., & Holland, E. (2020). Digital interventions with personalised feedback improve adherence in gestational diabetes management. *Journal of Medical Internet Research, 22*(4), e15515.

Kerns, J., Itriyeva, K., & Fisher, M. (2022). Etiology and management of amenorrhea in adolescent and young adult women. *Current Problems in Pediatric and Adolescent Health Care, 52*(5), 101184. DOI: 10.1016/j.cppeds.2022.101184 PMID: 35525789

Khalifa, A., & Hussein, R. (2025). Artificial Intelligence For 6P Medicine: Consolidating AI Needs of Predictive, Preventive, Personalized, Participatory, Precision, and Public Health Trajectories. Research Square *(*Research Square*)*. DOI: 10.21203/rs.3.rs-7402571/v1

Khan, R. H., Miah, J., Nipun, S. A. A., Islam, M., Amin, M. S., & Taluckder, M. S. (2023). Enhancing Lung Cancer Diagnosis with Machine Learning Methods and Systematic Review Synthesis. *2021 7th International Conference on Electrical, Electronics and Information Engineering (ICEEIE)*, 1. DOI: 10.1109/ICEEIE59078.2023.10334739

Kim, H., Lee, S., & Lee, M.-H.. (2019). Challenges in sustaining engagement with mobile health apps among women with gestational diabetes. *BMC Pregnancy and Childbirth, 19*, 108.

Kim, S. H., Kim, J. Y., Kim, G. B., Yu, J. J., & Choi, J. W. (2021). Diagnosis of coronary artery abnormalities in patients with Kawasaki disease according to established guidelines and Z score formulas. *Journal of the American Society of Echocardiography, 34*(6), 662–672. DOI: 10.1016/j.echo.2021.01.002 PMID: 33422668

Kirelli, Y., Arslankaya, S., Koçer, H. B., & Harmantepe, T. (2023). CNN-based deep learning method for predicting the disease response to the neoadjuvant chemotherapy (NAC) treatment in breast cancer. *Heliyon, 9*(6), e16812. DOI: 10.1016/j.heliyon.2023.e16812 PMID: 37303531

Krause, D. (2024). Addressing the challenges of auditing and testing for AI bias: A comparative analysis of regulatory frameworks. SSRN *Electronic Journal.* https://doi.org/DOI: 10.2139/ssrn.5050631

Kumar, A., Masud, M., Alsharif, M. H., Gaur, N., & Nanthaamornphong, A. (2025). Integrating 6G technology in smart hospitals: Challenges and opportunities for enhanced healthcare services. *Frontiers in Medicine, 12*, 1534551. DOI: 10.3389/fmed.2025.1534551 PMID: 40255587

Kumar, S. (2025). Patient-centered AI. *Frontiers in Digital Health, 7*, 1638098. Advance online publication. DOI: 10.3389/fdgth.2025.1638098 PMID: 40881731

Kunc, P., Fabry, J., Lucanska, M., & Pecova, R. (2020). Biomarkers of Bronchial Asthma. *Physiological Research*, •••, S29–S34. DOI: 10.33549/physiolres.934398 PMID: 32228009

Kyriako, D. N., Ricketts, V., Dyne, P. L., McCullough, M. D., & Talan, A. (1999). A 5-year time study analysis of emergency department patient care efficiency. *Annals of Emergency Medicine*, *34*(3), 326–335. DOI: 10.1016/S0196-0644(99)70126-5 PMID: 10459088

Lam, P. C., John, D. A., Galfalvy, H., Kunzel, C., & Lewis-Fernández, R. (2019). Oral health–related quality of life among publicly insured mental health service outpatients with serious mental illness. *Psychiatric Services (Washington, D.C.)*, *70*(12), 1101–1109. DOI: 10.1176/appi.ps.201900111 PMID: 31522632

Lau, P. L. (2025). *Rewriting the narrative of AI bias: A data feminist critique of algorithmic inequalities in healthcare*. Law, Technology and Humans., DOI: 10.5204/lthj.3845

Lazarus, R. S., & Folkman, S. (1984). *Stress, appraisal, and coping*. Springer. https://link.springer.com/book/10.1007/978-1-4419-1006-9

Le, L. K. D., Esturas, A. C., Mihalopoulos, C., Chiotelis, O., Bucholc, J., Chatterton, M. L., & Engel, L. (2021). Cost-effectiveness evidence of mental health prevention and promotion interventions: A systematic review of economic evaluations. *PLoS Medicine*, *18*(5), e1003606. DOI: 10.1371/journal.pmed.1003606 PMID: 33974641

Levy, R., Goldstein, B., & Trott, A. (1984). Approach to quality assurance in an emergency department: A one-year review. *Annals of Emergency Medicine*, *13*(3), 166–169. DOI: 10.1016/S0196-0644(84)80606-X PMID: 6696304

Li, D., Abhadiomhen, S. E., Zhou, D., Shen, X.-J., Shi, L., & Cui, Y. (2024). Asthma prediction via affinity graph enhanced classifier: A machine learning approach based on routine blood biomarkers. *Journal of Translational Medicine*, *22*(1), 100. DOI: 10.1186/s12967-024-04866-9 PMID: 38268004

Li, J. H., Tseng, Y. J., Chen, S. H., & Chen, K. F. (2025). Artificial Intelligence in Infection Surveillance: Data Integration, Applications and Future Directions. *Biomedical Journal*, •••, 100929. DOI: 10.1016/j.bj.2025.100929 PMID: 41205676

Li, J., Theng, Y. L., & Foo, S. (2020). Game-based digital interventions for depression therapy: A systematic review and meta-analysis. *Cyberpsychology, Behavior, and Social Networking*, *23*(8), 543–552. DOI: 10.1089/cyber.2019.0700 PMID: 24810933

Ling, Y.-L., Rascati, K. L., & Pawaskar, M. (2017). Direct and indirect costs among patients with binge-eating disorder in the United States. *International Journal of Eating Disorders*, *50*(5), 523–532. DOI: 10.1002/eat.22631 PMID: 27862132

Li, S., Ma, H., Zhang, Y., Wang, S., Guo, R., He, W., Xu, J., & Xie, Z. (2023). Emergency evacuation risk assessment method for educational buildings based on improved extreme learning machine. *Reliability Engineering & System Safety*, *238*, 109454. DOI: 10.1016/j.ress.2023.109454

Liu, B., Zhou, H., Tan, L., Siu, K. T. H., & Guan, X. (2024). Exploring treatment options in cancer: tumor treatment strategies [Review of *Exploring treatment options in cancer: tumor treatment strategies*]. *Signal Transduction and Targeted Therapy*, *9*(1), 175. Springer Nature. DOI: 10.1038/s41392-024-01856-7

Liu, N. H., Daumit, G. L., Dua, T., Aquila, R., Charlson, F., Cuijpers, P., Druss, B., Dudek, K., Freeman, M., Fujii, C., Gaebel, W., Hegerl, U., Levav, I., Munk Laursen, T., Ma, H., Maj, M., Elena Medina-Mora, M., Nordentoft, M., Prabhakaran, D., & Saxena, S. (2017). Excess mortality in persons with severe mental disorders: A multilevel intervention framework and priorities for clinical practice, policy and research agendas. *World Psychiatry; Official Journal of the World Psychiatric Association (WPA)*, *16*(1), 30–40. DOI: 10.1002/wps.20384 PMID: 28127922

Lombi, L., & Rossero, E. (2024). How artificial intelligence is reshaping the autonomy and boundary work of radiologists: A qualitative study. *Sociology of Health & Illness*, *46*(2), 200–218. DOI: 10.1111/1467-9566.13702 PMID: 37573551

Lu, L., & Huang, T. (2022). Effects of early nursing monitoring on pregnancy outcomes of pregnant women with gestational diabetes mellitus under the Internet of Things. *Computational and Mathematical Methods in Medicine*, *2022*(1), 8535714. DOI: 10.1155/2022/8535714 PMID: 35693264

Mahanta, P., Deuri, S. P., & Sobhana, H. (2021). Importance of Life Skills Education

Mahara, G., Tian, C., Xu, X., & Wang, W. (2023). Revolutionising health care: Exploring the latest advances in medical sciences. *Journal of Global Health*, *13*, 03042. Advance online publication. DOI: 10.7189/jogh.13.03042 PMID: 37539846

Mahendrakar, N. (2025). Adopting Technologies in Medical and Healthcare Systems. *International Journal for Research in Applied Science and Engineering Technology*, *13*(7), 1997–2009. DOI: 10.22214/ijraset.2025.73297

Mahmood, S., Hasan, R., Hussain, S., & Adhikari, R. (2025). An Interpretable and Generalizable Machine Learning Model for Predicting Asthma Outcomes: Integrating AutoML and Explainable AI Techniques. *WORLD (Oakland, Calif.)*, *6*(1), 15. DOI: 10.3390/world6010015

Maitra, A., & Chikhani, C. (1992). Patient satisfaction in an urban accident and emergency department. *International Journal of Clinical Practice*, *46*(3), 182–184. DOI: 10.1111/j.1742-1241.1992.tb10335.x PMID: 1286019

Malgaroli, M., Hull, T. D., Zech, J. M., & Althoff, T. (2023). Natural language processing for mental health interventions: A systematic review and research framework. *Translational Psychiatry*, *13*(1), 309. DOI: 10.1038/s41398-023-02592-2 PMID: 37798296

Mamandipoor, B., Bruno, R. R., Wernly, B., Wolff, G., Fjølner, J., Artigas, A., Pinto, B. B., Schefold, J. C., Kelm, M., Beil, M., Sigal, S., Leaver, S., De Lange, D. W., Guidet, B., Flaatten, H., Szczeklik, W., Jung, C., & Osmani, V. (2022). COVID-19 machine learning model predicts outcomes in older patients from various European countries, between pandemic waves, and in a cohort of Asian, African, and American patients. *PLOS Digital Health*, *1*(11), e0000136. DOI: 10.1371/journal.pdig.0000136 PMID: 36812571

Marais, D. L., & Petersen, I. (2015). Health system governance to support integrated mental health care in South Africa: Challenges and opportunities. *International Journal of Mental Health Systems*, *9*(1), 14. DOI: 10.1186/s13033-015-0004-z PMID: 25806085

Martinez, R. G., & van Dongen, D. M. (2023). Deep learning algorithms for the early detection of breast cancer: A comparative study with traditional machine learning. *Informatics in Medicine Unlocked*, *41*, 101317. DOI: 10.1016/j.imu.2023.101317

Maxwell, K., Rajabi, M., Esterle, J., Tivane, M., & Travassos, D. (2024). Spatial modelling and classification of altered coal using random forest- based methods at Moatize Basin, Mozambique. *Journal of African Earth Sciences*, *215*, 105279. DOI: 10.1016/j.jafrearsci.2024.105279

McCradden, M. D., Joshi, S., Mazwi, M., & Anderson, J. A. (2020). Ethical limitations of algorithmic fairness solutions in health care machine learning. *The Lancet. Digital Health*, *2*(5), e221–e223. DOI: 10.1016/S2589-7500(20)30065-0 PMID: 33328054

McLean, A. L. (2023, July 14). Towards Precision Medicine in Spinal Surgery: Leveraging AI Technologies. In *Annals of Biomedical Engineering* (Vol. 52, Issue 4, p. 735). Springer Science+Business Media. DOI: 10.1007/s10439-023-03315-w

McLeod, C., Jokwiro, Y., Gong, Y., Irvine, S., & Edvardsson, K. (2021). Undergraduate nursing student and preceptors' experiences of clinical placement through an innovative clinical school supervision model. *Nurse Education in Practice*, *51*, 102986. DOI: 10.1016/j.nepr.2021.102986 PMID: 33621926

McRae, S. (2021). Long-term forecasting of regional demand for hospital services. *Operations Research for Health Care*, *28*, 100289. DOI: 10.1016/j.orhc.2021.100289

Meczekalski, B., Podfigurna-Stopa, A., & Katulski, K. (2013). Long-term consequences of anorexia nervosa. *Maturitas*, *75*(3), 215–220. DOI: 10.1016/j.maturitas.2013.04.014 PMID: 23706279

Mergen, A., Çetin-Kılıç, N., & Özbilgin, M. F. (2025). Artificial intelligence and bias towards marginalised groups: Theoretical roots and challenges. In Vassilopoulou, J., & Kyriakidou, O. (Eds.), *International perspectives on equality, diversity and inclusion* (pp. 17–38). Emerald Publishing Limited., DOI: 10.1108/S2051-233320250000012004

Miao, K., Hounye, A. H., Su, L., Pan, Q., Wang, J., Hou, M., & Xiong, L. (2024). Exploring explainable machine learning and Shapley additive exPlanations (SHAP) technique to uncover key factors of HNSC cancer: An analysis of the best practices. *Biomedical Signal Processing and Control*, *89*, 105752. DOI: 10.1016/j.bspc.2023.105752

Ministry of Tribal Affairs, Government of India. (2013), *Annual Report.* https://tribal.nic.in/downloads/Statistics/AnnualReport/AR2013-14.pdf

Miremberg, H., Ben-Ari, T., & Betzer, T.. (2018). The impact of a smartphone-based daily monitoring system on care quality and glycaemic control in gestational diabetes. *American Journal of Obstetrics and Gynecology*, *218*(4), 448.e1–448.e7. DOI: 10.1016/j.ajog.2018.01.044 PMID: 29425836

Mitera, B., & Harasimowicz, K. (2024). Balancing Act: The Dual Impacts of AI and Healthcare Algorithms on Patient Welfare in Telemedicine. *European Research Studies*, *243*(2), 243–254. Advance online publication. DOI: 10.35808/ersj/3400

Mohindra, K. S., Narayana, D., Harikrishnadas, C., Anushreedha, S., & Haddad, S. (2010). Paniya Voices: A Participatory Poverty and Health Assessment among a marginalized South Indian tribal population. *BMC Public Health*, *10*(1), 149. Advance online publication. DOI: 10.1186/1471-2458-10-149 PMID: 20307290

Morales-Forero, A., Rueda Jaime, L., Gil-Quiñones, S. R., Barrera Montañez, M. Y., Bassetto, S., & Coatanea, E. (2024). An insight into racial bias in dermoscopy repositories: A HAM10000 data set analysis. *JEADV Clinical Practice*, *3*(3), 836–843. DOI: 10.1002/jvc2.477

Mordor Intelligence. (2024). *Latin America medical imaging software market size & share analysis – Growth trends & forecasts (2024–2029).* https://www.mordorintelligence.com/industry-reports/latin-america-medical-imaging-software-market-industry

Morley, J., & Floridi, L. (2020). An ethically mindful approach to AI for health care. *Lancet*, *395*(10220), 254–255. DOI: 10.1016/S0140-6736(19)32975-7 PMID: 31982053

Morrison-Koechl, J., Wu, S. A., Slaughter, S. E., Lengyel, C. O., Carrier, N., & Keller, H. H. (2021). Hungry for more: Low resident social engagement is indirectly associated with poor energy intake and mealtime experience in long-term care homes. *Appetite*, *159*, 105044. DOI: 10.1016/j.appet.2020.105044 PMID: 33227384

Moses, R. G., Wong, V. C., Lambert, K. A., & Morris, G. J. (2017). The management of gestational diabetes: Evidence gaps and emerging solutions. *The Medical Journal of Australia*, *207*(4), 152–158. PMID: 28814215

Msheik, B., Adda, M., Mcheick, H., Nasser, Y., & Dbouk, M. (2025). Developing Contextual Ontology for Chronic Diseases: AI-Enhanced Extension and Prediction in an Asthma Case Study. *Applied Sciences (Basel, Switzerland)*, *15*(8), 4353. DOI: 10.3390/app15084353

Munk, A. K., Jacomy, M., Ficozzi, M., & Jensen, T. E. (2024). Beyond artificial intelligence controversies: What are algorithms doing in the scientific literature? *Big Data & Society*, *11*(3), 20539517241255107. DOI: 10.1177/20539517241255107

Nadarzynski, T., Knights, N., Husbands, D., Graham, C. A., Llewellyn, C. D., Buchanan, T., Montgomery, I., & Ridge, D. (2024). Achieving health equity through conversational AI: A roadmap for design and implementation of inclusive chatbots in healthcare. *PLOS Digital Health*, *3*(5), e0000492. DOI: 10.1371/journal.pdig.0000492 PMID: 38696359

Najjar, R. (2024). Digital Frontiers in Healthcare: Integrating mHealth, AI, and Radiology for Future Medical Diagnostics. In *Biomedical engineering*. DOI: 10.5772/intechopen.114142

Nazer, L. H., Zatarah, R., Waldrip, S., Ke, J. X. C., Moukheiber, M., Khanna, A. K., Hicklen, R. S., Moukheiber, L., Moukheiber, D., Ma, H., & Mathur, P. (2023). Bias in artificial intelligence algorithms and recommendations for mitigation. *PLOS Digital Health, 2*(6), e0000278. DOI: 10.1371/journal.pdig.0000278 PMID: 37347721

Nerney, M. P., Chin, M. H., Jin, L., Karrison, T. G., Walter, J., Mulliken, R., Miller, A., Hayley, D. C., & Friedmann, P. D. (2001). Factors associated with older patients' satisfaction with care in an inner-city emergency department. *Annals of Emergency Medicine, 38*(2), 140–145. DOI: 10.1067/mem.2001.114304 PMID: 11468608

Nguyen, M. (2024). A scoping review of deep learning approaches for lung cancer detection using chest radiographs and computed tomography scans [Review of *A scoping review of deep learning approaches for lung cancer detection using chest radiographs and computed tomography scans*]. *Biomedical Engineering Advances, 9*, 100138. Elsevier BV. DOI: 10.1016/j.bea.2024.100138

Nohara, Y., Matsumoto, K., Soejima, H., & Nakashima, N. (2022). Explanation of machine learning models using shapley additive explanation and application for real data in hospital. *Computer Methods and Programs in Biomedicine, 214*, 106584. DOI: 10.1016/j.cmpb.2021.106584 PMID: 34942412

Nordin, N., Zainol, Z., Noor, M. H. M., & Chan, L. F. (2023). An explainable predictive model for suicide attempt risk using an ensemble learning and Shapley Additive Explanations (SHAP) approach. *Asian Journal of Psychiatry, 79*, 103316. DOI: 10.1016/j.ajp.2022.103316 PMID: 36395702

O'Malley, A., Veenhuizen, M., & Ahmed, A. (2024). Ensuring appropriate representation in artificial intelligence–generated medical imagery: Protocol for a methodological approach to address skin tone bias. *JMIR AI, 3*, e58275. DOI: 10.2196/58275 PMID: 39602221

Obermeyer, Z., Powers, B., Vogeli, C., & Mullainathan, S. (2019). Dissecting racial bias in an algorithm used to manage the health of populations. *Science, 366*(6464), 447–453. DOI: 10.1126/science.aax2342 PMID: 31649194

Ogbewele, E. G., Mbata, A. O., & Nwosu, N. T. (2024). Advancing pharmaceutical care in rural and underserved communities: Strategies for improving global healthcare access. *International Journal of Applied Research in Social Sciences, 6*(10), 2447–2461. DOI: 10.51594/ijarss.v6i10.1641

Olshaker, J. S., & Rathlev, N. K. (2006). Emergency department overcrowding and ambulance diversion: The impact and potential solutions of extended boarding of admitted patients in the emergency department. *The Journal of Emergency Medicine, 30*(3), 351–356. DOI: 10.1016/j.jemermed.2005.05.023 PMID: 16677993

Onyeaka, H., Ejiohuo, O., Taiwo, O. R., Nnaji, N. D., Odeyemi, O. A., Duan, K., Nwaiwu, O., & Odeyemi, O. (2024). The intersection of food security and mental health in the pursuit of Sustainable Development Goals. *Nutrients*, *16*(13), 2036. DOI: 10.3390/nu16132036 PMID: 38999784

P., U., S., A., M., K., & P., D. (2022). Potential Market-Predictive Features Based Bitcoin Price Prediction Using Machine Learning Algorithms: In A. Srinivasan (Ed.), *Advances in Computational Intelligence and Robotics* (pp. 233–245). IGI Global. DOI: 10.4018/978-1-7998-8892-5.ch014

Paleri, R. J., Meena, K. S. M., Sharma, M. K., Ravish, H., Krishnamurthy, L., Joshi, R. K., & Lepcha, R. (2023). Efficacy of video-based relaxation technique to minimize stress in young adults during the COVID-19 pandemic. *Journal of Neurosciences in Rural Practice*, *14*(3), 544–546. DOI: 10.25259/JNRP_68_2023 PMID: 37692799

Panch, T., Duralde, E., Mattie, H., Kotecha, G., Celi, L. A., Wright, M., & Greaves, F. (2022). A distributed approach to the regulation of clinical AI. *PLOS Digital Health*, *1*(5), e0000040. DOI: 10.1371/journal.pdig.0000040 PMID: 36812520

Panch, T., Mattie, H., & Atun, R. (2019). Artificial intelligence and algorithmic bias: Implications for health systems. *Journal of Global Health*, *9*(2), 020318. DOI: 10.7189/jogh.09.020318 PMID: 31788229

Panigutti, C., Beretta, A., Fadda, D., Giannotti, F., Pedreschi, D., Perotti, A., & Rinzivillo, S. (2023). Co-design of human-centered, explainable AI for clinical decision support. *ACM Transactions on Interactive Intelligent Systems*, *13*(4), 1–35. DOI: 10.1145/3587271

Pao, M., & Bosk, A. (2011). Anxiety in medically ill children/adolescents. *Depression and Anxiety*, *28*(1), 40–49. DOI: 10.1002/da.20727 PMID: 20721908

Papageorgiou, A., Fisher, C., & Cross, D. (2022). "Why don't I look like her?" How adolescent girls view social media and its connection to body image. *BMC Women's Health*, *22*(1), 261. DOI: 10.1186/s12905-022-01845-4 PMID: 35761231

Patel, V., Saxena, S., Lund, C., Kohrt, B., Kieling, C., Sunkel, C., Kola, L., Chang, O., Charlson, F., O'Neill, K., & Herrman, H. (2023). Transforming mental health systems globally: Principles and policy recommendations. *Lancet*, *402*(10402), 656–666. DOI: 10.1016/S0140-6736(23)00918-2 PMID: 37597892

Patria, D. G., & Ram, B. (2024). AI and Machine Learning in Biotechnology: A Paradigm Shift in Biochemical Innovation. *International Journal of Plant Animal and Environmental Sciences*, *14*(4). Advance online publication. DOI: 10.26502/ijpaes.4490166

Peacock, A. S., Lavery, J. A., & Farrell, C.. (2020). Hybrid telemedicine models reduce clinic burden while maintaining quality of gestational diabetes care. *Obstetrics and Gynecology, 135*(3), 583–591. PMID: 32028504

Peláez-Rodríguez, C., Torres-López, R., Pérez-Aracil, J., López-Laguna, N., Sánchez-Rodríguez, S., & Salcedo-Sanz, S. (2024). An explainable machine learning approach for hospital emergency department visits forecasting using continuous training and multi-model regression. *Computer Methods and Programs in Biomedicine, 245*, 108033. DOI: 10.1016/j.cmpb.2024.108033 PMID: 38278030

Petsis, S., Karamanou, A., Kalampokis, E., & Tarabanis, K. (2022). Forecasting and explaining emergency department visits in a public hospital. *Journal of Intelligent Information Systems, 59*(2), 479–500. DOI: 10.1007/s10844-022-00716-6

Pettman, D., O'Mahen, H., Blomberg, O., Svanberg, A. S., Von Essen, L., & Woodford, J. (2023). Effectiveness of cognitive behavioural therapy-based interventions for maternal perinatal depression: A systematic review and meta-analysis. *BMC Psychiatry, 23*(1), 208. DOI: 10.1186/s12888-023-04547-9 PMID: 36991389

Precedence Research. (n.d.). *AI in the medical imaging market.* https://www.precedenceresearch.com/ai-in-medical-imaging-market

Precedence Research. (n.d.). *PrecedenceQ.* https://www.precedenceresearch.com/precedenceq/

Precedence Research. (n.d.). *Sample report: AI in the medical imaging market.* https://www.precedenceresearch.com/sample/2380

Quon, S., Johanson, T. M., Wadhwa, R., Faiz, A., Flynn, A., Anderson, G. P., Cox, A. J., West, N. P., Menden, M. P., & Allan, R. S. (2025). Technological advances in the search for a CURE for asthma. *The Medical Journal of Australia, 223*(S10). Advance online publication. DOI: 10.5694/mja2.70084 PMID: 41241859

Qure.ai. (2025). *Qure.ai FY 2024–25 impact report.* https://www.qure.ai/impact-stories/qure-ai-fy-24-25-impact-report-global-ai-healthcare-innovations

Rahna, K. A., & Nithya, R. (2022). Psycho-social Issues Faced by Tribal Adolescents. IAHRW. *International Journal of Social Sciences Review, 10*(3), 379–381.

Rajan, S. I., & Zachariah, K. C. (2019). *Emigration and remittances: New evidences from the Kerala migration survey 2018.* Centre for Development Studies. https://cds.edu/wp-content/uploads/2019/03/KMSReport2018.pdf

Rajkomar, A., Dean, J., & Kohane, I. (2019). Machine learning in medicine. *The New England Journal of Medicine, 380*(14), 1347–1358. DOI: 10.1056/NEJMra1814259 PMID: 30943338

Rashdan, O., & Brodszky, V. (2020). Productivity loss in patients with chronic diseases: A pooled economic analysis of Hungarian cost-of-illness studies. *Value in Health Regional Issues, 22*, 75–82. DOI: 10.1016/j.vhri.2020.07.572 PMID: 32798838

Rawat, D., Sharma, S., & Bhadula, S. (2023). Deep Learning Techniques in Digital Clinical Diagnostic System for Lung Cancer. *2022 8th International Conference on Advanced Computing and Communication Systems (ICACCS)*, 1232. DOI: 10.1109/ICACCS57279.2023.10113055

Razavi, J., Dhafar, H. O., & BaHammam, A. S. (2025). Transforming health care with artificial intelligence: Regulations, challenges, and future directions. *Saudi Journal for Health Sciences, 14*(1), 11–22. DOI: 10.4103/sjhs.sjhs_26_25

Reich, M. R., Javadi, D., & Ghaffar, A. (2016). Introduction to the Special Issue on "Effective Leadership for Health Systems". *Health Systems and Reform, 2*(3), 171–175. DOI: 10.1080/23288604.2016.1223978 PMID: 31514592

Reis, J. S. D., Costa, R. L., Silva, F. D. D. S., De Souza, E. D. F., Cortes, T. R., Coelho, R. H., Velasco, S. R. M., Neves, D. J. D., Sousa Filho, J. F., Barreto, C. E. C., Cabral Júnior, J. B., Dos Reis, H. S., Mendes, K. R., Lins, M. C. C., Ferreira, T. R., Vanderlei, M. H. G. D. S., Alonso, M. F., Mariano, G. L., Gomes, H. B., & Gomes, H. B. (2025). Predicting Asthma Hospitalizations from Climate and Air Pollution Data: A Machine Learning-Based Approach. *Climate (Basel), 13*(2), 23. DOI: 10.3390/cli13020023

Rescher, N. (1997). *Predicting the future: An introduction to the theory of forecasting*. State University of New York Press.

Rigla, M., Martínez-Sarriegui, I., García-Sáez, G., Pons, B., & Hernando, M. E. (2018). Gestational diabetes management using smart mobile telemedicine. *Journal of Diabetes Science and Technology, 12*(2), 260–264. DOI: 10.1177/1932296817704442 PMID: 28420257

Riley, R. D., Debray, T. P. A., Collins, G. S., Archer, L., Ensor, J., van Smeden, M., & Snell, K. I. E. (2021). Minimum sample size for external validation of a clinical prediction model with a binary outcome. *Statistics in Medicine, 40*(19), 4230–4251. DOI: 10.1002/sim.9025 PMID: 34031906

Rockhill, C., Kodish, I., DiBattisto, C., Macias, M., Varley, C., & Ryan, S. (2010). Anxiety disorders in children and adolescents. *Current Problems in Pediatric and Adolescent Health Care, 40*(4), 66–99. DOI: 10.1016/j.cppeds.2010.02.002 PMID: 20381781

Rosenbacke, R., Melhus, Å., McKee, M., & Stuckler, D. (2024). How explainable artificial intelligence can increase or decrease clinicians' trust in AI applications in health care: Systematic review. *JMIR AI, 3*, e53207. DOI: 10.2196/53207 PMID: 39476365

Ruan, J., Cai, Y., & Stensaker, B. (2024). University managers or institutional leaders? An exploration of top-level leadership in Chinese universities. *Higher Education, 87*(3), 703–719. DOI: 10.1007/s10734-023-01031-x PMID: 37362758

Rubin, H. R., & Wu, A. W. (1991). *Patient satisfaction: Its importance and how to measure it. The Business of Medicine*. Elsevier.

Ryff, C. D., & Keyes, C. L. M. (1995). The structure of psychological well-being revisited. *Journal of Personality and Social Psychology, 69*(4), 719–727. DOI: 10.1037/0022-3514.69.4.719 PMID: 7473027

SAINI. (2025). Accelerating Drug Discovery: How Agentic AI and Multi-Agent Collaboration Transform BioPharma R&D. *Journal of Information Systems Engineering & Management, 10*(59s), 545–553. DOI: 10.52783/jisem.v10i59s.12898

Sakai, K., Iwama, N., & Nishigori, H.. (2019). Adherence to self-monitoring of blood glucose in women with gestational diabetes: Barriers and facilitators. *Journal of Diabetes Investigation, 10*(6), 1608–1617.

Salamonson, Y., Everett, B., Koch, J., Wilson, I., & Davidson, P. M. (2009). Learning strategies of first year nursing and medical students: A comparative study. *International Journal of Nursing Studies, 46*(12), 1541–1547. DOI: 10.1016/j.ijnurstu.2009.05.010 PMID: 19541308

Salehi, F. (2024). The transformative role of artificial intelligence in the healthcare industry: A comprehensive analysis. *Asian Journal of Research in Medicine and Medical Science, 6*(1), 62–70.

Santana, G. O., Couto, R. de M., Loureiro, R. M., Silva, B. C. R., Rother, E. T., Paiva, J. P. Q. de, & Correia, L. R. (2023). Economic Evaluations and Equity in the Use of Artificial Intelligence in Imaging Exams for Medical Diagnosis in People With Skin, Neurological, and Pulmonary Diseases: Protocol for a Systematic Review [Review of *Economic Evaluations and Equity in the Use of Artificial Intelligence in Imaging Exams for Medical Diagnosis in People With Skin, Neurological, and Pulmonary Diseases: Protocol for a Systematic Review*]. *JMIR Research Protocols, 12*. JMIR Publications. DOI: 10.2196/48544

Santhosh, C. S. (2024). Revolutionizing Healthcare: The Transformative Power of Artificial Intelligence. *International Journal for Research in Applied Science and Engineering Technology*, *12*(5), 1581–1586. DOI: 10.22214/ijraset.2024.61755

Saranya, T. S., Deb, S., Paul, D., & Deb, S. (2022). Untold and Painful Stories of Survival: The Life of Adolescent Girls of the Paniya Tribes of Kerala, India. In *Child Safety, Welfare and Well-being: Issues and Challenges* (pp. 185-194). Singapore: Springer Singapore. https://link.springer.com/chapter/10.1007/978-981-16-9820-0_11

Saravanakumar, A. R., & Devi, K. P. (2020). Realising life through life skills: An adolescents' perspective. *Journal of Critical Reviews*, *7*(18), 1277–1282. https://www.researchgate.net/profile/Dr-saravanakumar-2/publication/342834193

SARIYILDIZ. A. Y. (2022). New Approaches to Healthcare Marketing. *DergiPark (Istanbul University)*. https://dergipark.org.tr/tr/pub/ssd/issue/72835/1143346

Sarkar, A. (2023). The Impact and Potential of Artificial Intelligence in Healthcare: A Critical Review of Current Applications and Future Directions [Review of *The Impact and Potential of Artificial Intelligence in Healthcare: A Critical Review of Current Applications and Future Directions*]. *International Journal for Research in Applied Science and Engineering Technology, 11*(8), 2089. [IJRASET]. *International Journal for Research in Applied Science and Engineering Technology*. Advance online publication. DOI: 10.22214/ijraset.2023.55537

Schmidt, U. H., Claudino, A., Fernández-Aranda, F., Giel, K. E., Griffiths, J., Hay, P. J., Kim, Y.-R., Marshall, J., Micali, N., Monteleone, A. M., Nakazato, M., Steinglass, J., Wade, T. D., Wonderlich, S., Zipfel, S., Allen, K. L., & Sharpe, H. (2025). The current clinical approach to feeding and eating disorders aimed to increase personalization of management. *World Psychiatry; Official Journal of the World Psychiatric Association (WPA)*, *24*(1), 4–31. DOI: 10.1002/wps.21263 PMID: 39810680

Schor, B. G. S., Kallina, E., Singh, J., & Blackwell, A. (2024). Meaningful transparency for clinicians: Operationalising HCXAI research with gynaecologists. In *Proceedings of the 2024 ACM Conference on Fairness, Accountability, and Transparency* (pp. 1268–1281). ACM. DOI: 10.1145/3630106.3658971

Seema, G. B., & Kumar, G. V. (2018). Impact of social skills training on self-esteem among male and female adolescent students. *Indian Journal of Positive Psychology, 9*(1), 147–151. DOI: 10.15614/ijpp.v9i01.11761

Selbst, A. D. (2021). An institutional view of algorithmic impact assessments. *Harvard Journal of Law & Technology, 35*, 117.

Seyyed-Kalantari, L., Liu, G., McDermott, M., Chen, I. Y., & Ghassemi, M. (2020). CheXclusion: Fairness gaps in deep chest X-ray classifiers. In *Biocomputing 2021: Proceedings of the Pacific Symposium* (pp. 232–243). World Scientific. https://doi.org/DOI: 10.1142/9789811232701_0022

Shearer, C., Goss, H. R., Boddy, L. M., Knowles, Z. R., Durden-Myers, E. J., & Foweather, L. (2021). Assessments related to the physical, affective and cognitive domains of physical literacy amongst children aged 7–11.9 years: A systematic review. *Sports Medicine - Open, 7*(1), 1–40. DOI: 10.1186/s40798-021-00324-8 PMID: 34046703

Shijina, A. V. (2020). Role of Mobile technology in assisting decentralization process among Paniya tribes in Wayanad, Kerala. *Antrocom: Online Journal of Anthropology, 16*(2).

Silva Didier, L., Schildkamp, K., Visscher, A. J., & Bosker, R. J. (2025). Factors influencing the implementation of a teacher professional development program to improve teaching quality. *Frontiers in Education, 10*, 1546448. DOI: 10.3389/feduc.2025.1546448

Singhal, V., Shyam, R., Singhal, S., Tiwari, A., & Mangal, D. (2025). Healthcare and cutting-edge technology: Advancements, challenges, and future prospects. [Review of *Healthcare and cutting-edge technology: Advancements, challenges, and future prospects.*]. *PubMed, 196*, 110861. National Institutes of Health. DOI: 10.1016/j.compbiomed.2025.110861

Singhal, A., Neveditsin, N., Tanveer, H., & Mago, V. (2024). Toward fairness, accountability, transparency, and ethics in AI for social media and health care: Scoping review. *JMIR Medical Informatics, 12*(1), e50048. DOI: 10.2196/50048 PMID: 38568737

Sinha, R. K. (2024). The role and impact of new technologies on healthcare systems. *Discover Health Systems, 3*(1), 96. Advance online publication. DOI: 10.1007/s44250-024-00163-w

Slimi, H., Abid, S., & Sayadi, M. (2024). Advanced deep learning strategies for breast cancer image analysis. *Journal of Radiation Research and Applied Sciences, 17*(4), 101136. DOI: 10.1016/j.jrras.2024.101136

Soltan, A. A., Yang, J., Pattanshetty, R., Novak, A., Yang, Y., Rohanian, O., Beer, S., Soltan, M. A., Thickett, D. R., Fairhead, R., Zhu, T., Eyre, D. W., Clifton, D. A., Watson, A., Bhargav, A., Tough, A., Rogers, A., Shaikh, A., Valensise, C., & Muthusami, V. (2022). Real-world evaluation of rapid and laboratory-free COVID-19 triage for emergency care: External validation and pilot deployment of artificial intelligence-driven screening. *The Lancet. Digital Health, 4*(4), e266–e278. DOI: 10.1016/S2589-7500(21)00272-7 PMID: 35279399

Sonntag, H.-J., Filippi, S., Pipis, S., & Custovic, A. (2019a). Blood Biomarkers of Sensitization and Asthma. *Frontiers in Pediatrics, 7*, 251. DOI: 10.3389/fped.2019.00251 PMID: 31275911

Spear, J., Ehrenfeld, J. M., & Miller, B. J. (2023, November 17). Applications of Artificial Intelligence in Health Care Delivery. In *Journal of Medical Systems* (Vol. 47, Issue 1). Springer Science+Business Media. DOI: 10.1007/s10916-023-02018-y

Sprivulis, P. C., Da Silva, J. A., Jacobs, I. G., Jelinek, G. A., & Frazer, A. R. (2006). The association between hospital overcrowding and mortality among patients admitted via Western Australian emergency departments. *The Medical Journal of Australia, 184*(5), 208–212. DOI: 10.5694/j.1326-5377.2006.tb00203.x PMID: 16515429

Srivastava, R. (2011). Labour migration in India: Recent trends, patterns and policy issues. *The Indian Journal of Labour Economics : the Quarterly Journal of the Indian Society of Labour Economics, 54*(3), 411–440. https://www.researchgate.net/publication/319253996_Labour_migration_in_India_Recent_trends_patterns_and_policy_issues

Stanford Institute for Human-Centered Artificial Intelligence. (2025). *AI index report 2025.* https://hai.stanford.edu/ai-index/2025-ai-index-report

State Council of Educational Research and Training (SCERT). (2016). *A study on problems and challenges of tribal adolescents in Kerala.* SCERT.

Striegel Weissman, R., & Rosselli, F. (2017). Reducing the burden of suffering from eating disorders: Unmet treatment needs, cost of illness, and the quest for cost-effectiveness. *Behaviour Research and Therapy*, *88*, 49–64. DOI: 10.1016/j.brat.2016.09.006 PMID: 28110676

Subasree, R., Nair, A. R., & Ranjan, R. (2014). The Life Skills Assessment Scale: The construction and validation of a new comprehensive scale for measuring Life Skills. *Journal of the Humanities and Social Sciences*, *19*(1), 50–58. DOI: 10.9790/0837-19195058

Subtle Medical. (n.d.). *Subtle Elite.* https://subtlemedical.com/subtle-elite/

Sudarshan, V. K., Brabrand, M., Range, T. M., & Wiil, U. K. (2021). Performance evaluation of mergence Department patient arrivals forecasting models by including meteorological and calendar information: A comparative study. *Computers in Biology and Medicine*, *135*, 104541. DOI: 10.1016/j.compbiomed.2021.104541 PMID: 34166880

Sutton, R. T., Pincock, D., Baumgart, D. C., Sadowski, D. C., Fedorak, R. N., & Kroeker, K. I. (2020). An overview of clinical decision support systems: Benefits, risks, and strategies for success. *NPJ Digital Medicine*, *3*(1), 17. DOI: 10.1038/s41746-020-0221-y PMID: 32047862

Tan, C., Chen, H., Chen, M., & Lin, Z. (2024). Rapid identification of silk products by attenuated total reflection–mid-infrared spectroscopy and extreme learning machines. *Infrared Physics & Technology*, *139*, 105334. DOI: 10.1016/j.infrared.2024.105334

Tan, L., Nguyen, N., Lopez, E., Peverini, D., Shedd, M., Alismail, A., & Nguyen, H. (2025). Artificial Intelligence in the Management of Asthma: A Review of a New Frontier in Patient Care. *Journal of Asthma and Allergy*, *18*, 1179–1191. DOI: 10.2147/JAA.S535264 PMID: 40851769

Tanzer, J. R., Dufault, M., Rioux, L. R., Machan, J., Bergeron, K., & Napoli, A. (2023). "I Was Here First, Why Did They Go Before Me": Examining Patients' Perceptions of Priority in a Psychometric Study of Emergency Department Triage. *Journal of Emergency Nursing: JEN*, *49*(2), 294–304. DOI: 10.1016/j.jen.2022.09.017 PMID: 36567152

Tao, I.. (2023). A fusion deep learning framework based on breast cancer grade prediction. *Digital Communications and Networks.*

Tariq, S. (2023). AI and ethics: Interdisciplinary perspectives on algorithmic transparency and bias. *Multidisciplinary Research in Computer and Information Systems*, *3*(4), 256–266.

Tavares, D., Freire, T., & Faria, S. (2020). Internal and external factors underlying variations in adolescents' daily optimal experiences. *Journal of Research on Adolescence, 30*(1), 266–284. DOI: 10.1111/jora.12522 PMID: 31246377

Ter Beek, M., Wopereis, I., & Schildkamp, K. (2022). Don't Wait, Innovate! Preparing Students and Lecturers in Higher Education for the Future Labor Market. *Education Sciences, 12*(9), 620. DOI: 10.3390/educsci12090620

Thomas, L. R., Ripp, J. A., & Duncan, J. G. (2024). Graduate medical education well-being directors in the United States: Who are they, and what does the role entail? *BMC Medical Education, 24*(1), 254. DOI: 10.1186/s12909-024-05243-2 PMID: 38459448

Thomas, L., Rajeev, P. V., & Philip, S. (2020). Health crises and migrant vulnerabilities in Kerala: Lessons from COVID-19. *The Indian Journal of Social Work, 81*(4), 523–540. DOI: 10.1177/0020872820951150

Tibble, H., Sheikh, A., & Tsanas, A. (2025). Development and validation of a machine learning risk prediction model for asthma attacks in adults in primary care. *NPJ Primary Care Respiratory Medicine, 35*(1), 24. DOI: 10.1038/s41533-025-00428-8 PMID: 40268974

Tiotiu, A. (2018). Biomarkers in asthma: State of the art. *Asthma Research and Practice, 4*(1), 10. DOI: 10.1186/s40733-018-0047-4 PMID: 30598830

Tippur, A. (2023). AI-Powered Precision Oncology: Computational Insights Redefining Therapeutic Landscapes. *DHR Proceedings*. DOI: 10.47488/dhrp.v3iS1.95

Topol, E. J. (2019). High-performance medicine: The convergence of human and artificial intelligence. *Nature Medicine, 25*(1), 44–56. DOI: 10.1038/s41591-018-0300-7 PMID: 30617339

Torous, J., Bucci, S., Bell, I. H., Kessing, L. V., Faurholt-Jepsen, M., Whelan, P., Carvalho, A. F., Keshavan, M., Linardon, J., & Firth, J. (2021). The growing field of digital psychiatry: Current evidence and the future of apps, social media, chatbots, and virtual reality. *World Psychiatry; Official Journal of the World Psychiatric Association (WPA), 20*(3), 318–335. DOI: 10.1002/wps.20883 PMID: 34505369

Trzmielak, D., Lipka-Matusiak, I., & Oftedal, E. M. (2024). Responsible Innovation in E-Health Care: Empowering Patients with Emerging Technologies. *Marketing of Scientific and Research Organizations, 52*(2), 68–87. DOI: 10.2478/minib-2024-0010

Tsay, S. F., Chang, C. Y., Hung, S. S., Su, J. Y., Kuo, C. Y., & Mu, P. F. (2024). Pain prediction model based on machine learning and SHAP values for elders with dementia in Taiwan. *International Journal of Medical Informatics*, *188*, 105475. DOI: 10.1016/j.ijmedinf.2024.105475 PMID: 38743995

Turcatel, G., Xiao, Y., Caveney, S., Gnacadja, G., Kim, J., & Molfino, N. A. (2025). Predicting Asthma Exacerbations Using Machine Learning Models. *Advances in Therapy*, *42*(1), 362–374. DOI: 10.1007/s12325-024-03053-y PMID: 39556295

U.S. Food and Drug Administration. (2019). *Proposed regulatory framework for modifications to artificial intelligence/machine learning (AI/ML)-based software as a medical device (SaMD): Discussion paper and request for feedback.*

Udegbe, F. C., Ebulue, O. R., Ebulue, C. C., & Ekesiobi, C. S. (2024). The Role of Artificial Intelligence in Healthcare: A Systematic Review of Applications and Challenges [Review Of *The Role Of Artificial Intelligence In Healthcare: A Systematic Review Of Applications And Challenges*]. *International Medical Science Research Journal, 4*(4), 500. Fair East Publishers. DOI: 10.51594/imsrj.v4i4.1052

Umamaheswari, P., & Ramaswamy, V. (2024). Enhancing Rainfall Prediction Accuracy Through Fog Computing: Integration of Advanced Algorithms and Edge Analytics. In Revathy, G. (Ed.), (pp. 53–72). Advances in Systems Analysis, Software Engineering, and High Performance Computing. IGI Global., DOI: 10.4018/979-8-3693-1694-8.ch004

UNICEF. (2005). Life skills-Based Education in South Asia, A Regional Overview Prepared For: The South Asia Life Skills-Based Education Forum. *Paris: The United Nations Children's Fund (UNICEF).*

UNICEF. (2017*). Improving work outcomes for young people: What role for skills? Evidence review* (March 17, 004_edited_002). Retrieved from https://www.unicef.org/india/media/2571/file/Comprehensive-lifeskills-framework.pdf

Vallée, A. (2023). Digital twin for healthcare systems. *Frontiers in Digital Health*, *5*, 1253050. DOI: 10.3389/fdgth.2023.1253050 PMID: 37744683

Van der Velden, B. H., Kuijf, H. J., Gilhuijs, K. G., & Viergever, M. A. (2022). Explainable artificial intelligence (XAI) in deep learning-based medical image analysis. *Medical Image Analysis*, *79*, 102470. DOI: 10.1016/j.media.2022.102470 PMID: 35576821

Vats, K. (2024). Navigating the Digital Landscape: Embracing Innovation, Addressing Challenges, and Prioritizing Patient-Centric Care. *Cureus*. Advance online publication. DOI: 10.7759/cureus.58352 PMID: 38756283

Vayena, E., & Blasimme, A. (2018). Health research with big data: Time for systemic oversight. *The Journal of Law, Medicine & Ethics*, *46*(1), 119–129. DOI: 10.1177/1073110518766026 PMID: 30034208

Wang, C., & Fan, J. (2024). On the convergence of gradient descent for robust functional linear regression. *Journal of Complexity*, *84*, 101858. DOI: 10.1016/j.jco.2024.101858

Wang, J., Haq, A. U., Afzal, N., Khan, S., Alsolai, H., Alanazi, S. M., & Zamani, A. T. (2025). Developing an innovative lung cancer detection model for accurate diagnosis in AI healthcare systems. *Scientific Reports*, *15*(1), 22945. Advance online publication. DOI: 10.1038/s41598-025-03960-2 PMID: 40592932

Wang, Z., Liu, J., Shuai, H., Cai, Z., Fu, X., Liu, Y., Xiao, X., Zhang, W., Krabbendam, E., Liu, S., Liu, Z., Li, Z., & Yang, B. X. (2021). Mapping global prevalence of depression among postpartum women. *Translational Psychiatry*, *11*(1), 543. DOI: 10.1038/s41398-021-01663-6 PMID: 34671011

Wani, N. A., Kumar, R., & Bedi, J. (2023). DeepXplainer: An interpretable deep learning based approach for lung cancer detection using explainable artificial intelligence. *Computer Methods and Programs in Biomedicine*, *243*, 107879. DOI: 10.1016/j.cmpb.2023.107879 PMID: 37897989

Wegmann, E., Schiebener, J., & Brand, M. (2023). Social-networks use as adaptive or maladaptive strategy for coping with stress. *Scientific Reports*, *13*(1), 11895. DOI: 10.1038/s41598-023-39042-4 PMID: 37482602

Wei, W., Zhang, L., Ying, T., & Zheng, Y. (2025). Pet influencer marketing appeal in hotel booking: Exploring the power of message appeal and boundary conditions. *International Journal of Hospitality Management*, *126*, 104094. DOI: 10.1016/j.ijhm.2025.104094

Wheatley, H. (2022). Google Cloud's medical imaging suite to make AI-based diagnosis more accessible. *SiliconANGLE*. https://siliconangle.com/2022/10/04/google-clouds-medical-imaging-suite-make-ai-based-diagnosis-accessible/

Whicher, D., Ahmed, M., Israni, S. T., & Matheny, M. (2023). Artificial intelligence in health care: The hope, the hype, the promise, the peril.

Whitt, W., & Zhang, X. (2019). Forecasting arrivals and occupancy levels in an emergency department. *Operations Research for Health Care*, *21*, 1–18. DOI: 10.1016/j.orhc.2019.01.002

WHO. (2024). World Health Organization. Ethics and governance of artificial intelligence for health: WHO guidance. Geneva: World Health Organization; 2021. ISBN 9789240029200. Disponible sur https://iris.who.int/handle/10665/341996

Williams, D. R., & Mohammed, S. A. (2009). Discrimination and racial disparities in health: Evidence and needed research. *Journal of Behavioral Medicine*, *32*(1), 20–47. DOI: 10.1007/s10865-008-9185-0 PMID: 19030981

Willis, C. D., Saul, J. E., Bitz, J., Pompu, K., Best, A., & Jackson, B. (2014). Improving organizational capacity to address health literacy in public health: A rapid realist review. *Public Health*, *128*(6), 515–524. DOI: 10.1016/j.puhe.2014.01.014 PMID: 24923994

Wong, A., Otles, E., Donnelly, J. P., Krumm, A., McCullough, J., DeTroyer-Cooley, O., Pestrue, J., Phillips, M., Konye, J., Penoza, C., Ghous, M., & Singh, K. (2021). External validation of a widely implemented proprietary sepsis prediction model in hospitalized patients. *JAMA Internal Medicine*, *181*(8), 1065–1070. DOI: 10.1001/jamainternmed.2021.2626 PMID: 34152373

World Bank. (2016). *Making mental health a global development priority*. World Bank. https://documents1.worldbank.org/curated/en/270131468187759113/pdf/105052-WP-PUBLIC-wb-background-paper.pdf

World Health Organ World Health Organization. (2003). *Skills for Health Skills-Based Health Education Including Life Skills: An Important Component of a Child-Friendly/Health-Promoting School. Geneva: World Health Organ World Health Organization. (1997)*. Life Skills Education in Schools.

World Health Organization. (1994). *Life skills education for children and adolescents in schools. Pt. 3, Training workshops for the development and implementation of life skills programmes (No. WHO/MNH/PSF/93.7 B. Rev. 1)*. World Health Organization.

World Health Organization. (2021). *Comprehensive mental health action plan 2013–2030*. WHO. https://www.who.int/publications/i/item/9789240031029

World Health Organization. (2022). *Global report on effective access to assistive technology*. WHO. https://www.who.int/publications/i/item/9789240049451

Xu, Y., Wang, J., & Ma, M. (2023). Adapting to Lockdown: Exploring stress coping strategies on short video social media during the COVID-19 pandemic. *Psychology Research and Behavior Management*, *16*, 5273–5287. DOI: 10.2147/PRBM.S441744 PMID: 38170068

Yadav, C. P., Chakraborty, A., Price, D. B., Lim, L. H. M., Juang, Y. R., Beasley, R., Sadatsafavi, M., Janson, C., Siyue, M. K., Wang, E., Wechsler, M. E., Jackson, D. J., Busby, J., Heaney, L. G., Pfeffer, P. E., Mahboub, B., Perng, D.-W., Cosio, B. G., Perez-de-Llano, L., & Chen, W. (2025). Prediction Pathway for Severe Asthma Exacerbations. *Chest*, *168*(2), 301–316. DOI: 10.1016/j.chest.2025.04.046 PMID: 40398558

Yaqoob, H., Ju, X., Bibi, M., Anwar, S., & Naz, S. (2024). A systematic review of risk factors of postpartum depression. Evidence from Asian culture. *Acta Psychologica*, *249*, 104436. DOI: 10.1016/j.actpsy.2024.104436 PMID: 39142256

YouTube. (n.d.) Crying at 3AM and nobody knows why [Short video]. Available at: https://youtube.com/shorts/9Jfd7qq-2nI?si=GM64SqLEky1Kph4k (accessed 11 June 2025).

YouTube. (n.d.) Husband's response to postpartum meltdown [Short video]. Available at: https://youtube.com/shorts/n-wbQF67lEU?si=_WtWchCPUnQYB8SG (accessed 11 June 2025).

YouTube. (n.d.) Postpartum reality no one talks about [Short video]. Available at: https://youtube.com/shorts/QeCpZ_mQUcU?si=ybDTvSsnu5OcmN06 (accessed 11 June 2025).

YouTube. (n.d.) POV: New Mom's Daily Routine [Short video]. Available at: https://youtube.com/shorts/VwXAPNTdWiM?si=-kYP-PYZqrn-tn0o (accessed 11 June 2025).

YouTube. (n.d.) The things in-laws expect after childbirth! [Short video]. Available at: https://youtube.com/shorts/JnxaEpQ3JBk?si=EL-esARvdxhNVm8C (accessed 11 June 2025).

YouTube. (n.d.) When visitors say "You look tired!" after delivery [Short video]. Available at: https://youtube.com/shorts/v873qYRtkIk?si=U454jXB0mAi5P50 - (accessed 11 June 2025).

YouTube. (n.d.) You will sleep when baby sleeps they said [Short video]. Available at: https://youtube.com/shorts/MMZqHfWbog0?si=0__pnXZ1W8dvGJUA (accessed 11 June 2025).

Yu, J. Y., Xie, F., Nan, L., Yoon, S., Ong, M. E. H., Ng, Y. Y., & Cha, W. C. (2022). An external validation study of the Score for Emergency Risk Prediction (SERP), an interpretable machine learning-based triage score for the emergency department. *Scientific Reports*, *12*(1), 17466. DOI: 10.1038/s41598-022-22233-w PMID: 36261457

Zahidi, K., Obtel, M., & Naji, S. (2024). Healthcare Accessibility: Metrics, Assessment, Policies, and Barriers. In *IntechOpen eBooks*. IntechOpen. DOI: 10.5772/intechopen.1006821

Żak, A., Djakeli, K., & Bielińska-Dusza, E. (2024). Cross-Sector Partnerships and Relationship Marketing in Healthcare: The Example of Fairy Tale Therapy in Children's Hospitals in Poland. In Modern Healthcare Marketing in the Digital Era (pp. 164-192). IGI Global Scientific Publishing. REVISED

Zanella, E., & Lee, E. (2022). Integrative review on psychological and social risk and prevention factors of eating disorders including anorexia nervosa and bulimia nervosa: Seven major theories. *Heliyon*, *8*(11), e11422. DOI: 10.1016/j.heliyon.2022.e11422 PMID: 36406673

Zeb, S., Fnu, N., Abbasi, N., & Fahad, M. (2024). AI in Healthcare: Revolutionizing Diagnosis and Therapy. *International Journal of Multidisciplinary Sciences and Arts*, *3*(3), 118–128. DOI: 10.47709/ijmdsa.v3i3.4546

Zhang, S. (2023). Artificial Intelligence and Applications in Structural and Material Engineering. *Highlights in Science Engineering and Technology*, *75*, 240–245. DOI: 10.54097/9qknfc57

Zhang, X., Shen, H., Huang, T., Wu, Y., Guo, B., Liu, Z., Luo, H., Tang, J., Zhou, H., Wang, L., Xu, W., & Ou, G. (2024). Improved random forest algorithms for increasing the accuracy of forest aboveground biomass estimation using Sentinel-2 imagery. *Ecological Indicators*, *159*, 111752. DOI: 10.1016/j.ecolind.2024.111752

Zhang, Y., Zhu, J., Li, S., Huang, L., Fang, Q., & Zheng, X. (2023). The effectiveness of an internet-based support program on maternal self-efficacy, postpartum depression and social support for primiparous women during the COVID-19 pandemic: Randomized controlled trial. *Frontiers in Public Health*, *11*, 1035872. DOI: 10.3389/fpubh.2023.1035872 PMID: 36844811

Zhao, X., Lai, J. W., Ho, A. F. W., Liu, N., Ong, M. E. H., & Cheong, K. H. (2022). Predicting hospital emergency department visits with deep learning approaches. *Biocybernetics and Biomedical Engineering*, *42*(3), 1051–1065. DOI: 10.1016/j.bbe.2022.07.008

Zheng, D., Wu, S., & Hou, M. (2021). Fully connected deep network: An improved method to predict TOC of shale reservoirs from well logs. *Marine and Petroleum Geology*, *132*, 105205. DOI: 10.1016/j.marpetgeo.2021.105205

Zhou, C., Shuai, L., Hu, H., Ung, C. O. L., Lai, Y., Fan, L., Du, W., Wang, Y., & Li, M. (2025). Applications of machine learning approaches for pediatric asthma exacerbation management: A systematic review. *BMC Medical Informatics and Decision Making*, *25*(1), 170. DOI: 10.1186/s12911-025-02990-0 PMID: 40251545

Zhu, Z., Wang, H., Zhu, T., Wang, Z., Shen, Y., Xiong, C., & Jiang, H. (2025). Mental health service utilization among pregnant and postpartum women: Status, determinants, and insights from a mixed-methods study. *BMC Public Health*, *25*(1), 1942. DOI: 10.1186/s12889-025-23132-1 PMID: 40420041

About the Contributors

Kakhaber Djakeli is a Health Economist and Health Marketer. He wrote his PhD Thesis in Germany, being a Doctoral Student at Leibniz University Hannover (LUH) under the mentorship of the renowned German health Economist, Prof. Dr. Mathias Graf von der Schulenburg at IVBL. During 2006-2007, Kakhaber Djakeli was invited to Yale University's School of Public Health by Professor Hong Wang, where he worked on health reform concepts in the Soviet countries, particularly in Georgia. During 2007-2008, Kakhaber Djakeli was hired by the World Bank to assist the government of Georgia in developing the Health Reform Concept. With a team of Health Reformers, Kakhaber Djakeli elaborated the Concept of Georgian Healthcare Reform, which the government implemented. During 2008-2013, Georgia improved its Healthcare Potential, which was the result of reforms in the National Health System. Between 1998 and 2017, Kakhaber Djakeli was invited by DAAD to German universities for research on healthcare concept development. In 2017, Kakhaber Djakeli was a Visiting Professor at Kennesaw State University (USA). He currently works at the University of Georgia's School of Health Sciences, where he continues to study Healthcare Markets and Healthcare Reform opportunities in response to Global and Local Challenges. The digitalization and innovative information technologies implemented in the Healthcare Market and industry enable Professor Djakeli to study global and local challenges in national and international markets, promoting new concepts and ideas for better patient satisfaction. Kakhaber Djakeli has published numerous scientific articles and books on digitalization in the healthcare market. He continues to consult with Healthcare Companies, Hospitals, Healthcare Managers, and Marketers.

***

Mamatha A is working as Assistant Professor in Department of Computer Science and Engineering, Ramaiah Institute of Technology. Having a total of 1.5

decade of teaching experience. She is a member of ISTE and IAENG. Her areas of interest include Image Processing, Network Security, Artificial Intelligence and Machine Learning.

Wafaa Benkayba is a chemistry researcher specializing in electrochemistry and analytical chemistry. Her multidisciplinary work covers water treatment, pharmaceutical and cosmetic analysis, food authenticity, green nanomaterials, and the development of electrochemical sensors. She also contributes to research on antimicrobial resistance (AMR) and traditional medicine. Her research bridges analytical sciences, environmental sustainability, and public health, with a strong commitment to developing evidence-based, sustainable, and culturally informed solutions to address global health and environmental challenges.

Jince George is a Ph.D. Scholar in the Department of Social Work at Christ (Deemed to be University), Bengaluru. His research focuses on contemporary social issues and community development, with a particular interest in evidence-based social interventions and inclusive policy practices.

Smruthymol J An accomplished academician in the field of Commerce, this professional currently serves as an Assistant Professor in the Department of Commerce at Karpagam Academy of Higher Education . With a strong educational background that includes an M.Com from MA College, Ernakulam, and a B.Com from SNCAS, Udumbanchola under MG University, the individual has also qualified both the NET and SET examinations in Commerce, demonstrating a high level of subject mastery. A commitment to continuous development is evident through the completion of a PGDCA and several NPTEL courses, reflecting a proactive approach to enhancing academic and technical competence. The successful submission of a Ph.D. thesis marks a significant milestone in the ongoing research journey, further strengthened by seven Scopus-indexed publications achieved within the year—an indicator of strong research productivity and scholarly engagement. With analytical strength, interdisciplinary interest, and dedication to professional growth, this educator continues to contribute meaningfully to academia, combining effective teaching with a steadily expanding research profile.

K.Jothi working as an Associate Professor and Head, Department of E Commerce at KPR College of Arts Science and Research, Coimbatore. She completed her SLET and NET. To her credit she produced 10 Ph.D. Scholars and published more than 50 articles in various International Peer Reviewed Journals and Scopus Indexed Journals

Sunanda K is a Research Scholar and Teaching Assistant in the Department of English at SRC, SASTRA Deemed University, Tamil Nadu, India. Her research interests encompass cultural studies, hauntology, trauma theory, and the intersections of literature, identity, and social justice. She has presented and published several research papers in national and international peer-reviewed journals and conferences. Her academic work engages with contemporary literary theories, film studies, and pedagogical innovation in English language teaching. As an emerging scholar, she aims to bridge the gap between critical theory and classroom practice by exploring how literary theories and affect studies can reshape perspectives on narrative, memory, and identity. Her ongoing doctoral research focuses on spectrality, Hauntology, and social justice in Stephen graham Jones' trilogy particularly through the lens of Sadeq Rahimi and Avery Gordon's theoretical frameworks.

Sheeja Karalam is a dedicated faculty member in the Department of Social Work at Christ (Deemed to be University), Bengaluru. She brings extensive experience in social work education, research, and community engagement, with a strong commitment to promoting social justice, empowerment, and sustainable development through her academic and field initiatives.

S.Meganathan completed his Ph.D. in 2013 at SASTRA Deemed University. He works as an Associate Professor in the Department of Computer Science & Engineering at Srinivasa Ramanujan Centre, SASTRA Deemed University, Kumbakonam. Two research scholars have completed, and three scholars are pursuing a Ph.D. programme under his guidance in data mining and its applications. Their research focuses on tropical cyclone prediction, electrical consumption prediction based on climate data, patient diagnosis systems on medical data, and improved D.S.S. systems on medical database systems. There are 32 research articles published in SCOPUS-indexed journals and 8 in SCI/SCIE indexed journals. He has experience in consultancy projects in the area of Video and Image Analytics for the Mahamaham Festival 2016, held at Kumbakonam, Tamil Nadu. This project extended to various festivals conducted by the HR&CE departments and the Revenue Departments of the government of Tamil Nadu. The student projects for B.Tech, M.Sc., and M.C.A. programmes in meteorological data have been guiding for the past 20 years.

Umamaheswari Purushothaman holds a B.E. in Information Technology from Periyar Maniammai College of Engineering and Technology (2003), an M.B.A. from Alagappa University, Karaikudi, Tamil Nadu (2006), and an M.Tech in Computer Science from SASTRA Deemed University, Thanjavur, Tamil Nadu (2011). She earned her Ph.D. in Computer Science and Engineering from SASTRA Deemed

University. With two decades of experience, she has taught both undergraduate and postgraduate courses in Computer Science. She is currently an Assistant Professor in the Department of Computer Science and Engineering at SRC Campus, SASTRA University, Kumbakonam. Her research interests focus on Data Mining, Machine Learning, and Deep Learning. She has published numerous research papers in international conferences, SCI-indexed journals, Scopus, and book chapters.

R. Devika received the Ph.D. degree in Computer Science and Engineering from SASTRA Deemed University, Thanjavur, India. She received the M.Tech. degree in Computer Science and Engineering from SASTRA Deemed University, the M.Phil. degree in Computer Science from Alagappa University, and the M.Sc. degree in Computer Science (Gold Medalist) from Bharathidasan University, India.She is currently working as an Assistant Professor in the School of Computing, SASTRA Deemed University, and has 19 years of teaching experience. She has published several research articles in Scopus- and SCI-indexed journals and presented papers at reputed international conferences. She has also contributed book chapters in emerging areas of computing. Her research interests include text analytics, big data analytics, and social network analysis.

R.Sankar Ganesh, served in various reputed institutions. Currently employed as an Associate Professor in MBA Department and Manager in Office of Industry Relations at Vel Tech Rangarajan Dr. Sagunthala R&D Institute of Science and Technology, Chennai. His areas of specialisation are marketing and human resource management. He has 12 years of teaching experience and 4 years of industry experience. He has published Two design patent with IPR India. In addition to acting as a resource person in various conferences and FDPs, he has presented papers in many forums, participated in various national and international seminars and conferences, attended various faculty development programs, and published various research papers in Scopus, Web of Science, and UGC Care listed journals. He also guided Ph.D. scholars and postgraduate students in their research work. Taking care of School of management Industry related engegment and University.

R. Velmurugan is presently working as a Professor in the Department of Commerce at Karpagam Academy of Higher Education, Coimbatore. He began his career as a Project Fellow under a UGC-sponsored Major Research Project at NGM College, Pollachi. He has 19 years of teaching experience and 15 years of research experience. To his credit, he has successfully supervised 25 Ph.D. scholars and 5 M.Phil. scholars. At present, two scholars have submitted their theses, and six Ph.D. scholars are pursuing their research under his guidance. He has published 168 research articles in various international journals, of which 122 are in Scopus-indexed journals, 15 in Web of Science journals, and 76 in edited volumes. He has also participated in and presented 27 papers in international seminars/conferences and 54 papers in national seminars/conferences. He has served as an external examiner for numerous M.Phil. and Ph.D. viva voce examinations. He has been a Vice-Chancellor's nominee for Doctoral Committee meetings at Bharathiar University, Coimbatore, and Periyar University, Salem. He has also served as Chairperson at various national-level conferences. Furthermore, he has contributed as an expert in Syllabus Scrutiny Committees, Question Paper Scrutiny Committees, and Boards of Studies at several reputed colleges. In recognition of his meritorious contributions, he has received awards such as Best Paper Presenter, Best Research Supervisor, and Best Faculty Award from various research foundations and councils. He has also served as a resource person for 27 guest lectures, 30 workshops, and 10 faculty development programmes.

J.Sudarvel is an Associate Professor at Karpagam Academy of Higher Education, Coimbatore, with nine years of teaching and six years of research experience. Specializing in finance and marketing, he has supervised seven Ph.D. scholars, with six more currently under his guidance. He has published 111 articles, including 52 in Scopus Indexed Journals, 13 in the Web of Science, and 12 in edited volumes, and presented 36 papers at international conferences. He serves as a Doctoral Committee Expert at Periyar University, and as an expert on the Board of Studies for VLB College and Nallamuthu Gounder Mahalingam College. Recognized for his contributions, he has received awards like Best Paper Presenter and Best Faculty and has led workshops and guest lectures on research methodology.

A. Sumathi is working as an Assistant Professor in the Department of Computer Science and Engineering, SRC, SASTRA Deemed to be University, Kumbakonam, TN, India. Research areas include Data Mining, Machine Learning, Data Science, and Healthcare applications.

M. Siva Vidhya has been working as an Assistant Professor in the Department of English at SASTRA Deemed University since 2017. She completed her Ph.D. in 2023, with a research focus on imperialism and cultural exchange in Amitav Ghosh's Ibis Trilogy. Her current research interests extend to English Language Teaching, with a special focus on trauma-sensitive classrooms. Her article on "Visual English"—the use of humorous memes and reels for language enhancement and for addressing trauma—was selected as one of the featured papers at an international academic forum. She is deeply committed to academic growth and research development.

Index

A

B

C

D

E

F

H

I

L

M

N

P

R

S

T

W

www.ingramcontent.com/pod-product-compliance
Lightning Source LLC
LaVergne TN
LVHW060006031026
849161LV00025B/1525